VOLUME ONE HUNDRED AND TWENTY

INTERNATIONAL REVIEW OF NEUROBIOLOGY

The Neuropsychiatric Complications of Stimulant Abuse

INTERNATIONAL REVIEW OF NEUROBIOLOGY

VOLUME 120

SERIES EDITORS

R. ADRON HARRIS

Waggoner Center for Alcohol and Drug Addiction Research
The University of Texas at Austin
Austin, Texas, USA

PETER JENNER

Division of Pharmacology and Therapeutics
GKT School of Biomedical Sciences
King's College, London, UK

VOLUME ONE HUNDRED AND TWENTY

INTERNATIONAL REVIEW OF NEUROBIOLOGY

The Neuropsychiatric Complications of Stimulant Abuse

Edited by

PILLE TABA

Department of Neurology and Neurosurgery University of Tartu, Tartu, Estonia

ANDREW LEES

The National Hospital, Queen Square London, United Kingdom

KATRIN SIKK

Department of Neurology, North-Estonian Regional Hospital, Tallinn, Estonia

ELSEVIER

AMSTERDAM • BOSTON • HEIDELBERG • LONDON
NEW YORK • OXFORD • PARIS • SAN DIEGO
SAN FRANCISCO • SINGAPORE • SYDNEY • TOKYO

Academic Press is an imprint of Elsevier

Academic Press is an imprint of Elsevier
225 Wyman Street, Waltham, MA 02451, USA
525 B Street, Suite 1800, San Diego, CA 92101-4495, USA
125 London Wall, London, EC2Y 5AS, UK
The Boulevard, Langford Lane, Kidlington, Oxford OX5 1GB, UK

First edition 2015

Notices

Knowledge and best practice in this field are constantly changing. As new research and experience broaden our understanding, changes in research methods, professional practices, or medical treatment may become necessary.

Practitioners and researchers must always rely on their own experience and knowledge in evaluating and using any information, methods, compounds, or experiments described herein. In using such information or methods they should be mindful of their own safety and the safety of others, including parties for whom they have a professional responsibility.

To the fullest extent of the law, neither the Publisher nor the authors, contributors, or editors, assume any liability for any injury and/or damage to persons or property as a matter of products liability, negligence or otherwise, or from any use or operation of any methods, products, instructions, or ideas contained in the material herein.

ISBN: 978-0-12-802978-7
ISSN: 0074-7742

For information on all Academic Press publications
visit our website at http://store.elsevier.com/

CONTENTS

CONTRIBUTORS

Jenny Bearn
Addictions Clinical Academic Group, South London and Maudsley NHS Foundation Trust, Maudsley Hospital, and Institute of Psychiatry, Psychology and Neuroscience, King's College, London, United Kingdom

Atbin Djamshidian
Department of Neurology, Innsbruck Medical University, Innsbruck, Austria, and Reta Lila Weston Institute of Neurological Studies, University of London, London, United Kingdom

Małgorzata Filip
Laboratory of Drug Addiction Pharmacology, Institute of Pharmacology, Polish Academy of Sciences, and Department of Toxicology, Faculty of Pharmacy, Jagiellonian University, Krakow, Poland

Jaanus Harro
Division of Neuropsychopharmacology, Department of Psychology, University of Tartu, Tartu, Estonia

Mike Jay
Independent Scholar

Anti Kalda
Department of Pharmacology, Institute of Biomedicine and Translational Medicine, University of Tartu, Tartu, Estonia

Sulev Kõks
Department of Pathophysiology, University of Tartu, Tartu, Estonia

Andrew Lees
The National Hospital, Queen Square, London, United Kingdom

Andrew C. McCreary
Brains On-Line, Groningen, The Netherlands

Christian P. Müller
Department of Psychiatry and Psychotherapy, Friedrich-Alexander-University of Erlangen-Nuremberg, Erlangen, Germany

Matthew O'Brien
Addictions Clinical Academic Group, South London and Maudsley NHS Foundation Trust, Maudsley Hospital, London, United Kingdom

Nilesh B. Patel
Department of Medical Physiology, College of Health Sciences, University of Nairobi, Nairobi, Kenya

Nicolas Rasmussen
School of Humanities & Languages, University of New South Wales, Sydney, New South Wales, Australia

Juan Sanchez-Ramos
Ellis Endowed Chair of Neurology, University of South Florida, Tampa, Florida, USA

Katrin Sikk
Department of Neurology, North-Estonian Regional Hospital, Tallinn, Estonia

Iain Smith
The Kershaw Unit, Gartnavel Royal Hospital, Glasgow, Scotland, United Kingdom

Pille Taba
Department of Neurology and Neurosurgery, University of Tartu, Tartu, Estonia

Neil Vickers
Department of English Literature, King's College London, London, United Kingdom

Aleksander Zarkovski
Department of Pharmacology, Institute of Biomedicine and Translational Medicine, University of Tartu, Tartu, Estonia

Jolanta B. Zawilska
Department of Pharmacodynamics, Medical University of Lodz, and Institute of Medical Biology, Polish Academy of Sciences, Lodz, Poland

Alexander Zharkovsky
Department of Pharmacology, Institute of Biomedicine and Translational Medicine, University of Tartu, Tartu, Estonia

CHAPTER ONE

The Story of "Speed" from "Cloud Nine" to Brain Gain

Andrew Lees*[,1], Katrin Sikk[†], Pille Taba[‡]
*The National Hospital, Queen Square, London, United Kingdom
[†]Department of Neurology, North Estonian Regional Hospital, Tallinn, Estonia
[‡]Department of Neurology and Neurosurgery, University of Tartu, Tartu, Estonia
[1]Corresponding author: e-mail address: andrew.lees@ucl.ac.uk

Content

Abstract

The substituted amphetamines have had a checkered medical history intertwined with a sensational cultural history. Mankind's insatiable fascination with speed has led to widespread misuse sometimes with disastrous neurological and psychiatric consequences that may cause a permanent harm but their potential to enhance cognition should not be dismissed or forgotten. Further, smarter research could perhaps still lead to an expanded beneficial role for stimulant use in modern society.

Long before the advent of medicinal chemistry, Nature's Treasure Chest had revealed a diversity of tonics all of which would now be classified as stimulants. *Ma-huang*, the yellow hemp (*Ephedra sinica*) known to contain ephedrine and now banned in the United States was revered in Ancient China for its performance enhancement and used by its practitioners to induce perspiration and treat chest complaints. Quids of betel and khat leaves have been chewed for thousands of years in South East Asia and the Horn of Africa as a way to loosen the tongue and enhance gregariousness. Traces of nicotine from tobacco have been found on a Mayan vase dated 700 AD providing support for its early use as an entheogen by the shamen. The chewing of coca leaves mixed with lime can be traced back at least as far as the Moche period (600 AD). Among the Incas, coca was a divine practice and its leaves were revered by the Andean Indians as a means of assuaging hunger. By the fifteenth century AD, the beans of the coffee plant were being brewed in public places on the Arabian Peninsula as a pick me up for the exhausted.

International Review of Neurobiology, Volume 120
ISSN 0074-7742
http://dx.doi.org/10.1016/bs.irn.2015.03.001

When tea, coffee, and chocolate were brought from the new colonies by the great navigators the elite of Western Europe considered them sacred gifts and profane pleasures.

Following its extraction from *Erythroxylum coca* in the middle of the nineteenth century cocaine was soon adopted by the medical profession as a local anesthetic, nasal decongestant, and mistakenly as an effective treatment for morphinism. Sigmund Freud observed that it caused exhilaration and lasting euphoria and in 1885 Parke-Davis marketed it in the United States with the sensational but largely truthful slogan that it could, "supply the place of food, make the coward brave, the silent eloquent and render the sufferer insensitive to pain." At first, it was considered no more addictive than coffee or tea and was included as a vital ingredient in Coca-Cola. Mounting concerns about its addictive potential eventually led in 1914 to the U.S. Government decreeing that its unauthorized possession for recreational purposes was now a criminal offense.

Amphetamine and methylamphetamine were first synthesized around the same time as cocaine but little interest was shown in them until the 1930s when Smith Kline and French looking for a substitute for ephedrine launched Dexedrine inhalers for the relief of hay fever and asthma. During World War 2, amphetamine was widely used by the Allies to combat fatigue and increase bravado but concerns about the increasingly widespread use of "Mother's little helpers" in the 1960s led to its "off label" use being outlawed in Europe and North America. It was hardly surprising that a class of drugs reported to give limitless energy, increase vigilance, and improve sexual performance might prove attractive to human beings. Stockbrokers were able to stay up all night to play the international markets and be in the office the following morning fresh as daisies. Unscrupulous professional sportsmen got an edge on their adversaries broke records and achieved glory. Long distance truck drivers reached ever more demanding deadlines without falling asleep at the wheel. "Speed" offered a short cut to prosperity and bliss and fuelled the capitalist dream.

Advocates of responsible stimulant use pointed to the many well-known artists and intellectuals who attributed their creativity to amphetamine use. Jack Kerouac wrote *On The Road* in a "creative groove" working day and night for 3 weeks typing on a long roll of paper, chosen deliberately to avoid interrupting his rhythm.

> *Benny has made me see a lot. The process of intensifying awareness naturally leads to an overflow of old notions, and voila, new material wells up like water forming its proper level, and makes itself evident at the brim of consciousness.*

Amphetamines accelerated his thought processes and allowed him to write in "the now." He had found a new spontaneous way of writing that banished convention and communicated raw physical and emotional experience. "Speed" has also played a role in some of the youth culture movements of Generations X Y, and Z. First used by the Beats in the jazz scene "Bennies" and "Purple Hearts" helped the Mods gain their teenage rite of passage. Bronchipax (ephedrine) and Durophet black bombers (dexamphetamine) helped Northern Soul boys escape bleak post-industrial landscapes while "Ecstasy" brought a sense of emotional connection on the dance floor, increased appreciation of sound, color and touch, and a feeling of closeness to others.

The risk of physical dependence with cocaine and amphetamine is relatively low but heavy regular usage or overdosage can have serious medical consequences leading to accident and emergency hospital referral. Reckless behavior and feelings of invincibility lead to falls, fights, and road traffic accidents, and death can occur from malignant hyperthermia. Profound agitation and acute paranoid psychoses with morbid jealousy require urgent psychiatric referral and drug abstinence after long-term use can unmask chronic depression with suicidal risk. Chorea (crack dancing) abnormal stereotyped movements of the lips, mouth and tongue, and teeth grinding are underreported neurological complications. Complex stereotyped purposeless behaviors (punding) first described in Scandinavian and Californian bikers using high doses of intravenous amphetamine are also now recognized to occur with cocaine and are also seen in patients with Parkinson's disease treated with l-dopa, the natural precursor of dopamine. The sympathomimetic properties of stimulants can also lead to hypertension and an increased risk of stroke and heart failure.

The substituted amphetamines increase brain dopamine, serotonin, and noradrenaline release and inhibit reuptake at axonal synapses. Both cocaine and methamphetamine also act as substrates at vesicular and synaptic storage sites leading to competitive inhibition with monoamine transporters. It would seem reasonable therefore, to expect that they might be useful treatments for both depression and Parkinson's disease but so far the results have been modest at best. The brains of chronic methamphetamine users have been found to have significant (50–60%) reductions in dopamine but in contrast to the findings in Parkinson's disease caudate dopamine deficiency which in some cases approached that seen in Parkinson's disease was always greater than that found in the putamen. None of the methamphetamine addicts had developed Parkinson's disease during life and in contrast to

MPTP the unwanted by product of kitchen chemistry manufacture of the narcotic MPPP there was no evidence to suggest that it caused structural damage to dopamine neurones (Moszczynska et al., 2004). Further, evidence for permanent changes in striatal dopamine signaling, however, comes from functional imaging studies in abstinent methamphetamine addicts where dopamine receptor changes have been found (Volkow et al., 2001).

Amphetamine type stimulants comprise the second most widely used class of illicit drugs in the world. According to a national survey of recreational drug use in the United States carried out seventeen years ago 1 in 20 adults aged 35 years or older had used non-prescribed amphetamines at least once (mainly "crystal meths") (Office of Applied Studies, 1998). At least 4 million people (1.5% of the population) in the United States aged 12 and older have used methylphenidate at least once off label. Increasingly widespread use of "crystal meths" (methylamphetamine) has led to public health concerns that dopamine and serotonergic neurones could be "excited to death" in chronic high-dose users increasing the risk of depression and delayed Parkinson's disease (Guilarte, 2001).

Several retrospective case-control and population studies have provided backing for this notion. A 16-year follow-up cohort study involving California inpatient hospital episodes and death records in patients at least 30 years of age found an increased risk of Parkinson's disease in amphetamine users in an active comparator group of cocaine users and another control group with appendicitis. For every 10,000 meth/amphetamine users over 30 followed up for 10 years 21 cases of Parkinson's disease would be expected to occur compared with only 12 cases in the two control groups (Callaghan, Cunningham, Sykes, & Kish, 2012). In a telephone survey from three faculty practice clinics in San Francisco, there was an increase in Parkinson's disease but not peripheral neuropathy or amyotrophic lateral sclerosis in adult methamphetamine users with an Odds Ratio of 8.27. In the cases with Parkinson's disease, there was an average of 27 years between amphetamine exposure and the onset of bradykinesia and rigidity (Garwood, Bekele, McCulloch, & Christine, 2006).

Individuals with low-novelty-seeking personality traits, nonsmokers, and men who drink no caffeinated beverages are at greater risk of developing Parkinson's disease (Ascherio et al., 2004; Menza, Golbe, Cody, & Forman, 1993). These individuals are less likely to experiment with recreational drugs including cocaine and stimulants. Nevertheless, these findings provide support for the notion that there may be some individuals who would otherwise be considered at lower risk of developing Parkinson's disease who increase their chances of developing the disease from chronic use of high-dose methamphetamine (Guilarte, 2001). Although the mechanisms are completely different some the patients now in their sixties who were identified to have been exposed to subtoxic levels of MPTP have not yet gone on to develop Parkinsonism (Tetrud, Langston, Garbe, & Ruttenber, 1989).

Each new stimulant craze seems to last 30 or 40 years (cocaine, amphetamine, methylamphetamine, freebase cocaine, and MDMA). In the last few years, mephedrone (known on the street as "Meouw Meouw," "Bubble," "Vanilla Sky," "White Rush," "Impact," "White Dove," or "Drone") sometimes mixed with another stimulant methylone (Explosion) has started to replace Ecstasy as the favored party drug in the United Kingdom. It is a synthetic cathinone identical to one of the alkaloids present in khat and is sold on the Internet as crystals disguised as "bath salts" (internet names include "Purple Wave," "Zoom," and "Cloud Nine"). In the United Kingdom, substituted cathinones were made illegal in 2010 and khat widely used by Somali and Ethiopian immigrants and bought in markets has also been banned.

Although there is as yet no convincing evidence that methcathinone can lead to irreversible brain damage in humans, significant numbers of drug users in Russia, Estonia, Latvia, Ukraine, and Georgia who synthesizes methcathinone from pseudoepehedrine (Sudafed) nasal decongestants mixed with potassium permanganate and vinegar have developed a severe irreversible neurological syndrome (Sikk et al., 2007). Whether toxic levels of methcathinone in these "ephedrone" addicts compound the toxic damage of manganese related to the method of preparation remains to be determined.

"Designer psychostimulants" are also disguised as "plant food," "room deodorants," "fish food," or "computer screen cleaner." Some of these substances are relatively easily made without specific laboratory equipment and instructions for their manufacture are readily available on the web. Other "designer" cathinones include butylone (bk-MBDB), napthylpyrovalerone (NRG-1), and methylenedioxypyrovalerone (MPDV). A group of entactogens sometimes called 2C drugs similar in structure to Ecstasy, Benzo-fury (5and 6-APB) DMBA (Frenzy) and 4,4′-DMAR (Serotoni), and some piperazines are other stimulants currently in use. A methamphetamine-caffeine tablet known in Thailand as "yaba" (literal translation madness drug) is now beginning to be exported and used as a party drug by speed freaks in other countries. Some batches are adulterated with small amounts of heroin to boost the effect. These compounds are promoted as "legal highs" leading to the misapprehension that they are without risk.

The "uppers" epidemics have totally overshadowed the potential of substituted amphetamines for good and their use in medicine is now restricted to the treatment of sleep disorders including narcolepsy and hypersomnolence (amphetamine and modafinil), attention deficit hyperactivity disorder in children (amphetamines and methylphenidate) and as second line treatment for orthostatic hypotension due to autonomic failure (ephedrine). They are also sometimes used to counteract the sedative effects of opioids in palliative care and for legitimate non-medical uses such as to combat potentially fatal tiredness in military aviation and space flight.

Man's craving for excitement and exhilaration has resulted in an insatiable and so far unsatisfied quest for the perfect pick me up. Even though the regions of the brain now linked with pleasure are more clearly delineated Aldous Huxley's Brave New World "State prescribed happy pill" remains a pipe dream.

Although there is still considerable interest in the potential of stimulants to relieve chronic mental fatigue, suppress appetite and treat depression recent focus has been less on their powers of reinvigoration and more on their potential to improve vigilance and lay down long-term memories. On American university campuses some white males have replaced caffeine with methylphenidate, modafinil, and amphetamines as a way of helping them compensate for activities that are detrimental to their ability to pass competitive examinations. An online survey conducted by the Journal Nature on 1600 academics in 60 countries revealed that one in five had used pep pills for nonmedical reasons (Sahakian & Morein-Zamir, 2007).

Despite the substantial risks and hazards involved in nootropic research, it is to be hoped that neuroscientists and Pharma's psychiatric drug research departments will not give up on a group of drugs with the potential to improve society. If science can develop new stimulants that would safely allow human beings to repeat a whole conversation verbatim or increase their digit span from seven to twelve then smart drugs might no longer just be a privileged "Students little helper" but be used to enhance concentration and cognition in those from deprived socioeconomic backgrounds who "have been dealt a poor deck of cards."

REFERENCES

Ascherio, A., Weisskopf, M. G., O'Reilly, E. J., McCullough, M. L., Calle, E. E., Rodriguez, C., et al. (2004). Coffee consumption, gender, and Parkinson's disease mortality in the cancer prevention study II cohort: The modifying effects of estrogen. *American Journal of Epidemiology, 160*(10), 977–984.

Callaghan, R. C., Cunningham, J. K., Sykes, J., & Kish, S. J. (2012). Increased risk of Parkinson's disease in individuals hospitalized with conditions related to the use of methamphetamine or other amphetamine-type drugs. *Drug and Alcohol Dependence, 120*(1–3), 35–40.

Garwood, E. R., Bekele, W., McCulloch, C. E., & Christine, C. W. (2006). Amphetamine exposure is elevated in Parkinson's disease. *Neurotoxicology, 27*(6), 1003–1006.

Guilarte, T. R. (2001). Is methamphetamine abuse a risk factor in parkinsonism? *Neurotoxicology, 22*(6), 725–731.

Menza, M. A., Golbe, L. I., Cody, R. A., & Forman, N. E. (1993). Dopamine-related personality traits in Parkinson's disease. *Neurology, 43*(3 Pt 1), 505–508.

Moszczynska, A., Fitzmaurice, P., Ang, L., Kalasinsky, K. S., Schmunk, G. A., Peretti, F. J., et al. (2004). Why is parkinsonism not a feature of human methamphetamine users? *Brain, 127*(Pt 2), 363–370.

Office of Applied Studies. (1998). *National household survey on drug abuse,* Main findings. DHSS publication No SMA 00-381 Rockville, MD 2000. Substance abuse and mental health services administration, 32.

Sahakian, B., & Morein-Zamir, S. (2007). Professor's little helper. *Nature, 450*(7173), 1157–1159.

Sikk, K., Taba, P., Haldre, S., Bergquist, J., Nyholm, D., Zjablov, G., et al. (2007). Irreversible motor impairment in young addicts—Ephedrone, manganism or both? *Acta Neurologica Scandinavica, 115*(6), 385–389.

Tetrud, J. W., Langston, J. W., Garbe, P. L., & Ruttenber, A. J. (1989). Mild parkinsonism in persons exposed to 1-methyl-4-phenyl-1,2,3,6-tetrahydropyridine (MPTP). *Neurology, 39*(11), 1483–1487.

Volkow, N. D., Chang, L., Wang, G. J., Fowler, J. S., Ding, Y. S., Sedler, M., et al. (2001). Low level of brain dopamine D2 receptors in methamphetamine abusers: Association with metabolism in the orbitofrontal cortex. *The American Journal of Psychiatry, 158*(12), 2015–2021.

CHAPTER TWO

Amphetamine-Type Stimulants: The Early History of Their Medical and Non-Medical Uses

Nicolas Rasmussen[1]
School of Humanities & Languages, University of New South Wales, Sydney, New South Wales, Australia
[1]Corresponding author: e-mail address: N.Rasmussen@unsw.edu.au

Contents

Abstract

Amphetamine was discovered as a drug in the late 1920s, and its pharmacological effects on attention and cognition, emotions, and appetite were explored thoroughly in the 1930s and 1940s. By the late 1940s, it had achieved medical and market success as an antidepressant and was quickly gaining such success as a diet medication. In contrast, both careful testing and extensive military experience had left the impression that the drugs' benefits for attention and cognition were more subjective than real and that any objective benefits were explained mainly by the drug's mood-elevating effects. Because of its unpatentable status, methamphetamine had been introduced for all the same uses by drug firms competing with the holder of the amphetamine patent. The drugs were being widely used nonmedically and their abuse potential was becoming recognized by medicine, eventually leading to their strict control internationally around 1970.

International Review of Neurobiology, Volume 120
ISSN 0074-7742
http://dx.doi.org/10.1016/bs.irn.2015.02.001

1. INTRODUCTION

Amphetamine and related stimulants—including methamphetamine, methylphenidate, phentermine, and similar derivatives, the hallucinogenic methoxy derivates loosely grouped as "ecstasy," together with their natural congener ephedrine—are consumed in enormous quantities today. Some are mainly consumed on prescription for medically authorized purposes; others, both legally and illegally manufactured, mainly for recreational purposes; and others still in the broad grey zone between, encompassing both nonmedical use of prescribed drugs and unprescribed self-medication. All these stimulants have the same basic set of pharmacological actions on the central nervous system, which go far beyond "stimulation": they produce wakefulness and alter attention; they elevate mood and increase optimism and impulsiveness; they reduce appetite; and in many, they produce pleasure with its sequelae, including addictive behavior and eventually (after sufficiently heavy consumption) psychosis. All four of these different actions have been regarded at times, and by particular users, as the valuable action of the drug, and the other actions as "side effects." The first three actions were immediately noticed and deliberately explored by medical researchers in the commercial founder of the category, amphetamine, during the 1930s and 1940s. Amphetamine is still the commercially dominant drug of the family for the condition known today as "attention deficit," that is, for the first type of action. Many of the other psychostimulants widely used today are derivatives of amphetamine, developed in an effort to maximise one of the founder drug's other three types of action.

In this chapter, I will refer to the entire family of drugs as the "amphetamines" in preference to "psychostimulants," because this latter formulation foregrounds only the first type of action, making us forget, or minimize the others even if they are equally prominent. I will describe how the amphetamines were discovered as pharmacological agents, and the ways in which their various actions were exploited by medicine, the drug industry, the military, and (although I have insufficient space to say much here) also by recreational users up to about 1970, when the bad reputation they had earned brought them under international control and greatly reduced their medical use.

2. EARLY HISTORY OF THE AMPHETAMINES

The "discovery" of amphetamine is often traced to the 1880s, when the Romanian chemist Lazar Edeleano first synthesized the base. Like most organic chemists of his day, Edeleano was mainly interested in synthetic dyes and made no mention of any pharmacological activity (Edeleano, 1887). A more significant, contemporaneous event in amphetamine history stems from the work of Japanese chemists on the active components of the Chinese herbal medicine *Ephedra*. In particular, the Germany-trained chemist Nagayoshi Nagai isolated l-ephedrine as well r-pseudoephedrine along with several other pharmacologically active compounds, and this work became known to the Merck drug and chemical company in Germany. Nagai passed the compounds on to a colleague, K. Muira, who conducted a pharmacological analysis suggesting that ephedrine was too toxic for internal use but might be useful topically, for instance, as a mydriatic to dilate pupils (Anon., 1927; Lee, 2011; Miura, 1887). Pure ephedrine was not taken up in medicine at this time, but interest returned to the compound in the 'teens because of the similarity of its action to the hormone adrenaline, purified in the 1890s and introduced with great success to medicine in 1901. There was a commercial Japanese effort to market ephedrine as a mydriatic. In 1919, Japanese chemist Akira Ogata, as part of his effort to prove the structure of ephedrine, reported the synthesis of the closely related compound we now call methamphetamine, and this result was described in the Western literature (Amatsu & Kubota, 1913; Lee, 2011; Ogata, 1920). Soon afterward, building on the work of Karl Schmidt and K.K. Chen, ephedrine was marketed in the United States and Europe with great success, chiefly as a decongestant and asthma-relieving drug (major uses for the shorter acting, if more effective, adrenaline) in pill form, and also as a topical decongestant (Chen & Schmidt, 1923, 1926).

The net result was that ephedrine and its adrenaline-like actions on both the central and peripheral nervous system became well known by medicine in the late 1920s. Given the vigorous sales of the drug, there should be no surprise that amphetamine was discovered by the enterprising California chemist Gordon Alles (who worked in an allergist's practice) in a systematic search for adrenaline-like compounds superior for asthma to ephedrine. In 1932, Alles received a patent on amphetamine, specifying its use as a medicine, and in 1933, began extending its clinical testing beyond allergy through physician associates. In 1934, he assigned his patent to the Smith, Kline, and French (SKF) drug firm of Philadelphia, which from about 1935 oversaw its further clinical development and ensured that the compound had strong patent protection in Europe and elsewhere (Piness, Miller, & Alles, 1930; Rasmussen, 2008a, Chaps. 1–2; Rasmussen, 2008b). Soon, as I will shortly describe, under SKF's guidance amphetamine achieved market success, especially in psychiatry. As a result, when competitors began to consider emulating SKF's success in the late 1930s, they turned to methamphetamine, which had nearly indistinguishable effects but—because its synthesis together with its pharmacological characteristics was published before 1920—was free from patent encumbrance.

3. WAKEFULNESS, ATTENTION, AND COGNITIVE PERFORMANCE

When Alles conducted the first human trial with racemic amphetamine in 1929, by having himself injected with 50 mg, he noted "Nose cleared-dry," "Feeling of well-being—palpitation," and eventually "Rather sleepless night. Mind seemed to run from one subject to another." After unimpressive results with asthma and allergy, the "sleeplessness" and "well-being" effects (that is, wakefulness and mood actions) became the next obvious avenues for finding a profitable use for the drug. The first was explored around 1935 by some clinician friends of Alles, who successfully substituted amphetamine for ephedrine as a narcolepsy treatment. There was no large market here, nor for another early success with the drug, postencephalitic Parkinsonism, but the drug was readily adopted for these clinical indications (Doyle & Daniels, 1931; Nathanson, 1937; Prinzmetal & Bloomberg, 1935; Rasmussen, 2008a, Chaps. 1 and 2; Rasmussen, 2008b; Solomon, Mitchell, & Prinzmetal, 1937).

Closely related to the obvious alerting effects of amphetamine, many early users reported the sensation that their cognitive and working abilities were improved (as opposed to merely extended). Hospital staff serving as normal controls in early clinical studies reported this sense of efficiency along with "increased energy" and "pep"; perceived working performance on amphetamine may also have been enhanced by the increased talkativeness and assertiveness widely reported among both controls and patient subjects. To follow up on this promising lead, together with a prominent early trial at London's Maudsley clinic reporting that patients showed increased scores on standardized intelligence tests with amphetamine, SKF organized a particularly extensive, rigorous study on amphetamine's effects upon the personality, behavior, and work performance of normal adults by University of Pennsylvania psychologists William Turner and George Carl. Twenty-five different measures and tests were made with about 150 subjects, mainly women (nurses especially). They assessed effects on learning, primary intelligence indices, verbal and mathematical tasks, hand-eye tasks, emotional tone, and other mental states (Carl & Turner, 1939, 1940; Davidoff, 1936; Davidoff & Reifenstein,

1937; Myerson, 1936; Nathanson, 1937; Sargant & Blackburn, 1936; Solomon et al., 1937; Turner & Carl,1939).

When the findings were published in three massive papers, occupying between them 200 pages of journal space, they supported the following main conclusions: low-moderate doses of amphetamine boost psychomotor (hand-eye) output in simple tasks without changing accuracy, while higher doses impaired both; memory, arithmetical, and verbal task performance are not much affected at low-moderate doses (but, again, impaired by confusion at higher doses); and that the drug had no effect on intelligence measures. The measures of affect and attitude showed a pronounced drug effect, even at low doses (10 mg racemic): marked elevation of mood and talkativeness, and also a pattern of increased assertiveness and initiative—even a "devil-may-care" attitude—that today would be classed as impulsiveness. These alterations in mood and "personality," combined with physiological stimulation, explained why the drug improved efficiency in simple mental and psychomotor tasks, especially those requiring persistence and alertness. There was no enhancement to cognition, *per se* (Carl & Turner, 1939, 1940; Turner & Carl, 1939). Two SKF-supported early trials with learning-impaired children at about the same time—one the famous Bradley study cited decades later as the "discovery" of Attention Deficit Disorder—fit with these same conclusions, that the school performance of some students benefited with amphetamine, and that their psychiatric profiles taken together with their especially low baseline performance suggested that the mechanism was not cognitive but emotional: increased confidence during testing. Perhaps, because their new Benzedrine (amphetamine) tablets were already earning disrepute from their popularity as "pep pills" among American university students (and the "confidence drug" among British nonmedical users), SKF did not market the product for cognitive performance in adults or children (Bradley, 1937; Bromley, 2006; Editor, 1937a; Editor, 1937b; Molitch & Eccles, 1937; Molitch & Sullivan, 1937; Rasmussen, 2008a, Chap. 2; Rasmussen, 2008b; Singh, 2002).

4. MOOD ELEVATION

Among other potential applications of amphetamine, the obvious elevation of mood experienced by many early users—Alles' 1929 "well-being" or "exhilaration" for an asthma patient that year—quickly attracted the attention of psychiatrists. Before Benzedrine Sulfate's official marketing approval in December 1937, granted in those days by the American

(AMA) Council on Pharmacy, the drug had been tested particularly extensively by that psychiatry, which was selected by SKF's marketers as their most promising avenue. Amphetamine was tested as early as 1936 by asylum psychiatrists on major depressions and other serious conditions, and initial reports of the drug's value were mixed, in general finding that it was helpful in patients with less serious depressive illness, but of little or negative value with most suffering schizophrenia or anxious states. However, a champion for the product's use in milder (neurotic) depressions emerged that year in the person of Harvard professor Abraham Myerson, an authority on depression with an unconventional concept of the condition (Anderson, 1938; Davidoff & Reifenstein, 1937; Schube, McManamy, Trapp, & Myerson, 1937; Wilbur, MacLean, & Allen, 1937). For Myerson, anhedonia was the fundamental phenomenon of depression, both minor and major, rather than exhaustion and retardation (as the prevailing neurasthenia concept of depression had stressed). This concept especially fitted amphetamine's construal as an antidepressant, for its action in increasing the active pursuit of pleasures was reported by many subjects, both control and experimental. As soon as SKF received approval to market Benzedrine Sulfate in 1937, the emphasis in both general medicine and psychiatric journal advertising was on mild depression and that advertising drew heavily on Myerson's views (Fig. 1). As I have argued elsewhere, the success of this marketing effort and the consequent acceptance by medicine of amphetamine as the first "antidepressant" (a term that appears in SKF marketing material by the late 1940s) helped advance Myerson's theories and make anhedonia a cardinal feature of depression. In any event, by 1940 Benzedrine Sulfate had achieved medical acclaim and quickly growing sales as an antidepressant effective for milder forms of the condition, both in the United States and the United Kingdom. In Germany, the Temmler drug firm quickly copied SKF, marketing methamphetamine (again, unprotected by patents) tablets under the Pervitin brand, with claims that it restored "joy in work" in cases of mild depression around 1938 (Rasmussen, 2006; Steinkamp, 2006).

5. APPETITE SUPPRESSION

The third main clinically useful effect of amphetamine, appetite reduction, was also noted in some of the earliest trials with the drug. One of the first psychiatric studies, for example, reported in 1937 that many of the 40 patients and 80 hospital staff controls lost weight after several weeks (Nathanson, 1937). Practitioners of the somewhat dubious medical speciality of weight

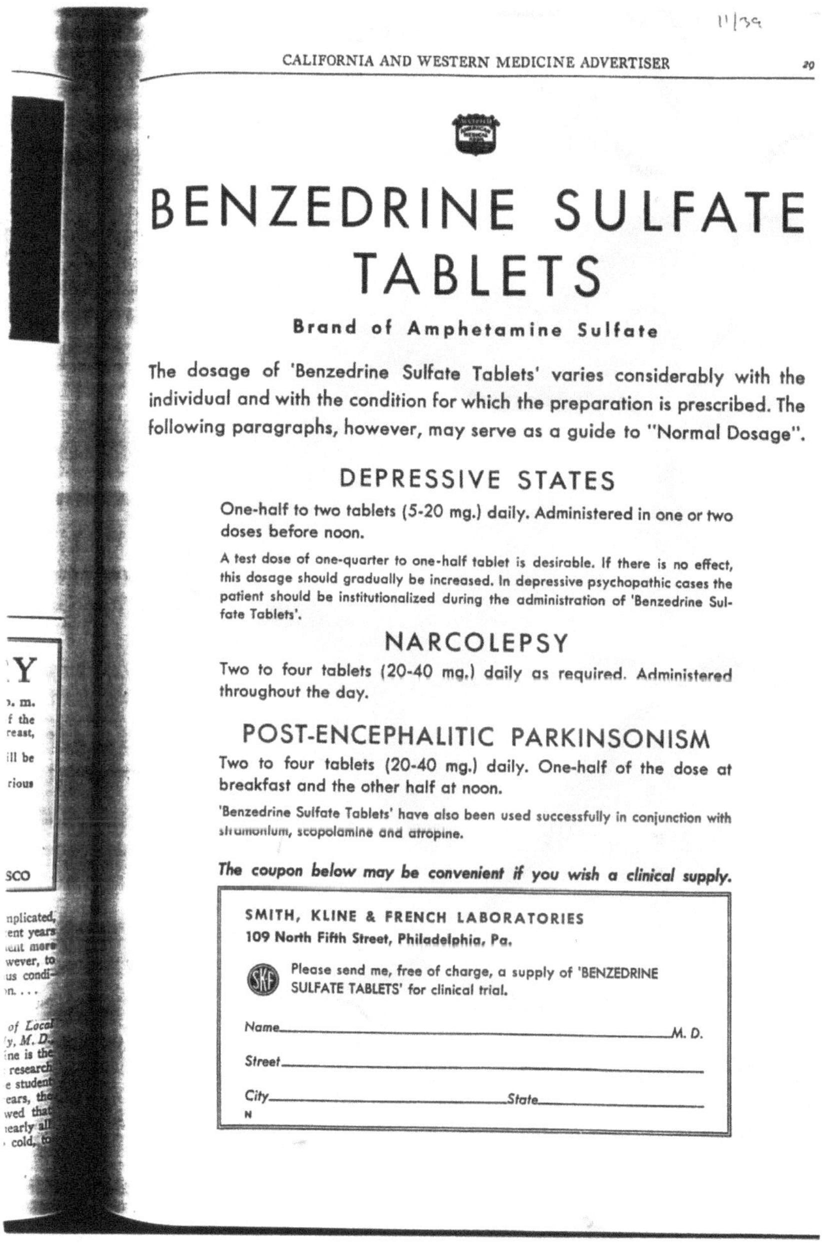

Figure 1 1939 advertisement for amphetamine tablets describing the earliest accepted indications. *California and Western Medicine.*

loss took note, spurred by attacks from the medical elite upon two diet drugs that were their old standbys, thyroid hormone, and dinitrophenol (the former working by speeding metabolism, the latter simply by poisoning—and both potentially lethal). As the diet doctors began to prescribe amphetamine more, this demand attracted enterprising small drugmakers (many deserving the label "fly-by-night") which, flaunting SKF's patents, began manufacturing both imitation Benzedrine Sulfate tablets and the brightly colored "rainbow" diet pills containing amphetamine and also, very often, thyroid hormone too. By late 1940, these patent infringers were producing enough amphetamine that SKF found that their Benzedrine Sulfate sales were no longer growing. SKF then investigated and sued the largest of these rivals, in 1945 eventually winning a judgment of unfair competition and having their patent (that is, Alles's) upheld (Cohen, Goday, & Swann, 2012; Rasmussen, 2008a, Chap. 4; Rasmussen, 2008b).

The diet pill makers promptly switched to methamphetamine. Meanwhile, during the war years, SKF had quietly sponsored clinical trials to establish amphetamine's effectiveness for weight loss, but did not pursue approval from the American Medical Association to market amphetamine for weight loss. This SKF finally did in 1947, on the strength of a study showing that amphetamine reduced weight by affecting brain centers responsible for appetite, rather than through metabolic or toxic effects. By the later 1960s, weight loss became the most common legitimate indication for amphetamine and methamphetamine, as the drugs' use as an antidepressant gradually declined through of competition from tricyclics and MAOIs (Harris, Ivy, & Searle, 1947; Rasmussen, 2008a, Chaps. 5–6; Rasmussen 2008b). But their use as a common (perhaps the most common) outpatient antidepressant did not die until the early 1970s, when amphetamines were scheduled as strictly controlled substances after the 1970 UN Convention on Psychotropics. This outcome can hardly be regarded as unjustified because, as the evidence noted below under "Abuse" showed, prescribed amphetamines had been established as major threat to public health. By this time, the United States' annual consumption of pharmaceutical amphetamines had reached the equivalent of about 50, 10 mg tablets per man, woman, and child (McAllister, 2000; Rasmussen, 2008b).

6. MILITARY USE: "COMBAT FATIGUE" AND THE SECOND WORLD WAR

When the Second World War broke out, amphetamine and methamphetamine had just been introduced in medicine, and the subjective impressions that the drugs enhanced work performance had not yet been subject to serious testing. Based upon such impressions, the German military conducted some rather casual trials of Pervitin at a military medicine facility on tasks like paperwork and marching among cadets, and on their basis, the *Wehrmacht* supplied its medical officers with the drug for use against fatigue. Men in the field quickly took to the drug. During the late 1939 and early 1940, *Blitzkrieg* German military usage reached levels over 10 million 3 mg methamphetamine tablets per month (for scale, consider that military divisions each contained very roughly 10,000 men, and Germany fielded about 100 divisions in the Western offensive, on the order of 1 million fighting men and thus about 10 pills/man/month in active theatres). This rather heavy usage was driven by demand among soldiers, as their were no special orders from above on how the drug should be used. Evidently, men felt the drug helped them fight. The combined amphetamine effects of increased alertness, physical activity, optimism, and impulsiveness must have contributed—as contemporary observations of "fearless and berserk" paratroopers behind Allied lines suggest—to the famous speed and ferocity of the German campaign. However, both the German medical profession and military officials quickly cooled on amphetamines, both due to widespread abuse among the troops and a mounting belief that the drug impaired efficiency and judgement at least with prolonged use. By the end of 1940, military consumption of Pervitin declined by an order of magnitude to little more than 1 million tablets/month and dropped again after the Reich restricted both methamphetamine and amphetamine to special prescriptions in mid-1941. In 1942, *Wehrmacht* consumption dropped still further when the drugs were listed as dangerously addictive narcotics, although the pills still remained available in the military for "emergency" use (Kemper, 2003; Noeldeke, 2003; Rasmussen, 2011; Snelders & Pieters, 2011; Steinkamp, 2006).

Ironically, just as the German military was deciding that its first optimistic assessments of amphetamines, resting on subjective impressions of enhanced performance, were seriously mistaken, the Allies were adopting the drugs. As I have described in detail elsewhere, top-level scientists carried out intensive testing of amphetamine effects for both British and American militaries, particularly with hand-eye and cognitive tasks related to flying but also other forms of work and cognition. The upshot of 2 years of carefully controlled studies comparing amphetamine, methamphetamine, and caffeine in rested and exhausted subjects, many conducted at simulated altitudes, was that in almost every quantifiable way the three drugs had the same objective effects. Caffeine produced significantly better work output and significantly worse hand tremor, and also required more frequent dosing to maintain alertness; otherwise, all three drugs were similarly superior to no drugs in exhausted subjects. (In general, they did not improve performance for rested subjects, except in some simple repetitive tasks.) However, by the time the elite scientists on both sides of the Atlantic reached these conclusions in the second half of 1942, both militaries had adopted amphetamine based on their own testing—not in controlled laboratory settings but in field exercises and combat (Rasmussen, 2011).

For example, one study by the RAF, influential in the United States as well as British military, involved the comparison of Benzedrine and placebo tablets for Bomber Command flight crews. The researcher, who went on 20 bombing sorties deep into Germany in late 1941 and early 1942, concluded that the amphetamine was valuable because "the drug may increase determination in circumstances of acute anxiety." These emotional effects made it the drug of choice over caffeine and also (he felt, without much evidence) methamphetamine. Men on amphetamine aggressively chose to bomb at lower altitudes and in heavier flak than others and would even swoop low to strafe anti-aircraft pits as if they were flying a fighter plane. RAF Bomber Command adopted routine use of the drug in mid-1942 because of such findings (in contrast to Fighter Command, whose missions were shorter and could not be planned). In the Middle East, the British Army similarly embraced the drug after General Montgomery found its effects valuable in his October 1942 offensive at El Alamein. General Eisenhower, also fighting Rommel's formidable *Afrika Korps*, followed suit in early 1943, and the US Marines found the drug valuable in their bloody amphibious landings in the Pacific from late that year. Essentially, I have argued, the Allied military supplied amphetamine for its tendency to promote aggression (or bravery, depending on perspective) and soldierly comportment; that is, for its "morale" or mood effects. There was a psychiatric rationale in that what was then called "war neurosis" or euphemistically "combat fatigue" (now PTSD) was regarded at the time as a depressive disorder aggravated by physical exhaustion, making the new antidepressant seems a plausible therapy (Kardiner, 1941; Pols, 2007; Rasmussen, 2011).

When nervous breakdown and panic in combat was the chief concern, any subtle objective effect on psychomotor performance was beside the point. But as the dark days of the Blitz receded and the drug's less favorable effects became more evident with experience (such as impaired judgment and impulsiveness especially under exhaustion), the British military reduced its amphetamine consumption in much the same way as the German military had. As a 1943 Air Ministry medical handbook warned, "Benzedrine has the effect of causing the individual to feel on top of things and able to carry on with his duties without rest: he feels that he is doing well, when in fact he is making all sorts of mistakes." Another RAF source suggested that in combat situations anxiety was the chief problem rather than physical exhaustion, so that amphetamine's use was counterproductive, and that there were better ways to maintain morale. The US military, on the other hand, continued consuming large quantities of amphetamines until the war's end, despite substantial evidence of its abuse in the service, and resumed soon afterward when the Korean conflict flared. Indeed, until the 1950s, when the specific attention effects of amphetamine attracted careful study, the US military's official explanation of how amphetamines "enhanced" performance in combat centered entirely on their mood effects (Davis, 1947; Rasmussen, 2011).

7. NONMEDICAL USE, ABUSE, AND DEPENDENCE

The legitimate, prescribed and officially condoned uses of the drug have never been successfully divorced from the dark side of the amphetamines: their seductive, deliberate use for pleasure, and their addictive properties when taken regularly either medically or nonmedically. In the United States, amphetamine was first released as a decongestant inhaler approved for direct to consumer sales and marketing in 1933, 4 years before the initial marketing of Benzedrine (amphetamine sulphate) tablets. SKF's Benzedrine Inhaler, containing 325 mg of nearly pure amphetamine base, was quickly discovered by marginal drug abusing populations, and by the late 1930s, its abuse—consuming the contents in a drink such as coffee—had become commonplace in venues such as jazz clubs and jails (Jackson, 1971; Rasmussen, 2008a, Chap. 4). The military's adoption of Benzedrine—both in pill form for "fatigue" (dispensed by medical officers, and available in emergency kits too), and also the decongestant inhaler (even more readily available)—seems to have spread amphetamine abuse. An investigation of widespread inhaler abuse in a military prison population around 1945 found that abusers were five times more likely than non-abusers to have been issued Benzedrine tablets by an officer. Thus, military service greatly magnified this previously marginal problem (Monroe & Drell, 1947; Rasmussen, 2008a, Chap. 4) (Fig. 2).

Although case reports of addiction and psychosis among American patients prescribed regular amphetamine doses had been accumulating since

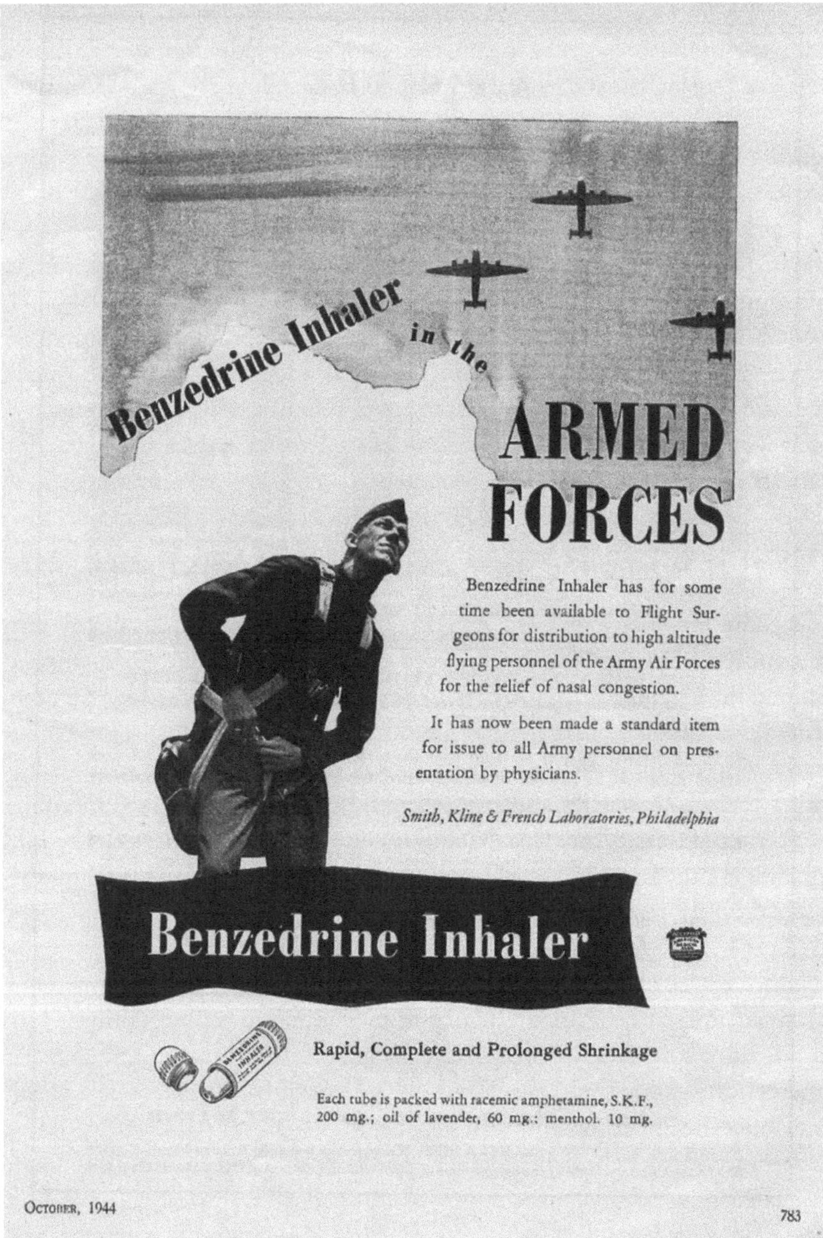
Benzedrine Inhaler in the
ARMED FORCES
Benzedrine Inhaler has for some time been available to Flight Surgeons for distribution to high altitude flying personnel of the Army Air Forces for the relief of nasal congestion.
It has now been made a standard item for issue to all Army personnel on presentation by physicians.
Smith, Kline & French Laboratories, Philadelphia
Benzedrine Inhaler
Rapid, Complete and Prolonged Shrinkage
Each tube is packed with racemic amphetamine, S.K.F., 200 mg.; oil of lavender, 60 mg.; menthol, 10 mg.
October, 1944
783

Figure 2 1944 advertisement for amphetamine base inhalants; abuse of this product was widespread in both military and civilian life by the end of the war years. *Minnesota Medicine.*

the 1930s, the first quantitative evidence gauging the abuse and dependency liability of medical amphetamine use came from Britain around 1960. A comprehensive set of studies on amphetamines prescribed in general practice in the city of Newcastle found that among this population—predominantly middle aged and female, given the drug in roughly equal proportions for weight loss, depression, and for other mostly psychiatric indications—about 10% of those prescribed the drug were dependent to some extent, a third of these "physically dependent" (Brandon & Smith, 1962; Kiloh & Brandon, 1962; Rasmussen, 2008a, Chap. 5 n. 52; Wilson & Beacon, 1964). Consistent with these findings Phillip Connell, the British psychiatrist responsible for drawing attention to the prevalence of amphetamine psychosis in the late 1950s, found that a third of the victims of this severe condition had first taken amphetamine by prescription (after which they became addicted and turned to less legitimate sources) (Connell, 1958, 1968). Quantitative evidence from later in the 1960s provides a picture of American abuse and dependence problems with prescribed amphetamines still more severe. In the most detailed study, based on a large statistically sophisticated sample of New York State residents, found that even among the roughly 5% of the population 14 years or older taking amphetamines by prescription in the past year (double the Newcastle prevalence), there was extensive nonmedical use of medically prescribed amphetamines. Indeed of the "regular" takers (six or more times in the past month) of amphetamine products lacking a sedative component, which would include those prescribed the drug for a psychiatric indication, nearly half reported that they used the drugs recreationally or socially, and conversely about half of those using the drugs nonmedically were supplied by prescription (Inciardi & Chambers, 1972; Rasmussen, 2008a, Chap. 6, n. 59–60; Rasmussen, 2008b). In this connection, it seems pertinent to note that a detailed analysis of stimulant abuse data from US national household drug surveys a decade ago that, despite the purportedly stricter control of these products under US Schedule II regulations, half of the 3.2 million past-year nonmedical users of stimulants in the United States used strictly non-methamphetamine psychiatric stimulants—that is, in today's pharmaceutical market, Attention Deficit medications. These abusers of Attention Deficit medications alone accounted for one-third of the approximately 300,000 Americans estimated to be amphetamine addicted (at the height of the public panic over "Meth") (Kroutil et al., 2006).

8. CONCLUSION

By the end of amphetamine's first official decade as a medicine in 1947, the three useful pharmacological actions of the drug class were well known and thoroughly explored in careful controlled trials: the effects on attention and cognitive performance, the appetite-suppressing effects, and the mood-elevating effects. The dextrorotatory optical isomer, dextro- or dexamphetamine, had been identified as the agent of all the valuable central effects, and had been introduced to the market by SKF during the War years as Dexedrine. By 1947, this product was starting to overshadow racemic Benzedrine for mainstream medical uses. Of the three uses, amphetamine's consumption for treatment of milder depression was expanding very rapidly, and after 1950 also for treatment of anxiety in combination with barbiturates (especially, the SKF product Dexamyl or Drinamyl). The mainstream use of amphetamine for weight loss only began in 1947, and this indication would also expand rapidly and eventually outstrip the psychiatric uses (thanks to competition from "minor tranquilisers" in the late 1950s and second generation antidepressants in the 1960s).

The amphetamines' effects on attention and perceived enhancement of work had also been explored carefully, both in civilian contexts and by the military for fatigued subjects. Perceived performance enhancement turned out to be more subjective than real in both testing programs, and amphetamine was not marketed along these lines. But despite this failure to find meaningful, objective performance benefits the United States and British militaries enthusiastically welcomed the drugs at first, because of their mood-elevating effects, while the German military had quickly adopted methamphetamine without extensive testing. By the end of the war, amphetamines had been largely abandoned by both the British and German militaries, because the crucible of combat had showed that they made more negative than positive contributions to real-world performance. The US military did not, evidently judging the "morale" effects to be more important. In the United States and in Germany (and Japan), the widespread wartime use of amphetamines led to large-scale postwar abuse that spread beyond veteran circles. Britain too suffered a postwar amphetamine abuse and addiction epidemic whose relation to military use has not been explored. Eventually, by the late 1960s, the abuse of amphetamines resulted in their strong control under narcotics laws internationally, and their use by mainstream medicine nearly went extinct (Alexander, 2013; Brill & Hirose,

1969; Jackson, 1971; Monroe & Drell, 1947; Rasmussen, 2008a, Chaps. 4 and 7; Rasmussen, 2008b; Snelders & Pieters, 2011; Steinkamp, 2006).

Ironically, the failed third indication for amphetamine in its first life cycle, cognitive performance enhancement, has made amphetamine a blockbuster drug again over the past two decades—as pediatric and adult Attention Deficit. In 2013, the United States reached approximately the same, once-scandalous per capita amphetamine consumption rate as at the height of the first amphetamine epidemic circa 1969, virtually all prescribed for Attention Deficit (Drug Enforcement Administration, 2013; Rasmussen, 2008b). History suggests that, as with military use in the Second World War, the reason the drugs may "work" not only in boosting perceived performance but also actual marks in schoolchildren impaired by anxiety, could have as much to do with the amphetamines' confidence-building emotional effects as any cognitive effects. Moreover, the leading product of this type—Shire Pharmaceutical's Adderall—contains levoamphetamine mixed with the centrally active dextroamphetamine component, very like SKF's original Benzedrine product. It is interesting to speculate that this inclusion of the isomer responsible for the drug's "buzz"-inducing peripheral side effects, and no useful central action, may contribute to the product's efficacy through the active placebo effect—enhancing confidence (already boosted via the drug's mood-elevating effects) by signaling that the drug is "working." The "confidence drug" has found its niche.

ACKNOWLEDGMENT

This work has been supported by the Australian Research Council.

REFERENCES

Alexander, J. W. (2013). Japan's *Hiropon* panic: Resident non-Japanese and the 1950s meth crisis. *The International Journal on Drug Policy*, *24*, 238–243.

Amatsu, H., & Kubota, S. (1913). Über die pharmakologische Wirkung des Ephedrins und Mydriatins. *Kyoto Igaka Zassi*, *10*, 301–309.

Anderson, E. W. (1938). Further observations on Benzedrine. *British Medical Journal*, *2*, 60–65.

Anon. (1927). Begrussung von Professor Dr. W. N. Nagai. *Berichte der Deutschen Chemischen Gesellschaft*, *60*, 167–175.

Bradley, C. (1937). The behavior of children receiving benzedrine. *American Journal of Psychiatry*, *94*, 577–585.

Brandon, S., & Smith, D. (1962). Amphetamines in general practice. *The Journal of the College of General Practitioners*, *5*, 603–606.

Brill, H., & Hirose, T. (1969). The rise and fall of a methamphetamine epidemic: Japan 1945–1955. *Seminars in Psychiatry*, *1*, 179–194.

Bromley, E. (2006). Stimulating a normal adjustment: Misbehavior, amphetamines, and the electroencephalogram at the Bradley Home for Children. *Journal of the History of the Behavioral Sciences*, *42*, 379–398.
Carl, G. P., & Turner, W. D. (1939). The effects of benzedrine sulfate (amphetamine sulfate) on performance in a comprehensive psychometric examination. *Journal of Psychology*, *8*, 165–216.
Carl, G. P., & Turner, W. D. (1940). A further report on Benzedrine Sulfate (amphetamine sulfate): Psycho-physical effects, and supplementary results from a fifth experimental group. *Journal of General Psychology*, *22*, 105–191.
Chen, K. K., & Schmidt, C. F. (1923). The action of ephedrine, an alkaloid from Ma Huang. *Proceedings of the Society for Experimental Biology and Medicine*, *21*, 351–354.
Chen, K. K., & Schmidt, C. F. (1926). The action and clinical use of ephedrine. *Journal of the American Medical Association*, *87*, 836–842.
Cohen, P. A., Goday, A., & Swann, J. P. (2012). The return of rainbow diet pills. *American Journal of Public Health*, *102*, 1676–1686.
Connell, P. H. (1958). *Amphetamine psychosis*. London: Oxford University Press.
Connell, P. H. (1968). Amphetamine dependence. *Proceedings of the Royal Society of Medicine*, *61*, 178–181.
Davidoff, E. (1936). A clinical study of the effect of benzedrine sulfate on self-absorbed patients. *Psychiatric Quarterly*, *10*, 652–659.
Davidoff, E., & Reifenstein, E. C. (1937). The stimulating action of benzedrine sulfate. *Journal of the American Medical Association*, *108*, 1770–1776.
Davis, D. R. (1947). Psychomotor effects of analeptics and their relation to 'fatigue' phenomena in aircrew. *British Medical Bulletin*, *5*, 43–45.
Doyle, B., & Daniels, L. E. (1931). Symptomatic treatment of narcolepsy. *Journal of the American Medical Association*, *96*, 1370–1372.
Drug Enforcement Administration (2013). Final adjusted aggregate production quotas for schedule I and II controlled substances and assessment of annual needs for the list I chemicals ephedrine, pseudoephedrine, and phenylpropanolamine for 2013. *Federal Register (USA)*, *78*, 48193–48197. available at, http://www.deadiversion.usdoj.gov/fed_regs/quotas/2013/fr0807.htm, accessed 16 October, 2014.
Edeleano, L. (1887). On a few derivatives of the phenylmeth-acrylic acid and of the phenyl-iso-butyric acid. *Berichte der Deutschen Chemischen Gesellschaft*, *20*, 616.
Editor (1937a). Benzedrine Sulfate 'pep pills'. *Journal of the American Medical Association*, *108*, 1973–1974.
Editor (1937b). The confidence drug. *The Pharmaceutical Journal*, *138*, 539.
Harris, S., Ivy, A. C., & Searle, L. (1947). The mechanism of amphetamine-induced loss of weight. *Journal of the American Medical Association*, *134*, 1468–1475.
Inciardi, J., & Chambers, C. (1972). The epidemiology of amphetamine use in the general population. *Canadian Journal of Criminology and Corrections*, *14*, 166–172.
Jackson, C. O. (1971). The amphetamine inhaler: A case study of medical abuse. *Journal of the History of Medicine and Allied Sciences*, *26*, 187–196.
Kardiner, A. (1941). *The traumatic neuroses of war*. Washington, D.C.: National Research Council, USA.
Kemper, W. (2003). Pervitin—Die endsieg-droge. In W. Pieper (Ed.), *Nazis on speed: Drogen im Dritten Reich* (pp. 122–133). Lohrbach: Gruene Kraft.
Kiloh, L. G., & Brandon, S. (1962). Habituation and addiction to amphetamines. *British Medical Journal*, *2*(5296), 40–43.
Kroutil, L. A., et al. (2006). Nonmedical use of prescription stimulants in the United States. *Drug and Alcohol Dependence*, *84*, 135–143.
Lee, M. R. (2011). The history of *Ephedra* (Ma-Huang). *The Journal of the Royal College of Physicians of Edinburgh*, *41*, 78–84.

McAllister, W. B. (2000). *Drug diplomacy in the twentieth century: An international history*. London: Routledge.
Miura, K. (1887). Vorläufige Mitteilung ueber Ephedrin, ein neues Mydriaticum. *Klinische Wochenschrift Berlin, 24*, 907–911.
Molitch, M., & Eccles, A. K. (1937). The effect of benzedrine sulfate on the intelligence scores of children. *American Journal of Psychology, 94*, 587–590.
Molitch, M., & Sullivan, J. P. (1937). The effect of benzedrine sulfate on children taking the New Stanford Achievement Test. *American Journal of Orthopsychiatry, 7*, 519–522.
Monroe, R., & Drell, H. (1947). Oral use of stimulants obtained from inhalers. *Journal of the American Medical Association, 135*, 909–915.
Myerson, A. (1936). Effect of benzedrine sulfate on mood and fatigue in normal and neurotic persons. *Archives of Neurology and Psychology, 36*, 816–822.
Nathanson, M. (1937). The central action of beta-aminopropylbenzene (benzedrine). *Journal of the American Medical Association, 108*, 528–531.
Noeldeke, H. (2003). Einsatz von Leistungssteigernden Medikamenten. In W. Pieper (Ed.), *Nazis on speed: Drogen im Dritten Reich* (pp. 134–142). Lohrbach: Gruene Kraft.
Ogata, A. (1920). Constitution of ephedrine—Desoxyephedrine. *Chemical Abstracts, 14*, 745, corresponding to Journal of the Pharmacological Society, Japan, 451, 751–754 (1919).
Piness, G., Miller, H., & Alles, G. (1930). Clinical observations on phenylethanolamine sulfate. *Journal of the American Medical Association, 94*, 790–791.
Pols, H. (2007). War neurosis, adjustment problems in veterans, and an ill nation: The disciplinary project of American psychiatry during and after World War II. *Osiris, 22*, 72–92.
Prinzmetal, M., & Bloomberg, W. (1935). The use of benzedrine for the treatment of narcolepsy. *Journal of the American Medical Association, 105*, 2051–2054.
Rasmussen, N. (2006). Making the first anti-depressant: Amphetamine in American medicine, 1929–1950. *Journal of the History of Medicine and Allied Sciences, 61*, 288–323.
Rasmussen, N. (2008a). *On speed: The many lives of amphetamine*. New York: New York University Press.
Rasmussen, N. (2008b). America's first amphetamine epidemic, 1929–1971: A quantitative and qualitative retrospective. *American Journal of Public Health, 98*, 974–985.
Rasmussen, N. (2011). On the military uses of scientific expertise: Amphetamine's adoption by the allies in the Second World War. *Journal of Interdisciplinary History, 42*, 205–233.
Sargant, W., & Blackburn, J. M. (1936). The effect of benzedrine on intelligence scores. *Lancet, 228*(5911), 1385–1387.
Schube, P. G., McManamy, M. C., Trapp, C. E., & Myerson, A. (1937). The effect of Benzedrine Sulfate on certain abnormal mental states. *American Journal of Psychiatry, 94*, 27–32.
Singh, I. (2002). Bad boys, good mothers, and the 'miracle' of Ritalin. *Science in Context, 15*, 577–603.
Snelders, S., & Pieters, T. (2011). Speed in the Third Reich: Methamphetamine (Pervitin) use and a drug history from below. *Social History of Medicine, 24*, 686–699.
Solomon, P., Mitchell, R., & Prinzmetal, M. (1937). The use of benzedrine sulfate in postencephalitic Parkinson's disease. *Journal of the American Medical Association, 108*, 1765–1770.
Steinkamp, P. (2006). Pervitin testing, use and misuse in the German Wehrmacht. In W. Eckart (Ed.), *Man, medicine, and the state: The human body as an object of government sponsored medical research in the 20th century* (pp. 61–71). Stuttgart: Franz Steiner Verlag.
Turner, W. D., & Carl, G. P. (1939). Temporary changes in affect and attitude following ingestion of various amounts of Benzedrine sulfate (amphetamine sulfate). *Journal of Psychology, 8*, 415–482.
Wilbur, D. L., MacLean, A. R., & Allen, E. V. (1937). Clinical observations on the effect of benzedrine sulfate. *Journal of the American Medical Association, 109*, 549–554.
Wilson, C. W. M., & Beacon, S. (1964). An investigation into the habituating properties of an amphetamine barbiturate mixture. *British Journal of Addiction, 60*, 81–92.

CHAPTER THREE

Miracle or Menace?

The Arrival of Cocaine 1860–1900

Mike Jay[1]
Independent Scholar
[1]Corresponding author: e-mail address: info@mikejay.net

Contents

Abstract

The arrival of cocaine was the formative episode in the modern understanding of the benefits and dangers of neurostimulants. European culture and medicine had historically been poor in stimulant plants and drugs. When coca and cocaine appeared in nineteenth-century Europe, doctors, pharmacists, and the public struggled to understand their benefits and risks, and to formulate a distinction between use and abuse.

> *It doth more speedily and readily refresh and invigorate the bodily strength than any other sustenance whatever...*
>
> ***Stubbe (1662, p. 97)***

Not cocaine, but chocolate. The claim was made by a seventeenth-century Spanish physician at the point when the trade in exotic stimulants such as chocolate, tea, and coffee was laying the foundations for the modern global economy. For early modern Europeans, these novel substances that imparted vigor and promoted wakefulness seemed miraculous. They straddled the boundary between medicine and luxury, as spices had before them; in modern parlance, they were not merely stimulants but cognitive enhancers, mood elevators, and "smart drugs." In Britain and the northern states, coffee spurred the minds of the urban business class to economic activity; in Spain, which held a monopoly on its trade, chocolate became the drink of scholars and artists on creative binges. It was particularly valued by preachers who burned the midnight oil to compose and deliver their sermons: it "repairs the exhausted spirits, and they ascertain that in addition it gives them ideas and fortifies the memory" (Juan Francisco Marañon, quoted in Norton, 2008, p. 197).

International Review of Neurobiology, Volume 120
ISSN 0074-7742
http://dx.doi.org/10.1016/bs.irn.2015.01.001

Europe was unusual among global cultures in having a native *materia medica* that was predominantly narcotic and sedative. Plant-derived stimulants were long-established elsewhere: *khat* and cola in Africa, ephedra in central Asia, betel from India to New Guinea, as well as coca in the Andes. But since classical times, European psychopharmacy had largely been confined to the dark spectrum of opium and the nightshades, from the "cold herbs" of Dioscorides (Gunther, 1934, pp. 456–478) to Shakespeare's "drowsy syrups" of "poppy and mandragora" (Shakespeare, 1603–1604, Act III Scene 3). The plant stimulants of the Enlightenment were more than new substances: they were a new idea, with profound medical and social consequences.

The coca leaf played no part in the stimulant culture of the Enlightenment, though its properties were described in an influential early study of New World botany, *Joyful Newes out of the New-found Worlde*, written by the Seville physician and botanist Nicolás Monardes and published in English in 1577. Monardes reported that the natives of the Andes used coca, especially while traveling, to suppress fatigue, hunger, and thirst, and that it gives its users "great contentment"; furthermore, when they chew it together with tobacco they "go out of their wittes" (quoted in Mortimer, 1901, pp. 151–152). But the habit proved resistant to transplantation. Unlike the successful stimulants, coca leaf needs to be fresh or well preserved to prevent its alkaloids from denaturing with heat and damp, or simply over time. Samples that made the early transatlantic crossing arrived more or less inactive.

It was not until the second half of the nineteenth century that coca preparations were successfully marketed in the west. They proved immediately popular in the form of tonics and digestive wines, of which the most enduring would of course be Coca-Cola. These stimulant beverages were sold in high street groceries and pharmacies as miraculous energy-boosters, much as caffeinated drinks had been two centuries before. By this time, however, the coca leaf had also become the source of the most potent stimulant drug known to science. Pure cocaine, isolated and extracted in 1860, was a neurostimulant and euphoriant of unprecedented potency, with a vastly expanded spectrum of benefits and dangers. It became the battleground on which the social and medical status of stimulants was contested.

Coca was introduced to nineteenth-century science by a young Italian doctor, Paolo Mantegazza, who practiced from 1855 to 1858 in Argentina and Paraguay where he came into contact with coca-chewing Indians. He experimented with the leaf and began using it regularly as an evening tonic to allow him to work after dinner, gradually chewing his way through larger doses to investigate their effects. When he returned to Italy in 1859, he published *On the Hygenic and Medicinal Virtues of Coca*, a monograph that combined physiological reporting with vivid descriptions of its effect on his mental state. Like most of the early texts on coca and cocaine, Mantegazza's work blurred science and enthusiastic promotion, advocating it equally as a medicine and the height of luxury: "God is unjust because he made man incapable of sustaining the effect of coca all life long" (Mantegazza, 1859, pp. 38–42). The leaf, he observed, aids digestion and has a central stimulant action on the nervous system. At low doses, this is barely noticeable, but at higher ones it impinges on consciousness to a marked degree. Muscular power is increased: "a new strength gradually drenches one's organism in every sense, as a sponge soaks itself with water," and "one feels stronger, more agile, and readier for any kind of work."

But there was more. By pushing his dose to the practical maximum, repeatedly chewing his way through an ounce of leaf at a time at top speed, Mantegazza was able to achieve "the delirium of coca intoxication." This was marked by a racing pulse, minor heart palpitations, a surge of "extraordinary happiness," and, in the mind's eye, "images that were more bizarre and splendid, in terms of color, than could ever be imagined." Mantegazza attempted to transcribe these, losing most of them through the labor of writing but struggling against "indescribable bliss" to record "a cave of lace through the entrance to which can be seen, toward the back, a golden tortoise seated on a throne made of soap. . .a ladder made of blotting paper lined with rattlesnakes from which several red rabbits with green ears come jumping down. . .looms made of matchsticks upon which cicadas are weaving pine trees made of sulphur. . ." (all *ibid.*). This was a state perhaps familiar to the peoples of the Andes, who had long used the leaf for divination; from a European perspective it can be recognized as a preview of the effects soon to be offered by cocaine.

Mantegazza's work brought coca into the purview of German pharmacists, who had for the previous 30 years been working systematically through the alkaloid chemistry of medicinal plants. In 1859, Professor Friedrich Wöhler of Göttingen University procured 25 kg of coca leaf from Lima, which he turned over to his young assistant Albert Niemann. Niemann isolated from them a crystalline organic base that was named, according to the convention established by morphine, "cocaïne." Niemann noted in his report that the new substance crystallized in "colorless transparent prisms" and had the bitter taste characteristic of an alkaloid; unusually, it left "a peculiar numbness, followed by a sense of cold when applied to the tongue" (Niemann, 1860).

Significant as this discovery may seem in retrospect, it attracted little interest at the time: cocaïne was added to the trade catalogue of Merck Pharmaceuticals in Darmstadt, where it joined many other plant alkaloids awaiting investigation. Coca, meanwhile, was at last penetrating the European consumer market, thanks to the Corsican pharmacist and entrepreneur Angelo Mariani who began in the 1860s to produce a potent tonic wine by steeping coca leaves in sweet burgundy. Mariani succeeded where others had failed by paying close attention to the potencies of different strains of coca leaf and refining techniques for its preservation and extraction. By the late 1880s, his product range would include Pâte Mariani (cocaine lozenges for catarrh), Thé Mariani (a concentrated coca tea recommended for long walks), and Pastilles Mariani (for coughing fits). Although presented in medical language as particularly suitable for convalescents and those with bronchial or nervous conditions, the claims for coca products also associated them more broadly with health, recreation, and enjoyment. Many of Mariani's rivals stressed the exotic provenance of the leaf, their labels featuring eye-catching tableaux of Incas and conquistadors. Like the stimulant beverages of the Enlightenment, coca tonics were aimed at an upmarket urban class looking for a smart alternative to alcohol: Coca-Cola advertised itself in 1886 as a "valuable brain tonic" and "intellectual beverage" (Prendergrast, 2013, p. 29).

Through the 1870s, however, the medical world remained skeptical about the efficacy of coca. In 1875, the Scottish toxicologist Sir Robert Christison, aged 78, proceeded to walk 6 miles round Edinburgh while chewing coca leaf before bounding up the stairs to his university chambers two at a time. He repeated the experiment on some of his students and noted the same results: "it not only removes extreme fatigue, but prevents it" (Christison, 1876, pp. 527–531). He took it again on the shores of Loch Lomond and marched rapidly to the summit. But Christison's positive findings were undermined the following year by a major study conducted by G.F. Dowdeswell at University College in London and published in *The Lancet*. Dowdeswell had his students chew a variety of leaf samples mixed with slaked lime before putting them through a battery of tests, measuring their pulse and temperature, and taking urine samples. He had trouble sourcing viable mail-order coca and his results were inconclusive. He concluded that "without asserting that it is positively inert. . .its action is so slight as to preclude the idea of its having any value either therapeutically or popularly"

(Dowdeswell, 1876, pp. 664–667). Medical reluctance to endorse claims for coca made the likes of Mariani more insistent and more persuasive to their growing ranks of satisfied customers.

The rapid ascent of cocaine in the 1880s also drew energy from this early medical resistance. The doctor who broke ranks most conspicuously was the young Sigmund Freud. He first encountered cocaine in a German medical paper by the military surgeon Theodor Aschenbrandt who had been testing its effects on his Bavarian recruits: he had added cocaine solution to their drinking water without telling them, claimed they had been better able to endure hunger, strain, fatigue, and heavy burdens, and concluded with alarming gusto that the drug might make it possible for troops to dispense with food for 8 days. Freud followed Aschenbrandt's potted history of coca back to the writings of Mantegazza, which impressed him greatly; checking for references to coca in the *Surgeon General's Index*, he found a scattering of American journal articles recommending it as a treatment for the new scourge of morphinism. One in the *Detroit Therapeutic Gazette*, an uncritical mouthpiece for pharmaceutical boosters, suggested that "one feels like trying coca with or without the opium habit. A harmless remedy for the blues..." (quoted in Musto, 1989, p. 59).

Freud ordered a sample of cocaine from Merck and took a small dose dissolved in water. He was immediately released from doubts about its efficacy, experiencing "a sudden exhilaration and a feeling of ease" (Freud, 1884, pp. 49–73). He offered it to friends and colleagues and noted similar reactions, although some required a larger dose and others experienced anxiety or discomfort. Over the next 6 months, he took it frequently (though always orally, and in modest doses of a tenth of a gram or less) and performed a battery of tests on himself under the influence.

Freud's enthusiasm for cocaine is often ascribed with hindsight to juvenile ambition or psychological addiction, but he had cause to believe it promised an important breakthrough. He had refuted the medical skepticism about coca and had discovered in cocaine a reliable centrally acting stimulant of unprecedented potency. The medicine of the day was rich in sedatives—opium and morphine had been joined by chloral hydrate, and a new generation of synthetic narcotics—but a reliable nervous stimulant might open up a new dimension of therapeutics. The first fruits of his exploration emerged in the summer of 1884 with his paper *Über Coca* (*On Coca*), a survey of coca's history and the metabolic and psychological properties of its alkaloid. But it also read as a work of advocacy, in part because of the force of his corrections to previous medical skepticism, which he refers to as "undeserved" and even "slander", but also because he adopted a literary style that aimed to reflect the euphoriant effects of the drug. He refers to a dose of cocaine as a "gift," and its effects as "the most gorgeous excitement": striking language that was effective in capturing attention but became a hostage to fortune when its less benign effects emerged.

The final sections of *Über Coca* offered a series of scenarios in which cocaine might prove medically useful, within which lay the seeds of the controversies to come. His first recommendation was for its stimulant effects "in those functional states which we now cover by the name neurasthenia" (wording that offers, perhaps, an early indication of the scale of his ambition). His second was for the treatment of indigestion, and his third "in the withdrawal of morphine." He concluded the list with the surmise that "some additional uses of cocaine, based on its anesthetic property, will probably be developed in the future" (all *ibid.*).

Freud's colleague Carl Koller was quick off the mark to develop this final suggestion, which led swiftly to cocaine's adoption in ophthalmology and surgery and vindicated the general claim that it had important medical applications. But the suggestion that it offered a cure for morphinism, which had not originated with Freud but would remain obstinately attached to him, exposed its dangers. Freud's mentor at Vienna's Physiological Institute, Ernst Fleischl von Marxow, was in the grip of such an addiction, provoked by chronic pain from an amputated thumb that been made worse by failed remedial surgery and experimental electrical stimulation of the nerves. He had resorted to morphine in spiraling doses; Freud offered cocaine, which initially seemed to sharpen Fleischl's mind and restore him to better health than he had enjoyed for years. But it was not long before Fleischl began to increase his doses of cocaine and switched to subcutaneous injection, revealing that large doses of the pure drug led to powerful cravings and tolerance, inability to eat or sleep, and paranoid hallucinations. Virtually overnight, Fleischl had gone from being one of the first patients cured of a morphine habit with cocaine to one of the first to present the terrifying symptoms of a full-scale addiction to it.

Freud had failed to spot cocaine's dangers not because he was reckless or addicted; rather the opposite. He himself had never taken it in anything other than small amounts, and never by the more compulsive methods of sniffing or injecting. He had personally never felt any craving—rather, as he observed in *Über Coca*, a "slight revulsion" at the idea of further or larger doses. Now, with cases like Fleischl's emerging from surgeries and clinics across Europe and America, the tenor of medical opinion turned violently against cocaine's advocates. The optimistic claims for cocaine, among which Freud's featured prominently, became a medical scandal. Cocaine made a rapid transit from a nostrum of dubious efficacy to, in the words of the leading German psychiatrist Albrecht Erlenmeyer, "the third scourge of mankind," after alcohol and opium (quoted in Freud, 1887, p. 172). Erlenmeyer's condemnation of the cocaine cure for morphinism was echoed by the toxicologist Louis Lewin, who predicted that "the only result would be a twin passion for the two drugs" (quoted in Nahas, 1989, p. 47).

Freud's "cocaine episode" is often taken to be the fulcrum on which medical perceptions of cocaine turned, but such clarity was only available with hindsight. In *Phantastica*, his influential compendium of 1924, Louis Lewin would remind his readers that he had "at once objected" in 1885 to "the unfortunate theory that morphinism could be cured by cocaine," predicting a "twofold craving": "this, and worse, is what in fact happened. Cocaine was soon used by itself as a pleasure-producing agent" (Lewin, 1998, p. 67). Yet Lewin in 1887, on a steamer bound for New York, recorded finding himself a little dizzy and with a headache: "Ah! I thought, cocaine! Out with you, prophylactic phial. . .0.05 gr. cocaine disappeared, dizziness and headache vanished magically; cheerfulness returned and I inhaled the refreshing sea breeze with delight" (Lewin, 2011, p. 2). The distinctions between medicine and pleasure, use and abuse, feeling better and feeling better than well, would remain difficult to draw.

By 1887, as the *British Medical Journal* noted, an "undeniable reaction against the extravagant pretensions advanced on behalf of this drug has already set in" (*British Medical Journal*, 1887, Vol. I, p. 1229). But the pendulum continued to swing. That year the leading American neurologist and former Surgeon-General Dr. William Hammond replied to the alarmists with a forceful essay on *Cocaine and the So-Called Cocaine Habit*. Hammond had been using cocaine medicinally for a spinal irritation and also as a general tonic; he had drunk it, injected it, experimented with large doses (a gram injected over 20 min) and prescribed large doses to others. His conclusion was that the cocaine habit was "similar to the tea or coffee habit" (Hammond, 1887, pp. 247–252). Unlike opiates, to which patients developed a physical dependence, Hammond maintained that there was not "a single instance of a well-pronounced cocaine habit" where the addict was unable to renounce the drug by simple willpower (Hammond, 1887). The debate was necessarily entangled with those surrounding the newly minted diagnosis of addiction, which was variously construed as a physical disease, a moral weakness, a hereditary taint, or the affliction of a pathological "type."

Medical opinion was hardening against cocaine, but supply and demand were both booming. Between 1884 and 1887, the wholesale price in the United States dropped from around 15 dollars a gram to 30 cents (Spillane, 1999, p. 23). The dozens of patent preparations and tonics jostling for Mariani's market share were now competing against "ethical" products, as pure pharmaceuticals were known, whose suppliers were no less extravagant in their claims. Parke, Davis, in their promotional brochure of 1885, offered cocaine in powders, solutions, tablets, lozenges, even cigars, and cheroots claiming the drug to be "the most important therapeutic discovery of the age, the benefits of which to humanity will be simply incalculable," and "as the facts recorded would now indicate, the long sought for specific for the opium habit" (Parke, Davis and Company, 1885, pp. 127–150). Their range expanded to include toothache drops, cocaine-impregnated bandages, hemorrhoid remedies, and, from the 1890s, asthma and catarrh inhalers that made use of cocaine's vasoconstrictive properties not only to dry up the nasal passages but also to increase its psychoactive effect. Assurances that cocaine "can supply the place of food, make the coward brave, the silent eloquent" (Parke, Davis and Company, 1885) ran alongside ads for smart pocket-sized steel cases containing cocaine, morphine, and miniature needles. Gone were the Incas and conquistadors: cocaine had escaped its perception as an exotic leaf and become a pure white drug, an exemplar of the miracles of modern pharmacy.

During this height of the cocaine boom—in retrospect, the euphoric high before the crash—the public was bombarded with miraculous claims and dire warnings. Each new shift in medical opinion was read as a sign of the times, in which some saw a new age of scientific marvels and others a chaos of dangerous fads and overstimulated neurotics. Consumers were obliged to negotiate an unregulated market of products, most of them without any reliable indication of dosage, and to discover by trial and error, the difference between strong and weak preparations, when and how they were best taken, and the consequences of taking too much. This process of negotiation can be observed in the two enduring literary characters to emerge from the cocaine boom, one dealing with it implicitly and the other explicitly: Dr. Jekyll and Sherlock Holmes.

In Robert Louis Stevenson's *The Strange Case of Dr. Jekyll and Mr. Hyde*, the drug that unleashes Mr. Hyde—"a large quantity of a particular salt" (Stevenson, 1886, p. 83)—is no more than a literary prop, but the spirit of cocaine lies behind the description of its effects and perhaps the writing process itself: Stevenson, who suffered from chronic nervous exhaustion, wrote the final version of the book over 3 days and nights after destroying his first draft. Jekyll's transformation into Hyde can be read not only as a heightened version of the mood swings that he experienced throughout his life but also as a cautionary fable for the new age of chemical stimulants. As Hyde's awakens to his new state—"there was something strange in my sensations. . .something indescribably new and, from its novelty, incredibly sweet. I felt younger, lighter, happier in body; within I was conscious of a heady recklessness" (Stevenson, 1886, p. 83)—he echoes Freud's euphoric descriptions in *Über Coca*.

Whether fable, metaphor or disguised confession, *Jekyll and Hyde* was prophetic of the ways in which the cocaine debate would be framed. Like Dr. Jekyll's drug, the "heady recklessness," it produced was experienced by its subject as the very essence of vitality and delight, but this sensation was precisely the root of its danger. In Stevenson's Calvinist rubric, evil is man's natural tendency: anything that eradicates fear and moral responsibility releases the atavistic and bestial self that is unrestrained human nature. Jekyll and Hyde would come to characterize the essential danger of cocaine: that in feeding egotism and the urge for instant gratification, it makes evil feel good. In the famous title of one of Stevenson's inspirations, the cocaine user becomes a justified sinner.

If *Jekyll and Hyde* offers an enduring metaphor for cocaine, Sherlock Holmes appears to present us directly with a habitué of the late 1880s, conceived by a physician who had become familiar with the drug in the course of his medical career. In the form in which he was originally conceived, the primary motivation of the world's most famous fictional detective is cocaine. "My mind," he tells us in the famous passage that opens *The Sign of Four* (1889), "rebels at stagnation. Give me problems, give me work, give me the most abstruse cryptogram. . .I can dispense then with artificial stimulants" (Doyle, Sir Arthur Conan, 1928a,b, p. 144). Part of Holmes' enduring appeal is that he is drawn to his profession not to do good, but to stave off boredom. What motivates him, and distinguishes him from the vast majority of subsequent fictional detectives, is his primary interest in pleasing himself. Ultimately, the only reason he bothers to solve crimes is to keep his mind active enough to dispense with his 7% solution.

The Sign of Four emerged in 1889, and it is this first period of Sherlock Holmes stories that is most liberally spiked with drug references. In the first published short story, *A Scandal in Bohemia*, we hear that Holmes "had risen out of his drug-created dreams, and was hot on the scent of some new problem" (Doyle, 1928, p. 4); in *The Five Orange Pips*, Watson describes him as a "self-poisoner by cocaine and tobacco" (Doyle, 1928, p. 103). But it is the exchange between Holmes and Watson at the beginning of *The Sign of Four* that most famously establishes Holmes' use and Watson's attitude to it. The story starts in Holmes' study, with the detective taking a syringe from a "neat morocco case" and injecting it into an arm "all dotted and scarred with innumerable puncture marks." Watson tells us that this has been going on "three times a day for many months," and remonstrates with Holmes about his habit (Doyle, Sir Arthur Conan, 1928a,b, p. 143–144).

Doyle had been immersing himself in the "yellow," decadent writings of Bloomsbury, and Holmes' cocaine use was part of his literary strategy to create a bohemian character with uncommon tastes. He had met Oscar Wilde at the famous dinner at the Langham Hotel in 1890 when *The Picture of Dorian Gray* was commissioned, and it is likely that he had Wilde partly in mind while conceiving his "pallid," "languid" detective. Holmes' other distinctive props—the violin, the Meerschaum pipe, and the bachelor apartment in the metropolis—are all intended to establish him as one of the new bohemians: eccentric, sophisticated, and tantalizingly immune to public opinion. His cocaine habit is not intended to be representative of its time, but to stand apart from it. Readers might imagine his supply of the drug being dispatched in sealed vials from Germany, and his hypodermic kit the bespoke creation of an exclusive pharmacist in Piccadilly or Mayfair.

The inner Holmes as well as the outer was faithfully conceived around the bohemian stereotype. He is solitary, haunted by an existential darkness: the "black moods" that come over him, his swings from insomnia or obsessive round-the-clock work to days and weeks "in the dumps," when he does not "open my mouth for days on end" (Doyle, Sir Arthur Conan, 1929a,b, p. 12). For a late Victorian doctor like Conan Doyle, these were the traits of the highly strung, "neurasthenic type," the febrile "brain-workers" who were identified as a high-risk group for drug addiction. In *The Sign of Four*, Doyle mirrors these mood swings by giving Holmes a dual dependence on morphine and cocaine, but morphine is never subsequently mentioned: perhaps, he felt that it carried rather too strong a whiff of the pathological addict, while cocaine remained an intriguing if reprehensible vice.

The rise and fall of Holmes' cocaine habit illustrate in microcosm the pressures that, by the end of the century, had tipped the public image of the drug from miracle to menace. Through the 1890s the great detective's career unfolded in parallel with a reversal in cocaine's public image. Concern about its dangers rose sharply throughout the 1890s, and by 1900 serious lobbying to control and prohibit it had begun. The cocaine addict—gaunt, unwashed, and manic, obsessively filling a syringe or poised on the edge of violence—was becoming familiar from sensation novels, lurid true-crime tales, and images of big-city vice. These anxieties were sharpest in the United States, where the "cocaine fiend" had an all too recognizable face: that of the young black male, denizen of the jazz club and after-hours bar, high on his "five-cent sniff," and, like Mr. Hyde, shameless in gratifying his animal instincts.

By the early 1900s, the Sherlock Holmes stories were finding huge success in America serialized to a large readership in *Collier's Weekly*. But by this point, many big-city pharmacies in the United States were refusing to sell cocaine to suspicious customers, and *Collier's* was running editorials about the "cocaine menace" and petitions for its licensed control. Doyle pruned back the references to Holmes' habit, limiting them to the occasional dark mention of his hero's "weakness." In 1903, Coca-Cola removed the cocaine from its product; in 1904, in *The Missing Three-Quarter*, Doyle removed it from his by announcing that Holmes had been "weaned" by Dr. Watson from the "drug mania" that had threatened to check his remarkable career (Doyle, 1928, p. 809). It was a narrative twist that undermined the coherence of his hero, requiring him to forget why he had become a detective in the first place. But it was congruent with the changing times: cocaine, having originally boosted Holmes' popularity, was now a liability that might destroy it.

The consumer of the late nineteenth century was presented with coca and cocaine preparations in a bewildering variety of forms and potencies, accompanied by a clamor of contested information and opinion, medical claim and counter claim. Though typically framed in medical terms, its use spanned strict medical applications, a general health tonic, an accessory to recreation, and, in its later stages, the untrammeled and self-destructive pursuit of pleasure. Although coca promoters such as Angelo Mariani were tireless in maintaining that the dangers were confined to the pure drug, the benefits and risks of cocaine and the milder herbal preparations were routinely conflated. The image of the "cocaine fiend" drew on wider anxieties that were also explored in popular fiction: the free availability of powerful stimulants in an anonymous and atomized urban society, and the disruptive subcultures that might coalesce around them.

In the years around the Great War, cocaine would be brought under statutory controls and its nonmedical use criminalized, codifying the change in its cultural status. But the consumer demand for stimulants was not so easily closed down. During the twentieth century, substitutes such as amphetamines would emerge and establish themselves in pharmacies before making cocaine's transit to controlled drug, and thereafter to a thriving illicit market. In the twenty-first century, western society is anything but stimulant poor. Coca and cocaine are now subsumed within a *materia medica* that encompasses pure caffeine powder and off-label modafinil, street methamphetamine and Ritalin, khat and mephedrone, and to which dozens of new "legal highs" are added each year. Global consumption of cocaine in 1900 was around 15 metric tons; today, the UN estimates it at 865 (United Nations, 2010, 2.3.1).

REFERENCES

Christison, R. (1876). Observations of cuca, or coca, the leaves of erythroxylon coca. *British Medical Journal, 1*, 527–531.

Dowdeswell, G. (1876). The coca leaf. *The Lancet, 1*, 631–633, 664–667.

Doyle, Sir Arthur Conan. (1928a). *Sherlock Holmes: Short stories*. Frome and London: John Murray and Jonathan Cape.

Doyle, Sir Arthur Conan. (1928b). *The sign of four*. Frome and London: John Murray and Jonathan Cape (in Sherlock Holmes: Long stories).

Freud, S. (1884). *Über Coca*. New York, 1974: Stonehill (English Trans. S. A. Edminster, reprinted in R. Byck (Ed.), *Cocaine papers: Sigmund Freud*).

Freud, S. (1887). *Craving for and fear of cocaine*. New York, 1974: Stonehill (English Trans. L. A. Freisinger, reprinted in R. Byck (Ed.), *Cocaine papers: Sigmund Freud*).

Gunther, R. (Ed.)., (1934). *Greek herbal of Dioscorides*. New York: Hafner Publishing.

Hammond, W. A. (1887). Cocaine and the so-called cocaine habit. In G. Andrews, & D. Solomon (Eds.), *The coca leaf and cocaine papers*. New York and London, 1975: Harcourt Brace Jovanovich.

Lewin, L. (1998). *Phantastica*. Rochester, VT: Park Street Press (1924, English Trans. P. H. A. Wirth, reprinted).

Lewin, L. (2011). *Across the USA and Canada in 1887: A German scientist experiences North America*. Bloomington IN: iUniverse (H. Jaffe and D. Sacks, Trans.).

Mantegazza, P. (1859). *On the hygenic and medicinal virtues of coca*. New York and London, 1975: Harcourt Brace Jovanovich (English excerpts Trans. L. Forti and G. Alhadeff, in G. Andrews and D. Solomon (Eds.), *The coca leaf and cocaine papers*).

Mortimer, W. G. (1901). *The divine plant of the Incas* (pp. 151–152). New York and London, 1975: Harcourt Brace Jovanovich (reprinted in G. Andrews and D. Solomon (Eds.), *The coca leaf and cocaine papers*).

Musto, D. F. (1989). America's first cocaine epidemic. *Wilson Quarterly, 13*(Summer), 59–64.

Nahas, G. (1989). *Cocaine: The great white plague*. Middlebury, VT: Paul S. Eriksson.

Niemann, A. (1860). On a new organic base in the coca leaves. *Archiv der Pharmazie, 153*, 2 (Wiley Online Library).

Norton, M. (2008). *Sacred gifts, profane pleasures: A history of tobacco and chocolate in the Atlantic world*. Ithaca, NY: Cornell (p/b ed. 2010).

Parke, Davis and Company. (1885). Coca erythroxolon and its derivatives. New York, 1974: Stonehill (reprinted in R. Byck (Ed.), *Cocaine papers: Sigmund Freud*).
Prendergrast, M. (2013). *For God, country and coca-cola.* New York: Basic Books.
Shakespeare, W. (1603–1604). *Tragedy of Othello.* London, 1622: Printed by N.O. for Thomas Walkley.
Spillane, J. F. (1999). *Making a modern drug: The manufacture, sale and control of cocaine in the United States, 1880–1920.* London and New York, 1999: Routledge (in P. Gootenberg (Ed.), *Cocaine: Global histories*).
Stevenson, R. L. (1886). *The strange case of Dr. Jekyll and Mr. Hyde.* London, 1979: Penguin Classics.
Stubbe, H. (1662). *The Indian nectar, or, a discourse concerning chocolata.* London: Printed by J.C. for Andrew Crooke.
United Nations. (2010). *World drug report.* http://www.unodc.org/documents/wdr/WDR_2010/World_Drug_Report_2010_lo-res.pdf.

CHAPTER FOUR

Psychostimulants: Basic and Clinical Pharmacology

Andrew C. McCreary*[,1], Christian P. Müller[†,1], Małgorzata Filip[‡,§,2]
*Brains On-Line, Groningen, The Netherlands
[†]Department of Psychiatry and Psychotherapy, Friedrich-Alexander-University of Erlangen-Nuremberg, Erlangen, Germany
[‡]Laboratory of Drug Addiction Pharmacology, Institute of Pharmacology, Polish Academy of Sciences, Krakow, Poland
[§]Department of Toxicology, Faculty of Pharmacy, Jagiellonian University, Krakow, Poland
[2]Corresponding author: e-mail address: mal.fil@if-pan.krakow.pl

Contents

Abstract

Substance use disorder, and particularly psychostimulant use disorder, has considerable socioeconomic burden globally. The psychostimulants include several chemical classes, being derivatives of benzoylecgonine, phenethylamine, phenylpropanolamine, or aminoaryloxazoline. Psychostimulant drugs activate the brain reward pathways of the mesoaccumbal system, and continued use leads to persistent neuroplastic and dysfunctional changes of a variety of structures involved in learning and memory, habit-forming learning, salience attribution, and inhibitory control. There are a variety of neurochemical and neurobehavioral changes in psychostimulant addiction, for

[1] Contributed equally.

International Review of Neurobiology, Volume 120
ISSN 0074-7742
http://dx.doi.org/10.1016/bs.irn.2015.02.008

example, dopaminergic, glutamatergic, serotonergic (5-HT-ergic), and γ-amino butyric acid (GABA) changes have all noted. In this chapter, we will review pharmacological changes associated with psychostimulant use and abuse in humans and animals, and on the basis of the best characterized and most widely abused psychostimulants (amphetamines, cocaine) discuss why use transitions into abuse and review basic science and clinical strategies that might assist in treating psychostimulant abuse.

1. INTRODUCTION

One of the leading health problems remains substance use disorder (SUD). "Drug addiction," now SUD, is a brain disease in which psychoactive drugs evoke clinically significant impairments or distress due to the continued pathological use. Using the current classification, the term *substance use disorder* includes *substance abuse* and *substance dependence/substance addiction* (DSM-5).

The most widely used psychoactive drugs are psychostimulants. A worldwide increase in their use is attributed to the positive (enhancing) effects on brain (Peroutka, Newman, & Harris, 1988). Here, we review the current knowledge pertaining to psychostimulants of different chemical classes, associated chemistry, and nonclinical and clinical pharmacology. Finally, we address the best characterized and most widely abused psychostimulants (amphetamines, cocaine) in the context of the neurobiology underling the transit from psychostimulant use to abuse and dependence and discuss approaches for the treatment of psychostimulant use disorder.

2. HUMAN AND ANIMAL EFFECTS OF PSYCHOSTIMULANTS

In humans, psychostimulants produce several effects. Low doses heighten alertness and increase energy, cognitive enhancement, locomotion, sociality, and mental attention, while they reduce fatigue, sexual stimulation, and appetite. In moderate doses, psychostimulants evoke euphoria, cognitive impairment, or in some cases hallucinations. High doses usually produce tremors, vomiting, tonic–clonic convulsions, agitation/anxiety, dizziness, psychoses (delusions and paranoia), restlessness, hyperthermia, and/or rapid muscle breakdown. Many of psychostimulants also share other adverse side effects such as cardiovascular or hematologic liability and the serotonin syndrome (Boutrel & Koob, 2004; Cami et al., 2000; Foley, 2005; Westfall,

2006). With repeated use at higher doses, some psychostimulants produce SUD in susceptible human individuals (Boutrel & Koob, 2004).

Basic research on psychostimulant actions concentrates primarily on modeling abuse–dependence symptoms using models of behavioral sensitization, conditioned locomotion, drug discrimination, conditioned place preference, drug self-administration, or variations in self-administration (de Wit & Stewart, 1981; Shippenberg & Koob, 2002; See, 2005).

3. CHEMISTRY AND PHARMACOLOGY OF PSYCHOSTIMULANTS

Psychostimulants belong to a various chemical classes, including benzoylecgonine, substituted phenethylamines, phenylpropanolamines, and aminoaryloxazolines (Table 1).

The benzoylecgonine derivatives include cocaine, a tropane alkaloid derived from the leaves of the coca plant.

The precursor of all synthetic amphetamines is ephedrine, the component derived from *Ephedra sinica* (yellow hemp, or *Ma huang* in Chinese traditional medicine). The diastereomer, pseudoephedrine, is also found naturally in this species. Both drugs are widely used for weight loss and to enhance performance; however, higher doses and protracted use are recognized as stimulants (Broadley, 2010). Ephedrine and pseudoephedrine are also precursors used in the synthesis of methamphetamine and have received regulatory control.

Amphetamine, sympathomimetic amine, is the prototypical structure of synthetic psychostimulants and possesses clinical anorexic and stimulant properties. Several of amphetamine derivatives have been synthesized including methamphetamine causing wakefulness and stronger euphoric effects that can lead to rapid abuse and addiction and other psychiatric consequences (Anglin, Burke, Perrochet, Stamper, & Dawud-Noursi, 2000). Other amphetamine-related drugs include bupropion, fenfluramine, methylphenidate, and phenylpropanolamine. Bupropion is used as an antidepressant and smoking cessation aid with low dependence liability. Fenfluramine has been used (with phentermine) as an appetite suppressant with amphetamine-like sympathomimetic. Methylphenidate is used for treatment of attention deficit hyperactivity disorder (ADHD), postural orthostatic tachycardia syndrome, and narcolepsy and possesses only moderate dependence liability, but which can result in SUD (Parran & Jasinski, 1991). Phenylpropanolamine is used as nasal decongestant

Table 1 Drugs That Evoke Brain Stimulation and (in High Doses) Lead to Euphoria

Drug	Other (Street) Names	Chemical Structure	Mechanism of Action
2C-B		2,5-Dimethoxy-4-bromophenethylamine	5-$HT_{2A/2C}$ partial agonist
2C-C		2,5-Dimethoxy-4-chlorophenethylamine	5-$HT_{2A/2C}$ partial agonist
2C-D	LE-25	2,5-Dimethoxy-4-methylphenethylamine	5-$HT_{2A/2C}$ partial agonist
2C-E	Europa	2,5-Dimethoxy-4-ethylphenethylamine	5-$HT_{2A/2C}$ partial agonist
2C-H		2,5-Dimethoxyphenethylamine	5-$HT_{2A/2C}$ partial agonist
2C-I	i	2,5-Dimethoxy-4-iodophenethylamine	5-$HT_{2A/2C}$ partial agonist
2C-T	4-Methylthio-2,5-DMPEA	2-(2,5-Dimethoxy-4-(methylthio)phenyl)-ethanamine	5-HT_{2A} agonist, MAO-A inhibitor
2C-T-2	T2	2,5-Dimethoxy-4-ethylthiophenethylamine	5-$HT_{2A/2C}$ partial agonist
2C-T-4	T4	2,5-Dimethoxy-4-isopropylthiophenethylamine	5-$HT_{2A/2C}$ partial agonist
2C-T-7	T7; 7th Heaven, Blue Mystic; Beautiful; Tripstacy; Tweety-Bird Mescaline; Belladona	2,5-Dimethoxy-4-propylthiophenethylamine	5-$HT_{2A/2C}$ partial agonist, MAO-A inhibitor
2C-T-19		2,5-Dimethoxy-4-butylthiophenethylamine	MAO-A inhibitor
2-FA		2-Fluoroamphetamine	Monoamine releaser
2-FMA		2-Fluoromethamphetamine	Monoamine releaser
2-MA	Ortetamine	2-Methylamphetamine	Monoamine releaser
3-FA		3-Fluoroamphetamine	Monoamine releaser

3-FEA		3-Fluoroethamphetamine	Monoamine releaser
3-FMA		3-Fluoromethamphetamine	Monoamine releaser
3-FMC		3-Fluoromethcathinone	Monoamine releaser
3-MA	PAL-314	3-Methylamphetamine	Monoamine releaser
4-FMA		4-Fluoromethamphetamine	Monoamine releaser
4-MA	PAL-313; Aptrol; *p*-TAP	4-Methylamphetamine	Monoamine releaser
4-MMA	PMMA	4-Methoxymethamphetamine	Monoamine releaser
4-MTA	Flatliner; Golden Eagle	4-Methylthioamphetamine	SRA, MAO-A inhibitor
4,4′-DMAR		4-Methyl-5-(-4-methylphenyl)-4,5-dihydrooxazol-2-amine = 4,4′-dimethylaminorex	Monoamine releaser
Amphepramone	Diethylpropion, Diethylcathinone	(*RS*)-2-Diethylamino-1-phenylpropan-1-one = α-methyl-β-keto-*N*,*N*-diethylphenethylamine	NRA > DRA > SRA
Amphetamine		(*RS*)-1-Phenylpropan-2-amine	TAAR1 agonist, VMAT2 inhibitor
Adrafinil	Prodrug to modafinil	(*RS*)-2-Benzhydrylsulfinylethanehydroxamic acid	α_1-adrenergic receptor agonist
Armodafinil		(−)-2-[(*R*)-(Diphenylmethyl)sulfinyl]acetamide = (−)-(*R*)-enantiomer of the racemic modafinil	DAT inhibitor, D2 receptor agonist
Bupropion	Amfebutamone	(±)-2-(*tert*-Butylamino)-1-(3-chlorophenyl)propan-1-one	NDRI

Continued

Table 1 Drugs That Evoke Brain Stimulation and (in High Doses) Lead to Euphoria—cont'd

Drug	Other (Street) Names	Chemical Structure	Mechanism of Action
Caffeine		1,3,7-Trimethylpurine-2,6-dione	A1/A2A/A2B/A3 receptor antagonist
Cocaine	Crack	Methyl(1*R*,2*R*,3*S*,5*S*)-3-(benzoyloxy)-8-methyl-8-azabicyclo[3.2.1]octane-2-carboxylate = metyl benzoylecgonine	Monoamine reuptake inhibitor
Dextroamphetamine		(2*S*)-1-Phenylpropan-2-amine	TAAR1 agonist, VMAT2 inhibitor
Dexfenfluramine		(*S*)-*N*-Ethyl-1-[3-(trifluoromethyl)phenyl]-propan-2-amine	SRI
DOET	DOE, Hecate	2,5-Dimethoxy-4-ethylamphetamine	5-$HT_{2A/2B/2C}$ receptor partial agonist, human TAAR1 agonist
DOI		2,5-Dimethoxy-4-iodoamphetamine	5-$HT_{2A/2B/2C}$ receptor partial agonist
DOM	STP (Serenity, Tranquility, and Peace)	2,5-Dimethoxy-4-methylamphetamine	5-$HT_{2A/2B/2C}$ receptor partial agonist
Ephedrine		(*R*,*S*)-2-(Methylamino)-1-phenylpropan-1-ol	NRA > DRA
Fenfluramine		3-Trifluoromethyl-*N*-ethylamphetamine	SRA/SRI
Lisdexamfetamine	LDX	L-Lysine-dextroamphetamine	TAAR1 agonist, VMAT2 inhibitor
MDA	Tenamfetamine, Sally, Sass, Sass-a-frass, Love Drug	3,4-Methylenedioxyamphetamine	DSRI

MDE	MDEA, *N*-ethyl MDA, Eve	3,4-Methylenedioxy-*N*-ethylamphetamine	Monoamine releaser
MDMA	Ecstasy, "E", "X", XTC, Adam, Mandy, Molly"	3,4-Methylenedioxymethamphetamine	Monoamine releaser/ reuptake inhibitor
MDMAR		3,4-Methylenedioxy-4-methylaminorex	Monoamine releaser
MDPV	Methylenedioxypyrovalerone	3,4-Methylenedioxypyrovalerone	NDRI
Mephedrone	4-Methylephedrone, 4-MMC, drone, M-CAT, meow meow	(*RS*)-2-Methylamino-1-(4-methylphenyl)propan-1-one = 4-methylmethcathinone	Monoamine releaser/ reuptake inhibitor
Methamphetamine	Desoxyn, ICE, Crank, Speed	D-Desoxyephedrine = *N*-methyl-1-phenylpropan-2-amine	TAAR1 agonist
Methcathinone	*N*-Methylcathinone, ephedrone, Jeff, mulka, cat, cosmos, Jee cocktail	(*RS*)-2-(Methylamino)-1-phenylpropan-1-one	NDRI > SRI
Methylone	M1, MDMC, bk-MDMA	3,4-Methylenedioxy-*N*-methylcathinone	Monoamine releaser/ reuptake inhibitor
Methylphenidate	MPH	Methylphenyl(2-piperidinyl)acetate	NDRI
MADA		1-(7-Methoxy-1,3-benzodioxol-5-y)-2-propanamine = 3-methoxy-MDA	SRA, 5-HT_{2A} receptor agonist
MAMMA		3-Methoxymethamphetamine	Monoamine releaser, TAAR1 agonist
Modafinil		2-Benzhydrylsulfinylacetamide	α_1-Adrenergic receptor agonist, DAT inhibitor

Continued

Table 1 Drugs That Evoke Brain Stimulation and (in High Doses) Lead to Euphoria—cont'd

Drug	Other (Street) Names	Chemical Structure	Mechanism of Action
Nephron	O-2482	1-Naphthalen-2-y-2-pyrrolidin-1-y-pentan-1-one	Monoamine reuptake inhibitor
NEA		*N*-Ethylamphetamine	TAAR1 agonist, VMAT2 inhibitor
N-hydroxy MDA	MDOH	*N*-Hydroxy-3,4-methylenedioxyamphetamine *N*-hydroxy-α-methyl-1,3-benzodioxole-5-ethanamine,monohydrochloride	NRI > SRI
N,*N*-DMA	Dimephenopan; dimephenopane; dimetamfetamine	Dimethylamphetamine	Monoamine releaser
Phenylpropanolamine	PPA	(1*S*,2*R*)-2-Amino-1-phenylpropan-1-ol = β-hydroxyamphetamine	α- and β_3-Adrenoceptor agonist, D1 receptor partial agonist
Pseudoephedrine	PSE	(*S*,*S*)-2-Methylamino-1-phenylpropan-1-ol	α- and β2-Adrenergic receptor agonist
TMA		1-(3,4,5-Trimethoxyphenyl)propan-2-amine	TAAR1 agonist, VMAT2 inhibitor

Abbreviations: 5-HT, serotonin; A, adenosine; D1, dopamine D1 receptor; DAT, dopamine transporter; DRA, dopamine-releasing agent; DSRI, dopamine/serotonin reuptake inhibitor; MAO-A, monoamine oxidase type A; NDRI, noradrenalin/dopamine reuptake inhibitor; NRA, noradrenaline-releasing agent; NRI, noradrenaline reuptake inhibitor; SRA, serotonin-releasing agent; SRI, serotonin reuptake inhibitor; TAAR1, trace amine-associated receptor 1; VMAT2, vesicular monoamine transporter 2.

(Fossberg, Beisland, & Lundgren, 1983), and as an appetite suppressor (Weintraub, Masek, & Billingham, 1985), presumably through β_3-adrenoceptor stimulation (Collins & Surwit, 2001).

Other amphetamine-like drugs of abuse are popular recreational illegal substances with hallucinogenic properties include the entactogens 3,4-methylenedioxymethamphetamine (MDMA, ecstasy), 3,4-methylenedioxyethamphetamine (MDEA), and their metabolite 3,4-methylenedioxyamphetamine (MDA; Condon & Smith, 2003). A marked increase in the popularity of MDMA use (Landry, 2002) is attributed to its positive effects on mood, well-being, and perceived safety (Peroutka et al., 1988), despite the fact that adverse health effects including serotonin neurotoxicity, psychiatric disorders, renal failure, malignant hyperthermia, rhabdomyolysis, and disseminated intravascular coagulation (Skrinska & Gock, 2005). 4,4′-DMAR and MDMAR (see Table 1) have recently appeared on the illicit market and share psychostimulant properties similar to those of amphetamine and MDMA, but users are prone to sudden death.

Another series of designer psychostimulants producing combination of stimulant and hallucinogenic effects is listed in Table 1 (Kerrigan et al., 2014).

Beta-cathinone derivatives or "designer" recreational drugs have been recently described and bear structural homology with amphetamine. They appeared as intermediates in the synthesis of ephedrine analogs; however, the parent, sympathomimetic amine, *S*-(−)-cathinone, possesses euphoric amphetamine-like properties (Kalix & Braenden, 1985). The most popular beta-cathinones include mephedrone, naphyrone, and MDPV (see Table 1). In humans, they evoke stimulation (so-called flying euphoria) followed by a period of feeling of invincibility, increased libido, and physical desire. Chronic abuse of beta-cathinones leads to the development of tolerance and dependence. The most common adverse effects reported in beta-cathinone users are neurological, psychiatric, cardiovascular, and hematologic disturbances.

Psychostimulant use is widespread and occurs in both recreational and clinical settings. They include drugs with (i) a high potential for abuse and no accepted medical use (e.g., beta-cathinones, MDMA), (ii) a high potential for abuse which may lead to severe psychological or physical dependence and accepted for medical use with severe restrictions (e.g., amphetamine, cocaine, methamphetamine, methylphenidate), (iii) a low potential for abuse which may lead to limited physical dependence or psychological dependence with accepted medical use (e.g., armodafinil, dexfenfluramine, dextromethylphenidate, modafinil), and (iv) unscheduled (e.g., adrafinil, bupropion).

Almost all psychostimulants display abuse potential, and it should be underlined that recreational doses are generally much larger than those prescribed by clinicians for therapeutic applications, and therefore carry a far greater risk of serious side effects.

The primary mechanism of action of psychostimulants varies, yet common, or overlapping, mechanisms of action are extensively described:

(1) release of neuronal catecholamines (amphetamines, fenfluramine, methylone, methylphenidate);
(2) inhibition of monoamine uptake (amphetamines, beta-cathinones, cocaine, fenfluramine, methylone, methylphenidate);
(3) inhibition of monoamine oxidase (amphetamine);
(4) binding to extracellular receptors: adrenoceptors (adrafinil, armodafinil, ephedrine, modafinil, phenylpropanamine, pseudoephedrine), serotonin (5-HT) receptors (e.g., 5-$HT_{2A/2C}$ series "hallucinogens," DOI, DOM), and adenosine receptors (caffeine).

A particular psychostimulant can have multiple mechanisms of actions (Table 1). For example, amphetamines inhibit the transporter proteins for the dopamine, norepinephrine, and 5-HT neurotransmitters via trace amine-associated receptor 1, release these neurotransmitters from synaptic vesicles via vesicular monoamine transporter 2 (Riddle, Topham, Haycock, Hanson, & Fleckenstein, 2002; Sitte et al., 1998), and impair dopamine metabolism by inhibiting monoamine oxidase (Ramsay & Hunter, 2002).

A hallmark of psychostimulants, which possess different primary mechanisms of action, is the increased dopaminergic neurotransmission within the mesolimbic or so-called reward system (Filip, Alenina, Bader, & Przegalinski, 2010; Sulzer, 2011). This reward pathway is composed of dopaminergic neurons projecting from the ventral tegmental area to several cortical and subcortical structures. The terminus of the mesolimbic dopaminergic pathway, the nucleus accumbens, is the key structure executing reward processes and serves to regulate motivation and learning processes (Di Chiara et al., 1999). It should be underlined that although impairment evoked by the abuse of addictive drugs starts in brain areas processing reward, the long-term drug intake disrupts the whole brain leading to dysfunctions of emotions, motivations, learning, memory, executive control, and cognitive awareness (Volkow, Fowler, & Wang, 2003) and appears to be under control of glutamatergic neurotransmission (reviewed by Kalivas, 2004; Pomierny-Chamioło et al., 2014; Tzschentke & Schmidt, 2003). Glutamate is a key mediator of synaptic plasticity, learning and memory processes, and the current notion of addiction, indicating that aberrant forms of drug-induced synaptic plasticity and learning drive compulsive relapsing behaviors (Dacher & Nugent, 2011).

4. PSYCHOSTIMULANT USE VERSUS ABUSE

Psychostimulant use and addiction cannot be fully explained on the basis of the pharmacological properties of the drugs, and it was suggested that psychostimulant use disorder is always anteceded by a period of controlled psychostimulant use. To view controlled drug use as driven by the pharmacological reinforcing effects of the drug may be an oversimplification of the complex processes driving these behaviors. While drug addiction constitutes a maladaptive behavior, the nonaddicted controlled use of psychostimulant drugs might, under certain circumstances, have beneficial effects on life goals, performance, or well-being (Hagen et al., 2009; Lende & Smith, 2002; Müller & Schumann, 2011a, 2011b).

Developmentally humans are not programmed to establish drug consumptive behavior. Thus, it may be assumed that the expression of this behavioral trait over generations is based on the capability to learn this trait (Hopitt & Laland, 2013; Müller, 2015; Müller et al., 2012). However, the ability to modify food consumption according to nonnutritional needs may be the phylogenetic origin of psychostimulant drug consumption (Müller & Schumann, 2011a, 2011b). This capability is in evolutionary terms established in various species (Huffman, 2003; Rodriguez & Wrangham, 1993). The learning of this kind of consummatory behavior may then involve either learning by trial-and-error events (newly emerging substances) or cultural inheritance (Dean, Kendal, Schapiro, Thierry, & Laland, 2012; Hassan et al., 2013).

Epidemiological data suggest that the majority of people who consume psychoactive drugs are not addicts and will never become addicted (O'Malley & Johnston, 2002; Zinberg & Jacobson, 1976). Among the 22.5 million illicit drugs "users" (previous month use) in the United States, approximately only 28.9% are addicts (SAMHSA, 2011), statistics echoed in the European Union (20% EMCDDA, 2012). This parallels epidemiological studies, suggesting that cumulative risk (at age <54) to meet criteria for cocaine dependence was 21% (Wagner & Anthony, 2002). Overall, risk estimates and trajectory research support this view, indicating that the majority of psychostimulant users are not addicts, nor will they ever become addicts, but do develop a regular well-controlled consumption pattern (Smirnov et al., 2013; Swendsen et al., 2012). While this should not underestimate the socioeconomic burden of psychostimulant addiction, it does show that considerable psychoactive drug use is not related to addiction *per se*.

When interviewed, nonaddicted drug users acknowledge subjectively perceived psychological benefits of drug consumption (Chick, 1999) related to moderate and noncompulsive, i.e., nonaddictive, consumption. There is evidence for beneficial effects of psychostimulant use on everyday function (Singh, Müller, & Vicknasingam, 2014). Thereby, the overwhelming majority of nonaddicted humans consume psychoactive drugs as an activity of normal daily living (O'Malley & Johnston, 2002; Skogen, Harvey, Henderson, Stordal, & Mykletun, 2009). Their drug usage appears highly organized and context- and task-specific, e.g., attending social events. Nonaddicted users may take these drugs because the subsequent effects can be used for the attainment of personal goals in a highly systematic way (Müller & Schumann, 2011a, 2011b). It was proposed that psychoactive drugs can be *instrumentalized*. Thereby, *drug instrumentalization* refers to a two-step behavioral complex consisting of two interlinked processes. In the *A-process*, a psychoactive drug is sought and consumed in order to change the mental state of a person into a previously learned mental state. In the *B-process*, the induced mental state allows for a better performance of another, previously established behavior (Müller & Schumann, 2011a, 2011b). An *instrument* may generally be conceived as something that helps to achieve a goal, which would not be achievable or require higher workload without the use of the instrument (Müller & Schumann, 2011a). A *goal* is defined here as the outcome of an already established, nondrug-related behavior. In the case of drug instrumentalization, the instrument is the effect of the drug on *mental state*. The nervous system of human beings displays different modes of action, which can be conceived as internal, affective or synonymously, mental states. Mental states are the working modes of the brain which are held stable over longer periods of time during which they provide the functional setting for fast computational processes. Mental states control subjective perception, memory retrieval, and autonomic and behavioral responses (White, 1996). The mental states of the brain are determined by the different functional states of the modulatory transmitter systems, such as the dopaminergic, 5-HT-ergic, acetylcholinergic, noradrenergic, and various neuropeptidergic systems, which control information processing in diencephalic and telencephalic regions of the brain (Castren, 2005; Müller et al., 2011). These systems display different modes of basal activity depending on various external factors and internal factors, such as glucose, oxygen, or hormone levels (Müller & Jacobs, 2010; Sarter, Hasselmo, Bruno, & Givens, 2005). The mental state of the brain predisposes an organism's responses to environmental stimuli which, in turn, determine the efficacy of an organism in performing established instrumental behaviors and, thus, how effectively goals are achieved. Importantly, when an organism pursues specific goals, there are particular mental states permissive to the behavior. Using this framework, nonaddicted psychoactive drug consumption is more complex than simple reinforcement-driven behavior. The full extent of the behavioral complex needs not only to consider the *set* of the organism, its surrounding *settings* (Zinberg, 1984), but importantly *subsequent* behaviors and their outcomes that follow the ensuing mental state change (Müller & Schumann, 2011a).

Settings prone for drug instrumentalization can be identified by asking nonaddicts why and under which circumstances they consume psychoactive drugs. Numerous mechanisms of psychoactive drug use have been described in terms of unique instrumentalization goals (Chick, 1999). These instrumentalization goals are extensive, but at a simplistic level might reflect (learnt) coping strategies to what might seem like normal life events.

4.1 Improved Social Interaction

Psychostimulant drugs are among those drugs that can change mental states in a way facilitating the transition from a professional to more private behavioral repertoire. It is not the pharmacological effect of the drug alone that enhances social behavior, but rather the interaction with social stimuli. Psychostimulant drugs, such as cocaine, amphetamine, methylphenidate, methamphetamine, and MDMA, are also used in a social context as a "social lubrication" (Britt & McCance-Katz, 2005; Ramo, Grov, Delucchi, Kelly, & Parsons, 2011) and appear effective at low–medium dose ranges (Morgan, Noronha, Muetzelfeldt, Fielding, & Curran, 2013). In addition to arousal and increased attention, people become more disinhibited and self-confident, while fatigue is suppressed, facilitating prolonged social interaction (Fischman & Schuster, 1980). An increase in aggression after psychostimulant consumption (Emley & Hutchinson, 1983) may result in dominating in social gatherings and the "competition" for partners, which can further enhance the beneficial effects (King, Johnson, & Van Vugt, 2009).

4.2 Facilitated Sexual Behavior

Much of the same rules controlling social interactions restrict occasions for sexual behavior. Thus, a "scheduled" and time-dependent (Patrick & Maggs, 2008) transition from professional to private environments may significantly enhance the chances of finding a partner and/or increase the frequency of sexual behavior. The latter may also account for established couples to escape daily routine. It may, therefore, not be surprising that psychostimulant drugs like amphetamines, MDMA, and cocaine instrumentalized to improve social interactions can also facilitate sexual behavior. However, psychostimulants serve to improve chances for sexual behavior, although they may interfere with physical performance during sexual intercourse in males (Waldorf, Reinarman, & Murphy, 1991).

4.3 Improved Cognitive Performance and Counteracting Fatigue

Highly developed societies put a high cognitive demand on individuals in education and work environments (Arria & Wish, 2006). Having the means to "artificially" prolong cognitive capacity may appear beneficial for the individual. While little is known about whether drugs can actually increase cognitive performance in a normal healthy person with full mental capacity, there is considerable evidence, suggesting that mild impairments due to exhaustion, fatigue, or mood swings can be compensated with psychoactive drugs (Morgan et al., 2013). In this case, no other mental state is desirable, but the maintenance of a baseline state becomes the driver. This may also refer to tasks with a low cognitive load and the wish to enhance "everyday functioning" and "quality of life" (Padwa et al., 2014; Singh et al., 2014). Psychostimulant drugs have been widely used to increase cognitive performance over long periods of time, in particular to improve concentration, vigilance, wakefulness, studying, etc. (Arria & Wish, 2006; Eickenhorst, Vitzthum, Klapp, Groneberg, & Mache, 2012; Grinspoon & Hedblom, 2005; McCabe, Knight, Teter, & Wechsler, 2005). Psychostimulants effectively increase arousal and learning attention in humans for long periods of time at doses inducing only a short lasting "high," with no signs of dysphoria (Higgins et al., 1990; Stillman, Jones, Moore, Walker, & Welm, 1993). Attention deficits induced by sleep deprivation can be ameliorated by low/medium doses of cocaine (Fischman & Schuster, 1980). Long-term regular use of these drugs, however, can induce tolerance for the cognitive effects and even lead to cognitive and social cognition deficits (Hulka et al., 2014; Preller et al., 2014).

4.4 Facilitated Recovery and Coping with Psychological Stress

Modern societies demand constant high cognitive and physical performance, and they also allow decreasingly little time for the individual to recover from periods of high workload. Using drugs to accelerate recovery and to enhance coping, thus, increases the success of many other behaviors (Morgan et al., 2013).

There are a number of different drugs that are instrumentalized to facilitate recovery and coping with psychological stress (Müller & Schumann, 2011a), including psychostimulant drugs (Waldorf et al., 1991). Chronic exaggerated drug use for this instrumentalization goal may result in restlessness and a hyperanxious state during withdrawal, and compulsive drug use to overcome this state.

4.5 Sensory Curiosity—Expanded Perception Horizon and Boredom

The search for novelty is a driving force to expose an individual to stimuli and environments where new stimulus-reward contingencies exist and which can be learned (Kelley, Cador, & Stinus, 1990; Thiel, Müller, Huston, & Schwarting, 1999). As such, a qualitatively and/or quantitatively altered cognitive performance (Stillman et al., 1993) may also count as novelty. Novelty and new sensations can be considered as primary reinforcers in humans and animals (Weil, 1998; Zuckerman, 1990). Psychoactive drugs, by definition, change mental states. This constitutes a novelty effect on the first consumption episodes for each drug. It is unique to particular substances and reflected in the discriminative stimulus properties of a drug (Stolerman, 1992). After repeated exposure, the discriminative stimulus properties still exist, but are not novel anymore and something other than the novelty effects are needed to motivate continuation of drug use. However, in a "boring" environment, where the drug-induced change in mental state is among the only ways to provide entertainment and distraction, this consummatory reason may prevail for longer periods of time. A particular group of psychoactive drugs used to change sensation and perception of the external world and to increase self-understanding and self-discovery are hallucinogens and psychostimulants with a hallucinogenic profile (Morgan et al., 2013; Nichols, 2004). The entactogen, MDMA, induces a unique feeling of "divine oneness" with the world (Halberstadt & Nichols, 2010). Several drugs can be used to change mental state in a way that environmental stimuli and the self are perceived in a new fashion, without significant effects on euphoria or on the incentive properties of the stimuli. Exaggerated drug use for this instrumentalization goal may result in dangerous activities and schizophrenia-like psychoses.

4.6 Euphoria, Hedonia, and High

These concepts describe an intense feeling of well-being. The pursuit of euphoria or happiness—as either a series of short-lasting feelings or a long-lasting mental state—is probably the greatest desire in human life (Marcuse, 1984; Tatarkiewicz, 1976). The human brains work toward linking this subjective feeling with either the receipt of a primary or secondary reward, or the change in reward contingencies, i.e., when a formerly meaningless stimulus now predicts reward availability or a formerly useless behavior now yields a reward. While the biological function of the subjective perception of euphoria is far from clear, it appears that the degree of euphoria we perceive is related to well-being. It was argued that mood enhancement alone is a psychological benefit gained from psychoactive drug use (Lende & Smith, 2002). An enhanced mood by itself, i.e., one without an impact on physical health and behavior, however, would rather constitute a mock benefit. Alternatively, enhanced mood can be seen as one instance of a mental state change, facilitating efficient performance of goal-directed behaviors. Psychostimulant drugs like cocaine, amphetamine, methamphetamine, methylphenidate, and MDMA can induce a potent feeling of euphoria and an emotional "high" (e.g., Javaid, Fischman, Schuster, Dekirmenjian, & Davis, 1978; Resnick, Kestenbaum, & Schwartz, 1977) and are used for this reason by nonaddicts (Boyd, McCabe, Cranford, & Young, 2006). Euphoria is probably the easiest to accept instrumentalization goal for psychoactive drugs. Nevertheless, euphoria is not the most predominant and sought after effect during most psychoactive drug taking occasions in nonaddicts. For those drugs, which are classically associated with euphoria effects, euphoria requires a considerably higher dose than the use of the drug effects for other instrumentalization goals. Nevertheless, the mental state of a mild euphoria can be useful for many other instrumentalization goals as well, e.g., for social or sexual behavior. Chronic overinstrumentalization of euphoria-inducing drugs may result in tolerance to the euphoria effects, and in an escalation of intake. Acute withdrawal effects are characterized by dysphoria and a depression-like mental state (Heilig & Koob, 2007; Koob & Le Moal, 1997).

There are more behavioral complexes reported to benefit from psychoactive drug action. However, psychostimulant drugs may not serve all of them alike (Müller & Schumann, 2011a, 2011b).

5. STRATEGIES FOR THE TREATMENT OF PSYCHOSTIMULANT USE DISORDER: CLINICAL AND NONCLINICAL APPROACHES, EVOLVING TARGETS

Several pharmacological and pharmacokinetic strategies have been tested for the development of pharmacotherapy for psychostimulant addiction.

5.1 Pharmacological Strategies

5.1.1 Dopamine-Based Strategies

One potential way of reducing substance use is to provide a treatment that works like an "agonist" or "mimetic" to the consumed psychostimulant drug, or substitutes for it, but more long acting with less pronounced peak responses (Forray & Sofuoglu, 2014; Potenza, Sofuoglu, Carroll, & Rounsaville, 2011). In particular, substances that mimic or restore dopaminergic action were tested and yielded treatment potential (Perez-Mana, Castells, Vidal, Casas, & Capella, 2011).

5.1.1.1 L-DOPA

L-DOPA is the precursor of dopamine biosynthesis. L-DOPA therapy proved to be effective in the treatment of dopamine deficiency disorders like Parkinson's disease. It was suggested that it may also have beneficial effects in the treatment of psychostimulant addiction, which is also associated with a dopamine deficiency. The effects of L-DOPA (plus carbidopa) were tested in combination with clinical management (CM), cognitive behavioral therapy (CBT), or CM + CBT + voucher-based reinforcement therapy (VBRT) in treatment-seeking cocaine-dependent individuals in a 12-week randomized, placebo-controlled, double-blind trial. L-DOPA showed beneficial effects on the number of cocaine-negative urine samples, but only in combination with CM + CBT + VBRT, suggesting that L-DOPA pharmacotherapy may be an option for cocaine dependence when combined with behavioral therapies (Schmitz et al., 2008). Ropinirole acted as, albeit a weak, reinforcer in nonhuman primates (Freeman, Heal, McCreary, & Woolverton, 2012), which partly supports clinical data, suggesting that ropinirole marginally reduced craving in humans (Meini et al., 2012) and reduced the subjective intensity for the "cocaine rush" (Maremmani et al., 2011). Treatment with another dopamine D_2 agonist, pramipexole, caused perseverated responding in a reversal learning task, which was associated with stimulant dependence, rather than compulsive measures, suggesting additional efficacy for the potential treatment of SUD (Ersche et al., 2011). Together, these data support the dopamine replacement hypotheses, suggesting that clinically approved dopaminomimetic compounds might have clinical utility.

5.1.1.2 Dexamphetamine

Oral dexamphetamine was used to substitute for aggressive amphetamine use (Shearer et al., 2001). Increased retention was found in a randomized controlled trial with oral sustained-release dexamphetamine treatment for 12 weeks in methamphetamine-dependent individuals. Generally, dexamphetamine appears to reduce psychostimulant withdrawal, craving, dependency, and criminal activity. Interestingly, urine or hair cocaine or methamphetamine levels remained unaffected (Longo et al., 2010; Shearer, Wodak, van Beek, Mattick, & Lewis, 2003). However, dexamphetamine was also effective in cocaine- and heroin-dependent individuals stabilized with methadone together with reduced cocaine use as measured by cocaine-negative urine samples (Grabowski et al., 2004).

5.1.1.3 Methylphenidate

Methylphenidate is a monoamine-reuptake inhibitor, which has functional agonistic effects resembling psychostimulants, and is marketed for the treatment of ADHD and attention deficit disorder. Methylphenidate reduced the positive subjective effects of cocaine in nontreatment-seeking cocaine-dependent individuals. It is tolerated well and does not affect the acute physiological effects of cocaine (Winhusen et al., 2006). However, in a small open-label study with cocaine abusers without ADHD, methylphenidate did not affect cocaine use (Gawin, Riordan, & Kleber, 1985). Also a double-blind, placebo-controlled study did not find an effect of the methylphenidate versus placebo on retention and number of positive urine screens (Grabowski et al., 1997). Psychostimulant dependence occurs frequently with comorbid ADHD, which is routinely treated with methylphenidate. Methylphenidate was shown to reduce ADHD symptoms, but not affect cocaine use or craving in a 12-week double-blind, placebo-controlled trial (Schubiner et al., 2002). Furthermore, the cardiovascular and positive subjective responses to cocaine were unaffected in cocaine abusers with ADHD versus those without ADHD (Collins, Levin, Foltin, Kleber, & Evans, 2006). Maintenance on sustained-release methylphenidate for 3 weeks decreased some of the positive subjective effects of cocaine in abusers with ADHD (Collins et al., 2006). Sustained-release methylphenidate treatment for 14 weeks was effective in reducing probability of cocaine-positive urine samples in treatment-seeking adults with ADHD and cocaine dependence in a double-blind, placebo-controlled treatment study (Levin, Evans, Brooks, & Garawi, 2007). Methylphenidate treatment (20 weeks) was also tested in a randomized, placebo-controlled trial in Finnish amphetamine/methamphetamine-dependent patients; results showed reduced percentage of amphetamine-positive urine samples, and methylphenidate was therefore suggested as a potential substitution therapy (Tiihonen et al., 2007). A later parallel-group, double-blind, randomized, placebo-controlled study in amphetamine/methamphetamine-dependent outpatients administered methylphenidate for 22 weeks, but did not find a superior effect of methylphenidate over placebo in positive urine samples, drug use, or craving (Miles et al., 2013). Overall, psychostimulant medications only occasionally work as replacement therapies and may need patient collectives to be further differentiated for a more personalized treatment (Perez-Mana, Castells, Torrens, Capella, & Farre, 2013).

5.1.1.4 Selegiline

Selegiline is an MAO-type B inhibitor, which can increase monoamine (dopamine) levels in the brain and could therefore potentially reverse monoamine deficits in psychostimulant addicts. Transdermal selegiline was tested in a double-blind, placebo-controlled trial in cocaine-dependent subjects which reported no superior effect of selegiline to placebo on self-reported cocaine use or benzoylecgonine-free urine samples, which may suggest that MAO-B inhibitors may only have a limited application to treat psychostimulant addiction (Elkashef et al., 2006). The related compound rasagiline, used for the treatment of Parkinson's disease, has not been tested in nonclinical or clinical pharmacological analyses.

5.1.1.5 Bupropion

This drug is a noradrenaline and dopamine reuptake inhibitor which may mimic some of the effects of psychostimulants in the mesolimbic system and serve to "replace" the psychostimulant drug (Rothman, 1990). Bupropion does not alter the acute subjective and cardiovascular effects of cocaine in cocaine consumers (Oliveto et al., 2001). Using it as a treatment may, therefore, be based at the assumption that it may restore disrupted monoamine levels after chronic psychostimulant consumption. However, this appears not to be the case in methadone-maintained cocaine-dependent individuals (Margolin et al., 1995). Bupropion treatment when combined with contingency management, however, did reduce cocaine consumption in methadone-maintained opiate-dependent cocaine abusers (Poling et al., 2006). Nonetheless, negative results for bupropion in combination with CBT in cocaine-dependent outpatients have been reported (Shoptaw et al., 2008). Also multicenter, placebo-controlled, randomized, double-blind trials in treatment-seeking methamphetamine-dependent outpatients did not indicate an improvement. However, this study identified a subgroup of patients in which bupropion was actually effective: male patients with low-to-moderate methamphetamine consumption (Elkashef et al., 2008). A retrospective analysis of these two studies suggested that bupropion may be effective in patients with only moderate baseline methamphetamine use. Thereby, the failure to provide at least two negative urine samples in the first three weekly tests would confer an enhanced risk of treatment failure (Brensilver, Heinzerling, Swanson, & Shoptaw, 2012). However, abstinence was significantly higher in those individuals with high medication adherence compared to those with low adherence in a patient population with low methamphetamine abuse (Heinzerling et al., 2014). Together, these findings suggest that a high degree of personalization and management is needed (Brensilver, Heinzerling, & Shoptaw, 2013). A trial in adolescent methamphetamine abusers/dependent individuals did support bupropion as a treatment for this subpopulation of patients (Heinzerling et al., 2013).

5.1.1.6 Modafinil

Modafinil is an α_1-adrenergic receptor agonist and DAT inhibitor used as a wake-promoting agent. It is usually well tolerated and has a low abuse potential (Dackis, Kampman, Lynch, Pettinati, & O'Brien, 2005). Experimental studies suggest that it may attenuate positive subjective and cardiovascular effects of psychostimulants in a laboratory setting (Martinez-Raga, Knecht, & Cepeda, 2008). A double-blind, placebo-controlled trial in cocaine-dependent patients receiving modafinil or placebo together with CBT for 8 weeks showed superior action of modafinil versus placebo in the reduction of benzoylecgonine-positive urine samples and achievement of protracted abstinence periods. A subsequent double-blind, placebo-controlled trial in only cocaine-dependent individuals showed no effect on benzoylecgonine-positive urine samples, nor in secondary measures, such as craving and withdrawal (Dackis et al., 2012). Similarly, modafinil did not moderate the effects of baseline abstinence rates in cocaine-dependent individuals on treatment outcome of a pharmacological and behavioral therapy (Schmitz et al., 2014). In methamphetamine-dependent individuals, modafinil was ineffective (Anderson et al., 2009; Heinzerling et al., 2010; Shearer et al., 2009), while positive urine samples were reduced, but not significantly (Shearer et al., 2009). However, potential beneficial effects of modafinil in subgroups of patients, such as those with high-frequency baseline methamphetamine use, were suggested (Heinzerling et al., 2010). However, modafinil may increase retention in treatment trials and, thus, adherence to combined psychotherapy (McElhiney, Rabkin, Rabkin, & Nunes, 2009). It was also suggested that modafinil treatment effects may be genotype dependent (Heinzerling et al., 2013), which needs further research in order to become a guiding variable.

5.1.1.7 Disulfiram

Disulfiram is a dopamine-β-hydroxylase inhibitor that catalyzes the conversion of dopamine to noradrenaline in noradrenergic cells. Clinical trials suggested that disulfiram treatment may reduce cocaine consumption in methadone-maintained opiate addicts (Petrakis et al., 2000) and in combined cocaine- and alcohol addicts (Carroll et al., 2000; Grassi, Cioce, Giudici, Antonilli, & Nencini, 2007). Disulfiram appears to show a gender-specific effect with men having better treatment outcomes than women (Nich et al., 2004). A randomized, placebo-controlled trial in cocaine-dependent outpatients confirmed that a 12-week disulfiram treatment in combination with CBT was superior to a placebo treatment in reducing frequency of cocaine use and of cocaine-positive urine samples. This effect was most pronounced in those individuals who were not alcohol dependent or who abstained from drinking during the treatment period (Carroll et al., 2004). A double-blind, placebo-controlled trial in combined cocaine- and alcohol-dependent individuals showed that 11-week disulfiram treatment resulted in highest rates of combined cocaine and alcohol abstinence, without having significant effects on each drug alone. If disulfiram was combined with naltrexone, highest rates of 3 consecutive weeks of abstinence from cocaine and alcohol were achieved (Pettinati et al., 2008). Testing disulfiram in cocaine- and opiate-dependent individuals who were initially stabilized with methadone suggested that potential beneficial effects of disulfiram were highly dose dependent. While low-to-medium doses of disulfiram (62.5 and 125 mg) in an 11-week treatment actually increased cocaine consumption, the high dose (250 mg) reduced it (Oliveto et al., 2011). Another treatment approach seeks to antagonize the effects of psychostimulants, which would decrease their reinforcing action and possibly reduce consummatory episodes (Forray & Sofuoglu, 2014; Potenza et al., 2011). Studies are ongoing in opioid-dependent cocaine addicts (clinicaltrials.gov; http://ClinicalTrials.gov/show/NCT00580827).

5.1.1.8 Antipsychotics

Classical and atypical antipsychotic drugs generally blunt mesocorticolimbic output. The new generation antipsychotic aripiprazole is a partial dopamine D_2-like receptor agonist, 5-HT_{1A} receptor agonist, and antagonist at the 5-HT_{2A} receptor and was tested in a randomized, placebo-controlled trial in amphetamine/methamphetamine dependent patients. Surprisingly, aripiprazole treatment dramatically enhanced the percentage of amphetamine-positive urine samples (Tiihonen et al., 2007). A randomized, placebo-controlled study in methamphetamine-dependent subjects tested the effects of 12-week aripiprazole or placebo treatment on methamphetamine-positive urine samples. While the positive samples declined in the course of the study, aripiprazole had no superior effect versus placebo, but did also not enhance consumption (Coffin et al., 2013). Other atypical antipsychotics, like risperidone, olanzapine, or reserpine, were no more effective in reducing psychostimulant consumption than placebo when considered in a meta-analysis (Grabowski et al., 2004; Kishi, Matsuda, Iwata, & Correll, 2013). Similar conclusions were reached when antipsychotics were considered as a treatment of cocaine addiction in schizophrenic patients (Sabioni, Ramos, & Galduroz, 2013).

5.1.2 5-HT-Based Strategies

Neuroadaptations in the 5-HT-ergic system are increasingly recognized as a major factor inducing and maintaining psychostimulant addiction (Müller & Homberg, 2015). Given the huge complexity of the 5-HT system (Müller & Jacobs, 2010), numerous targets to treat psychostimulant addiction have been investigated.

The lowering of serotonergic tone by low-tryptophan diet can reduce the acute subjective effects of cocaine and cocaine craving in subjects diagnosed for cocaine dependence (Aronson et al., 1995; Satel, Krystal, Delgado, Kosten, & Charney, 1995). However, no beneficial effects were found in a double-blind study (Chadwick, Gregory, & Wendling, 1990). Lowering

5-HT availability may reduce some acute cocaine effects in addicts, but no efficacy in the treatment of addiction has emerged as of yet. Enhancing 5-HT activity with the selective 5-HT reuptake inhibitor, escitalopram, acutely decreased attentional bias to cocaine-related words in nontreatment-seeking cocaine-dependent subjects. This effect, however, was not consistent during chronic escitalopram treatment (Liu et al., 2013). Grabowski et al. (1995) reported a transient reduction of cocaine consumption in fluoxetine-treated cocaine-dependent patients. Crack cocaine-dependent outpatients did not find reduced cocaine use or cocaine craving after fluoxetine treatment (Batki, Washburn, Delucchi, & Jones, 1996). In contrast, Covi, Hess, Kreiter, and Haertzen (1995) reported increased cocaine consumption in patients treated with a high dose of fluoxetine for 12 weeks. In patients dually dependent on cocaine and opioids, fluoxetine treatment plus a voucher incentive was less effective in reducing cocaine use than placebo plus voucher in an outpatient clinical trial (Winstanley, Bigelow, Silverman, Johnson, & Strain, 2011). The effects of citalopram in combination with behavioral therapy and contingency management were investigated in cocaine-dependent patients (Moeller et al., 2007). Citalopram-treated subjects showed higher abstinence rates as measured by a reduction of cocaine-positive urine samples. Similar effects were found when another selective 5-HT reuptake inhibitor sertraline in combination with CBT was tested in a double-blind, placebo-controlled clinical trial in cocaine-dependent volunteers with depressive symptoms. During 12 weeks of treatment, the sertraline-treated group showed significantly more days before first and second cocaine-positive urine samples. Depression scores decreased in both groups, but were unrelated to the treatment (Oliveto et al., 2012). Given that depression is common comorbidity among individuals with methamphetamine dependence, it has been investigated whether selective 5-HT reuptake inhibitors are effective in treating the disorder. However, chronic treatment with sertraline had no significant effect (Shoptaw et al., 2006), or actually increased methamphetamine craving and use (Zorick, Sugar, Hellemann, Shoptaw, & London, 2011). Together, treatments based on selective 5-HT reuptake inhibition did not yet yield convincing results in the treatment of psychostimulant addiction, but subgroups of patients with other comorbidities may still benefit from such drugs. Also, a combination with supportive behavioral therapy may enhance efficacy of this treatment.

Since atypical and newer generation antipsychotics bind to 5-HT receptors (above), including, but not limited to, 5-HT_{2A}, 5-HT_{1A}, and 5-HT_6

receptors (Müller & Homberg, 2015), and 5-HT plays an important role in the control of impulsivity and establishment of compulsive behaviors, drugs targeting these 5-HT receptors are of special interest as targets to treat psychostimulant use and/or abuse (Cunningham & Anastasio, 2014; Müller & Homberg, 2015). However, studies using the nonspecific 5-HT_2 receptor ligand ritanserin failed to reduce cocaine craving in addicts (Cornish et al., 2001; Ehrman, Robbins, Cornish, Childress, & O'Brien, 1996). The 5-HT_{2C} receptor, however, does appear critically involved, and data have suggested that the progression to relapse and/or addiction may be related to a single nucleotide polymorphism in HTR2C gene encoding for the conversion of cysteine to serine at codon 23 (Ser23 variant) (Anastasio et al., 2014). Agonist actions at 5-HT_{2C} receptors may reduce cocaine reinforcement, based on nonclinical data (see Cunningham et al., 2011; Müller & Homberg, 2015 for detailed review), but the addition of 5-HT_{2A} receptor antagonism with 5-HT_{2C} agonist moieties may also be beneficial (Howell & Cunningham, 2015). Positive allosteric modulation of the 5-HT_{2C} receptor also has efficacy (Ding et al., 2012). Many antipsychotic agents also possess 5-HT_{1A} receptor (partial) agonist properties (Jones & McCreary, 2008; McCreary & Jones, 2010). Clinically, buspirone, a 5-HT_{1A} receptor partial agonist, also possessing affinity at dopamine D_2-like receptor was assessed in a double-blind multicenter placebo-controlled study in SUD. However, no overall benefits were seen, and buspirone was not able to prevent cocaine relapse; actually, buspirone may have actually worsened relapse in female subjects (Winhusen et al., 2014). 5-HT_3 receptors undergo adaptations during chronic psychostimulant administration (for review see Müller & Homberg, 2015), suggesting that targeting them might have beneficial effects in addicts. It was investigated whether the 5-HT_3 receptor antagonist ondansetron would be superior to placebo in reducing methamphetamine use in methamphetamine-dependent patients. In this multisite, randomized, double-blind, placebo-controlled study, ondansetron was given for 8 weeks in combination with CBT. Although ondansetron was well tolerated, there was no significant difference in the number of methamphetamine-free study weeks assessed by drug-free urine samples between the ondansetron and the placebo-treated groups (Johnson et al., 2008). 5-HT_6 receptor antagonists have a key role in mnemonic processes and therefore are under intense nonclinical and clinical investigation for the treatment of the cognitive anomalies, like those seen in schizophrenia and Alzheimer's disease (Mitchell & Neumaier, 2005). However, the role of this receptor in SUD warrants further attention. The first report that 5-HT_6

receptors were of relevant demonstrated that augmented accumbal expression of 5-HT_6 receptors blocked the rewarding, but not psychomotor actions of cocaine (Ferguson, Mitchell, & Neumaier, 2008). There is evidence that application of 5-HT_6 receptor antagonists reduced the development and expression of nicotine-induced behavioral sensitization (de Bruin, Kloeze, & McCreary, 2011), reduced ethanol and nicotine seeking (de Bruin et al., 2013), altered cocaine, maintained self-administration, and reinstated cocaine-seeking behavior and the expression of conditioned place preference (Fijał et al., 2010; van Gaalen, Schetters, Schoffelmeer, & De Vries, 2010).

5.1.3 GABA-Based Strategies

GABA is the major inhibitory neurotransmitter in the brain having a pivotal role in dorsal and ventral striatal circuitry and mesocorticolimbic function, modulating the influence of local dopaminergic inputs and glutamatergic neurotransmission (Schoffelmeer et al., 2000; Sesack & Pickel, 1990).

5.1.3.1 Gabapentin

This is a GABA-ergic modulator that enhances GABA levels in the brain and is marketed for the treatment of chronic neuropathic pain conditions. A randomized, double-blind, placebo-controlled trial in cocaine-dependent individuals, who received gabapentin for 12 weeks, did not find superior effects versus placebo when all patients were considered together. A subgroup analysis, however, suggested that gabapentin may be useful in reducing cocaine consumption specifically in the low-use group (Bisaga et al., 2006). No such subgroup effect was found in a clinical trial in methamphetamine-dependent individuals (Heinzerling et al., 2006). There was also no beneficial gabapentin effect on cocaine use in cocaine- and opiate-dependent individuals on methadone maintenance (Gonzalez et al., 2007).

5.1.3.2 Tiagabine

Tiagabine, being a GABA reuptake inhibitor, did not alter the acute subjective and cardiovascular effects of oral or intranasal cocaine in nontreatment-seeking cocaine users (Lile, Stoops, Allen, et al., 2004; Lile, Stoops, Glaser, Hays, & Rush, 2004). Conversely, tiagabine treatment for 10 weeks increased the number of cocaine-free urine samples in cocaine- and opiate-dependent individuals on methadone maintenance in a double-blind, placebo-controlled study (Gonzalez et al., 2007).

5.1.3.3 Vigabatrin

γ-Vinyl gamma-aminobutyric acid (vigabatrin) is an antiepileptic drug that increases GABA levels in the brain, by inhibiting GABA-transaminase activity. Vigabatrin treatment in humans was safe and without severe side effects in the treatment of psychostimulant dependence (Brodie, Figueroa, & Dewey, 2003; Brodie, Figueroa, Laska, & Dewey, 2005). A randomized, double-blind, placebo-controlled trial in treatment-seeking individuals with cocaine dependence showed beneficial effects in retention and full end-of-trial abstinence rates, which may suggest further exploration of vigabatrin to treat psychostimulant addiction (Brodie et al., 2009).

Among three subtypes of GABA receptors, accumulating data over the past decades clearly supports a role of $GABA_B$ receptors in mediating long-term neuroplastic changes which are the consequences of SUD-like behavior (Filip & Frankowska, 2008; Filip et al., 2015).

5.1.3.4 Baclofen

The $GABA_B$ receptor agonist baclofen was tested to treat cocaine dependence in the clinic and showed a favorable outcome versus placebo by increasing the probability of benzoylecgonine-free urine samples. Baclofen did not increase retention or lower craving for cocaine (Shoptaw et al., 2003). In experimental trials in nontreatment-seeking cocaine-dependent individuals, baclofen decreased cocaine choice. In cocaine- and opiate-dependent individuals on methadone maintenance, baclofen reduced craving for cocaine. In both groups, there was no effect of baclofen on the acute positive subjective effects of cocaine (Haney, Hart, & Foltin, 2006). A multisite, double-blind, placebo-controlled study tested the baclofen treatment in patients with severe cocaine dependence. Compared to placebo, baclofen did not show superior effects on self-reported cocaine use or benzoylecgonine-positive urine samples (Kahn et al., 2009). A randomized, double-blind, placebo-controlled trial in methamphetamine-dependent individuals found no statistically significant treatment effects. However, there was an indication for potential beneficial action of baclofen in those participants reporting high medication adherence (Heinzerling et al., 2006).

In light of these data, it will be interesting to test the influence of $GABA_B$-positive allosteric modulators in SUD. Such drugs have the advantage over classical agonists, like baclofen, that desensitization will not be observed following continued treatment and have fewer side effects, such as myorelaxation, hyperthermia, and cognitive dysfunction (Filip et al.,

2015). Evidence suggests that the $GABA_B$-positive allosteric modulators abrogate ethanol, cocaine, or nicotine-induced locomotor activity in mice, did not reduce the expression of cocaine or ethanol sensitization, while there was reduction in the development of cocaine sensitization. Moreover, the augmentation of ethanol sensitization did not influence the stimulus effects of cocaine. More extensive studies exploring the effects in self-administration and the reinstatement of cocaine, ethanol, and nicotine seeking behavior yielded positive results (see review Filip et al., 2015).

5.1.4 Glutamate-Based Strategies

Glutamate is the primary excitatory neurotransmitter in the brain and is involved in a variety of neuropsychiatric conditions. There are extensive data supporting a role for this neurotransmitter in SUD. Repeated administration of psychostimulant drugs dysregulates brain glutamatergic systems in preclinical models (Pomierny-Chamioło et al., 2014). In clinical trials, ketamine, memantine, and *N*-acetylcysteine were/are currently being tested in psychostimulant use disorder.

5.1.4.1 Ketamine

Ketamine, an NMDA receptor antagonist and a recreational drug (Uosukainen et al., 2014). Apart from being a potential treatment for major depressive disorder (Dutta, McKie, & Deakin, 2014), it is also being explored in cocaine dependence (clinicaltrials.gov; http://ClinicalTrials.gov/show/NCT01535937). The study designed to assess ketamine treatment on mindfulness-based cocaine relapse prevention and abstinence rates is still running, and no data are reported.

5.1.4.2 Memantine

The voltage-dependent noncompetitive NMDA receptor antagonist memantine, which has received marketing approval for the treatment of Alzheimer's disease, reduces cocaine self-administration in rats and the reinstatement of cocaine-seeking behavior in rodents (Bespalov, Zvartau, Balster, & Beardsley, 2000; Hyytiä, Bäckström, & Liljequist, 1999), cocaine conditioned locomotion (Bespalov, Dravolina, Zvartau, Beardsley, & Balster, 2000), place preference (Kotlińska & Biała, 2000), and sensitization (Li, White, & Wolf, 2000). However, human studies have not supported a role for memantine in reducing cocaine self-administration in humans (Collins, Vosberg, Ward, Haney, & Foltin, 2007); however, the stratification of these patients may not have been optimal (Bisaga et al., 2010).

Recently, clinical placebo-controlled study on memantine (40 mg/day) exploring weekly cocaine intake and abstinence was completed (clinicaltrials.gov; http://ClinicalTrials.gov/show/NCT00134901), although not released.

5.1.4.3 *N*-Acetylcysteine

N-Acetylcysteine is a cystine–glutamate exchange activator which reduced the desire for cocaine, cocaine-cue reactivity, and cocaine craving in clinical experimental settings (Amen et al., 2011; LaRowe et al., 2007) as well as cocaine reinstatement in animal studies (Amen et al., 2011). Recently, the potential utility of *N*-acetylcysteine to reduce cocaine seeking enhanced by coexisting depression was demonstrated (Frankowska et al., 2014). These findings suggest a potential treatment option for long-term application (Asevedo, Mendes, Berk, & Brietzke, 2014; McClure, Gipson, Malcolm, Kalivas, & Gray, 2014), although further studies will be needed to test this hypothesis.

Glutamatergic neurotransmission is mediated not only via ionotropic (NMDA, AMPA, and kainate) but also via eight subtypes of metabotropic-like receptors ($mGluR_{1-8}$) (Pomierny-Chamioło et al., 2014). So far, clinical studies have addressed the density of $mGluR_5$ receptors using $[^{18}F]$SP203 using PET in dependent individuals (clinicaltrials.gov; http://ClinicalTrials.gov/show/NCT00951314), data not available. Clinical data on mGluR ligands have been restricted to the use of receptor-selective agents which have been developed for use in schizophrenia. The $mGluR_{2/3}$ receptor agonist pomaglumetad methionil (LY2140023) has been extensively studied in schizophrenic patients (Patil et al., 2007). Nonetheless, nonclinical studies have extensively assessed effects of mGluR antagonists in psychostimulant abuse/dependence models (Pomierny-Chamioło et al., 2014). These data strongly support the significance of $mGluR_1$ and $mGluR_5$ antagonists to diminish psychostimulant addictive behavior, as the $mGluR_1$ antagonism attenuated drug-reinstatement of drug-seeking behavior evoked by cocaine and methamphetamine or the subjective effects of cocaine and the methamphetamine-induced substitution to the cocaine stimulus in squirrel monkeys (Achat-Mendes, Platt, & Spealman, 2012), but not in rats (Besheer et al., 2009), while the $mGluR_5$ receptor blockade via negative allosteric modulation or competitive antagonism reduced cocaine or amphetamines' rewarding, subjective, and seeking effects (for detailed review, see Pomierny-Chamioło et al., 2014). More extensive pharmacological proof-of-principal (clinical) validation is needed.

5.1.5 "Other" Target-Based Strategies

5.1.5.1 Acamprosate

Acamprosate is considered to be effective in the treatment of alcohol addiction (Spanagel & Kiefer, 2008). While its mechanism of action is still largely unclear, its beneficial effects may arise from enhancing Ca^{2+} supply (Spanagel et al., 2014). Acamprosate treatment was tested in cocaine-dependent patients in a double-blind, placebo-controlled pilot trial with 8 weeks' treatment. Although tolerated well, acamprosate did not have superior effects versus placebo on retention, percent positive urine screens for cocaine, cocaine craving, or withdrawal in this study (Kampman et al., 2011).

5.1.5.2 Galantamine

Galantamine is a reversible acetylcholine esterase inhibitor and enhanced reaction time and accuracy in a rapid visual information processing task in recently abstinent cocaine users (Sofuoglu, Waters, Poling, & Carroll, 2011). The mechanism of galantamine may strengthen impulse control and cognitive and social abilities, which are attenuated by long-term psychostimulant consumption (Hulka et al., 2014; Preller et al., 2014). Galantamine was also found to have some efficacy in reducing cocaine consumption in methadone-maintained cocaine- and opiate addicts in an 8-week double-blind, placebo-controlled clinical trial (Sofuoglu & Carroll, 2011).

5.1.5.3 Naltrexone

The drug is an opiate receptor antagonist that can effectively block acute subjective effects of opiates. A randomized, double-blind, placebo-controlled trial investigated the effects of a naltrexone implant for 10 weeks in heroin- and amphetamine-dependent outpatients. Naltrexone treatment resulted in higher retention rate and decreased heroin and amphetamine use as measured by drug-free urine. It also improved the global clinical condition of the patients. This study suggested naltrexone use as an option for treating polydrug dependence with psychostimulant drugs (Tiihonen et al., 2012). However, in other studies, no beneficial effects of naltrexone were reported in cocaine- and alcohol-dependent outpatients when combined with psychotherapy or drug counseling (Schmitz, Stotts, Sayre, DeLaune, & Grabowski, 2004).

5.1.5.4 Varenicline

Varenicline, being a partial agonist at the $\alpha_4\beta_2$ nicotinic acetylcholine receptors, and which enhances the DA neurotransmission, has been marketed as a smoking cessation aid. However, the use of this compound in reducing the consumption of other drugs warrants extended research. Poling, Rounsaville, Gonsai, Severino, and Sofuoglu (2010) tested varenicline in cocaine- and opiate-dependent individuals on methadone maintenance in a placebo-controlled pilot study. Varenicline, however, was no more effective than placebo in reducing cocaine consumption; cigarette smoking was reduced. Thus, its use may be more appropriate and efficacious in treating nicotine- rather than psychostimulant use and dependence. However, a small placebo-controlled, double-blind test trial in cocaine-dependent subjects suggested varenicline treatment for 9 weeks to be effective in reducing the number of benzoylecgonine-positive urine samples and cocaine reward (Plebani et al., 2012).

Recently, treatment modalities impacting food intake have been proposed for SUD. In fact, the regulation of food and psychostimulant pathways shares common neurobiological substrates (Engel & Jerlhag, 2014; Müller & Schumann, 2011a, 2011b); therefore, compounds impacting food intake at a mesoaccumbal level might (e.g., ghrelin, GHS-R1A receptors) impact putative reward pathways and have the potential to treat SUD (Engel & Jerlhag, 2014); parallels can be drawn, with the endocannabinoid system. The endocannabinoids 2-arachidonoyl glycerol (2-AG) and anandamide appeared increased in the limbic forebrain when animals were food deprived, and when 2-AG was injected in the shell of the nucleus accumbens food consumption increased (Kirkham, Williams, Fezza, & Di Marzo, 2002). CB_1 receptor involvement is strongly indicated in these effects and parallels cocaine studies demonstrating a role in reward and relapse to cocaine seeking (Adamczyk et al., 2012; De Vries et al., 2001; Filip et al., 2006). Such strategies should therefore be investigated more extensively.

5.2 Pharmacokinetic/Immuno Strategies

In pharmacokinetic approaches, treatments were developed strive to reduce psychostimulant concentration. Several ways were tested which can achieve this effect, such as immunotherapies or a stimulation of metabolism (Bagasra, Forman, Howeedy, & Whittle, 1992; Forray & Sofuoglu, 2014).

High levels of anticocaine antibodies can sequester blood cocaine, which facilitates cocaine inactivation before entering the brain. Since less cocaine reaches the brain, cocaine-induced acute euphoria was attenuated.

An open-label study suggested that treatment with the human cocaine vaccine TA-CD when reaching a high antibody titer response enhanced the likelihood of maintaining cocaine-free urine (Martell, Mitchell, Poling, Gonsai, & Kosten, 2005). Martell et al. (2009) demonstrated the efficacy of vaccinations with succinylnorcocaine linked to recombinant cholera toxin B-subunit protein in enhancing the number of cocaine-free urine. However, only those patients attaining a high IgG anticocaine antibody showed effect (Martell et al., 2009). However, further refinement will be needed clinically, such as the addition of adjuvants, or even with the addition of cocaine enzymes (for recent review, see Orson et al., 2014).

6. CONCLUDING REMARKS

SUD, and particularly that relating to psychostimulants, is considered a global health concern with significant socioeconomic burden to society. In the twenty-first century, the list of drugs with putative psychostimulant properties includes over 60 compounds belonging to different chemical classes. Psychostimulants are used in both recreational and clinical settings; a majority of them display a high potential for abuse. The reasons for the development of SUD have multifactorial components ranging from: impulse control phenomena, social lubrication, sexual reward, anxiogenic avoidance during withdrawal, secondary reinforcement of drug paired cues, parallels with food consummator behavior, and of course euphoria all have a role in driving the switch from use to abuse with sometimes drastic consequences. Experimentally, a variety of approaches are under clinical and nonclinical investigation, e.g., dopaminergic, glutamatergic, 5-HT-ergic, and GABA-ergic strategies. Generally, however, clinical data remain disappointing; nonetheless, a multifaceted approach employing cognitive behavioral approaches with novel pharmacological strategies appears to be the best course of action and the realization of the importance of the differing psychiatric sequelae of abuse and the targets that can be used to treat these symptoms may assist in better stratification of patients, and therefore the pharmacological and cognitive behavioral therapeutic treatment of these patients. SUD, and particularly psychostimulant use disorder, remains a key health concern; therefore, combined nonclinical, psychiatric, psychological collaboration from academic, industrial, and regulatory bodies will be needed to make inroads.

REFERENCES

Achat-Mendes, C., Platt, D. M., & Spealman, R. D. (2012). Antagonism of metabotropic glutamate 1 receptors attenuates behavioral effects of cocaine and methamphetamine in squirrel monkeys. *The Journal of Pharmacology and Experimental Therapeutics*, *343*, 214–224.

Adamczyk, P., Miszkiel, J., McCreary, A. C., Filip, M., Papp, M., & Przegaliński, E. (2012). The effects of cannabinoid CB1, CB2 and vanilloid TRPV1 receptor antagonists on cocaine addictive behavior in rats. *Brain Research*, *1444*, 45–54.

Amen, S. L., Piacentine, L. B., Ahmad, M. E., Li, S. J., Mantsch, J. R., Risinger, R. C., et al. (2011). Repeated *N*-acetyl cysteine reduces cocaine seeking in rodents and craving in cocaine-dependent humans. *Neuropsychopharmacology*, *36*, 871–878.

Anastasio, N. C., Stutz, S. J., Fox, R. G., Sears, R. M., Emeson, R. B., Dileone, R. J., et al. (2014). Functional status of the serotonin 5-HT2C receptor (5-HT2CR) drives interlocked phenotypes that precipitate relapse-like behaviors in cocaine dependence. *Neuropsychopharmacology*, *39*, 370–382.

Anderson, A. L., Reid, M. S., Li, S. H., Holmes, T., Shemanski, L., Slee, A., et al. (2009). Modafinil for the treatment of cocaine dependence. *Drug and Alcohol Dependence*, *104*, 133–139.

Anglin, M. D., Burke, C., Perrochet, B., Stamper, E., & Dawud-Noursi, S. (2000). History of the methamphetamine problem. *Journal of Psychoactive Drugs*, *32*, 137–141.

Aronson, S. C., Black, J. E., McDougle, C. J., Scanley, B. E., Jatlow, P., Kosten, T. R., et al. (1995). Serotonergic mechanisms of cocaine effects in humans. *Psychopharmacology*, *119*, 179–185.

Arria, A. M., & Wish, E. D. (2006). Nonmedical use of prescription stimulants among students. *Pediatric Annals*, *35*, 565–571.

Asevedo, E., Mendes, A. C., Berk, M., & Brietzke, E. (2014). Systematic review of *N*-acetylcysteine in the treatment of addictions. *Revista Brasileira de Psiquiatria*, *36*, 168–175.

Bagasra, O., Forman, L. J., Howeedy, A., & Whittle, P. (1992). A potential vaccine for cocaine abuse prophylaxis. *Immunopharmacology*, *23*, 173–179.

Batki, S. L., Washburn, A. M., Delucchi, K., & Jones, R. T. (1996). A controlled trial of fluoxetine in crack cocaine dependence. *Drug and Alcohol Dependence*, *41*, 137–142.

Besheer, J., Grondin, J. J., Salling, M. C., Spanos, M., Stevenson, R. A., & Hodge, C. W. (2009). Interoceptive effects of alcohol require mGlu5 receptor activity in the nucleus accumbens. *The Journal of Neuroscience*, *29*, 9582–9591.

Bespalov, A. Y., Dravolina, O. A., Zvartau, E. E., Beardsley, P. M., & Balster, R. L. (2000). Effects of NMDA receptor antagonists on cocaine-conditioned motor activity in rats. *European Journal of Pharmacology*, *390*, 303–311.

Bespalov, A. Y., Zvartau, E. E., Balster, R. L., & Beardsley, P. M. (2000). Effects of *N*-methyl-D-aspartate receptor antagonists on reinstatement of cocaine-seeking behavior by priming injections of cocaine or exposures to cocaine-associated cues in rats. *Behavioral Pharmacology*, *11*, 37–44.

Bisaga, A., Aharonovich, E., Cheng, W. Y., Levin, F. R., Mariani, J. J., Raby, W. N., et al. (2010). A placebo-controlled trial of memantine for cocaine dependence with high-value voucher incentives during a pre-randomization lead-in period. *Drug and Alcohol Dependence*, *111*, 97–104.

Bisaga, A., Aharonovich, E., Garawi, F., Levin, F. R., Rubin, E., Raby, W. N., et al. (2006). A randomized placebo-controlled trial of gabapentin for cocaine dependence. *Drug and Alcohol Dependence*, *81*, 267–274.

Boutrel, B., & Koob, G. F. (2004). What keeps us awake: The neuropharmacology of stimulants and wakefulness-promoting medications. *Sleep*, *27*, 1181–1194.

Boyd, C. J., McCabe, S. E., Cranford, J. A., & Young, A. (2006). Adolescents' motivations to abuse prescription medications. *Pediatrics*, *118*, 2472–2480.

Brensilver, M., Heinzerling, K. G., & Shoptaw, S. (2013). Pharmacotherapy of amphetamine-type stimulant dependence: An update. *Drug and Alcohol Review*, *32*, 449–460.

Brensilver, M., Heinzerling, K. G., Swanson, A. N., & Shoptaw, S. J. (2012). A retrospective analysis of two randomized trials of bupropion for methamphetamine dependence: Suggested guidelines for treatment discontinuation/augmentation. *Drug and Alcohol Dependence*, *125*, 169–172.

Britt, G. C., & McCance-Katz, E. F. (2005). A brief overview of the clinical pharmacology of "club drugs" *Substance Use and Misuse*, *40*, 1189–1201.

Broadley, K. J. (2010). The vascular effects of trace amines and amphetamines. *Pharmacology & Therapeutics*, *125*, 363–375.

Brodie, J. D., Case, B. G., Figueroa, E., Dewey, S. L., Robinson, J. A., Wanderling, J. A., et al. (2009). Randomized, double-blind, placebo-controlled trial of vigabatrin for the treatment of cocaine dependence in Mexican parolees. *The American Journal of Psychiatry*, *166*, 1269–1277.

Brodie, J. D., Figueroa, E., & Dewey, S. L. (2003). Treating cocaine addiction: From pre-clinical to clinical trial experience with gamma-vinyl GABA. *Synapse*, *50*, 261–265.

Brodie, J. D., Figueroa, E., Laska, E. M., & Dewey, S. L. (2005). Safety and efficacy of gamma-vinyl GABA (GVG) for the treatment of methamphetamine and/or cocaine addiction. *Synapse*, *55*, 122–125.

Cami, J., Farré, M., Mas, M., Roset, P. N., Poudevida, S., Mas, A., et al. (2000). Human pharmacology of 3,4-methylenedioxymethamphetamine ("ecstasy"): Psychomotor performance and subjective effects. *Journal of Clinical Psychopharmacology*, *20*, 455–466.

Carroll, K. M., Fenton, L. R., Ball, S. A., Nich, C., Frankforter, T. L., Shi, J., et al. (2004). Efficacy of disulfiram and cognitive behavior therapy in cocaine-dependent outpatients: A randomized placebo-controlled trial. *Archives of General Psychiatry*, *61*, 264–272.

Carroll, K. M., Nich, C., Ball, S. A., McCance, E., Frankforter, T. L., & Rounsaville, B. J. (2000). One-year follow-up of disulfiram and psychotherapy for cocaine-alcohol users: Sustained effects of treatment. *Addiction*, *95*, 1335–1349.

Castren, E. (2005). Is mood chemistry? *Nature Reviews. Neuroscience*, *6*, 241–246.

Chadwick, M. J., Gregory, D. L., & Wendling, G. (1990). A double-blind amino acids, L-tryptophan and L-tyrosine, and placebo study with cocaine-dependent subjects in an inpatient chemical dependency treatment center. *The American Journal of Drug and Alcohol Abuse*, *16*, 275–286.

Chick, J. (1999). Can light or moderate drinking benefit mental health? *European Addiction Research*, *5*, 74–81.

Coffin, P. O., Santos, G. M., Das, M., Santos, D. M., Huffaker, S., Matheson, T., et al. (2013). Aripiprazole for the treatment of methamphetamine dependence: A randomized, double-blind, placebo-controlled trial. *Addiction*, *108*, 751–761.

Collins, S. L., Levin, F. R., Foltin, R. W., Kleber, H. D., & Evans, S. M. (2006). Response to cocaine, alone and in combination with methylphenidate, in cocaine abusers with ADHD. *Drug and Alcohol Dependence*, *82*, 158–167.

Collins, S., & Surwit, R. S. (2001). The beta-adrenergic receptors and the control of adipose tissue metabolism and thermogenesis. *Recent Progress in Hormone Research*, *56*, 309–328.

Collins, E. D., Vosberg, S. K., Ward, A. S., Haney, M., & Foltin, R. W. (2007). The effects of acute pretreatment with high-dose memantine on the cardiovascular and behavioral effects of cocaine in humans. *Experimental and Clinical Psychopharmacology*, *15*, 228–237.

Condon, J., & Smith, N. (2003). Prevalence of drug use: Key findings from the 2002/2003 British Crime Survey. *Findings*, *229*, 1–5.

Cornish, J. W., Maany, I., Fudala, P. J., Ehrman, R. N., Robbins, S. J., & O'Brien, C. P. (2001). A randomized, double-blind, placebo-controlled study of ritanserin pharmacotherapy for cocaine dependence. *Drug and Alcohol Dependence, 61*, 183–189.

Covi, L., Hess, J. M., Kreiter, N. A., & Haertzen, C. A. (1995). Effects of combined fluoxetine and counseling in the outpatient treatment of cocaine abusers. *The American Journal of Drug and Alcohol Abuse, 21*, 327–344.

Cunningham, K. A., & Anastasio, N. C. (2014). Serotonin at the nexus of impulsivity and cue reactivity in cocaine addiction. *Neuropharmacology, 76*(Pt B), 460–478.

Cunningham, K. A., Fox, R. G., Anastasio, N. C., Bubar, M. J., Stutz, S. J., Moeller, F. G., et al. (2011). Selective serotonin 5-HT(2C) receptor activation suppresses the reinforcing efficacy of cocaine and sucrose but differentially affects the incentive-salience value of cocaine- vs. sucrose-associated cues. *Neuropharmacology, 61*, 513–523.

Dacher, M., & Nugent, F. S. (2011). Opiates and plasticity. *Neuropharmacology, 61*, 1088–1096.

Dackis, C. A., Kampman, K. M., Lynch, K. G., Pettinati, H. M., & O'Brien, C. P. (2005). A double-blind, placebo-controlled trial of modafinil for cocaine dependence. *Neuropsychopharmacology, 30*, 205–211.

Dackis, C. A., Kampman, K. M., Lynch, K. G., Plebani, J. G., Pettinati, H. M., Sparkman, T., et al. (2012). A double-blind, placebo-controlled trial of modafinil for cocaine dependence. *Journal of Substance Abuse Treatment, 43*, 303–312.

Dean, L. G., Kendal, R. L., Schapiro, S. J., Thierry, B., & Laland, K. N. (2012). Identification of the social and cognitive processes underlying human cumulative culture. *Science, 335*, 1114–1118.

de Bruin, N. M., Kloeze, B. M., & McCreary, A. C. (2011). The 5-HT$_6$ serotonin receptor antagonist SB-271046 attenuates the development and expression of nicotine-induced locomotor sensitisation in Wistar rats. *Neuropharmacology, 61*, 451–457.

de Bruin, N. M., McCreary, A. C., van Loevezijn, A., de Vries, T. J., Venhorst, J., van Drimmelen, M., et al. (2013). A novel highly selective 5-HT6 receptor antagonist attenuates ethanol and nicotine seeking but does not affect inhibitory response control in Wistar rats. *Behavioural Brain Research, 236*, 157–165.

De Vries, T. J., Shaham, Y., Homberg, J. R., Crombag, H., Schuurman, K., Dieben, J., et al. (2001). A cannabinoid mechanism in relapse to cocaine seeking. *Nature Medicine, 7*, 1151–1154.

de Wit, H., & Stewart, J. (1981). Reinstatement of cocaine-reinforced responding in the rat. *Psychopharmacology, 75*, 134–143.

Di Chiara, G., Tanda, G., Bassareo, V., Pontieri, F., Acquas, E., Fenu, S., et al. (1999). Drug addiction as a disorder of associative learning. Role of nucleus accumbens shell/extended amygdala dopamine. *Annals of the New York Academy of Sciences, 877*, 461–485.

Ding, C., Bremer, N. M., Smith, T. D., Seitz, P. K., Anastasio, N. C., Cunningham, K. A., et al. (2012). Exploration of synthetic approaches and pharmacological evaluation of PNU-69176E and its stereoisomer as 5-HT2C receptor allosteric modulators. *ACS Chemical Neuroscience, 3*, 538–545.

Dutta, A., McKie, S., & Deakin, J. F. (2014). Ketamine and other potential glutamate antidepressants. *Psychiatry Research, 225*, 1–13. http://dx.doi.org/10.1016/j.psychres.2014.10.028.

Ehrman, R. N., Robbins, S. J., Cornish, J. W., Childress, A. R., & O'Brien, C. P. (1996). Failure of ritanserin to block cocaine cue reactivity in humans. *Drug and Alcohol Dependence, 42*, 167–174.

Eickenhorst, P., Vitzthum, K., Klapp, B. F., Groneberg, D., & Mache, S. (2012). Neuroenhancement among German university students: Motives, expectations, and relationship with psychoactive lifestyle drugs. *Journal of Psychoactive Drugs, 44*, 418–427.

Elkashef, A., Fudala, P. J., Gorgon, L., Li, S. H., Kahn, R., Chiang, N., et al. (2006). Double-blind, placebo-controlled trial of selegiline transdermal system (STS) for the treatment of cocaine dependence. *Drug and Alcohol Dependence*, *85*, 191–197.

Elkashef, A. M., Rawson, R. A., Anderson, A. L., Li, S. H., Holmes, T., Smith, E. V., et al. (2008). Bupropion for the treatment of methamphetamine dependence. *Neuropsychopharmacology*, *33*, 1162–1170.

EMCDDA (2012). European monitoring center for addictive drugs, state of the drug problem 2012. http://www.emcdda.europa.eu/publications/annual-report/2012.

Emley, G. S., & Hutchinson, R. R. (1983). Unique influences of 10 drugs upon post-shock biting attack and preshock manual responding. *Pharmacology, Biochemistry, and Behavior*, *19*, 5–12.

Engel, J. A., & Jerlhag, E. (2014). Role of appetite-regulating peptides in the pathophysiology of addiction: Implications for pharmacotherapy. *CNS Drugs*, *28*, 875–886.

Ersche, K. D., Roiser, J. P., Abbott, S., Craig, K. J., Müller, U., Suckling, J., et al. (2011). Response perseveration in stimulant dependence is associated with striatal dysfunction and can be ameliorated by a D(2/3) receptor agonist. *Biological Psychiatry*, *70*, 754–762.

Ferguson, S. M., Mitchell, E. S., & Neumaier, J. F. (2008). Increased expression of 5-HT6 receptors in the nucleus accumbens blocks the rewarding but not psychomotor activating properties of cocaine. *Biological Psychiatry*, *63*, 207–213.

Fijał, K., Pachuta, A., McCreary, A. C., Wydra, K., Nowak, E., Papp, M., et al. (2010). Effects of serotonin (5-HT)6 receptor ligands on responding for cocaine reward and seeking in rats. *Pharmacological Reports*, *62*, 1005–1014.

Filip, M., Alenina, N., Bader, M., & Przegalinski, E. (2010). Behavioral evidence for the significance of serotoninergic (5-HT) receptors in cocaine addiction. *Addiction Biology*, *15*, 227–249.

Filip, M., & Frankowska, M. (2008). GABA(B) receptors in drug addiction. *Pharmacological Reports*, *60*, 755–770.

Filip, M., Frankowska, M., Sadakierska-Chudy, A., Suder, A., Szumiec, L., Mierzejewski, P., et al. (2015). GABA receptors as a therapeutic strategy in substance use disorders: Focus on positive allosteric modulators. *Neuropharmacology*, *88*, 36–47.

Filip, M., Gołda, A., Zaniewska, M., McCreary, A. C., Nowak, E., Kolasiewicz, W., et al. (2006). Involvement of cannabinoid CB1 receptors in drug addiction: Effects of rimonabant on behavioral responses induced by cocaine. *Pharmacological Reports*, *58*, 806–819.

Fischman, M. W., & Schuster, C. R. (1980). Cocaine effects in sleep-deprived humans. *Psychopharmacology*, *72*, 1–8.

Foley, K. F. (2005). Mechanism of action and therapeutic uses of psychostimulants. *Clinical Laboratory Science*, *18*, 107–113.

Forray, A., & Sofuoglu, M. (2014). Future pharmacological treatments for substance use disorders. *British Journal of Clinical Pharmacology*, *77*, 382–400.

Fossberg, E., Beisland, H. O., & Lundgren, R. A. (1983). Stress incontinence in females: Treatment with phenylpropanolamine. A urodynamic and pharmacological evaluation. *Urologia Internationalis*, *38*, 293–299.

Frankowska, M., Jastrzębska, J., Nowak, E., Białko, M., Przegaliński, E., & Filip, M. (2014). The effects of *N*-acetylcysteine on cocaine reward and seeking behaviors in a rat model of depression. *Behavioural Brain Research*, *266*, 108–118.

Freeman, K. B., Heal, D. J., McCreary, A. C., & Woolverton, W. L. (2012). Assessment of ropinirole as a reinforcer in rhesus monkeys. *Drug and Alcohol Dependence*, *125*, 173–177.

Gawin, F., Riordan, C., & Kleber, H. (1985). Methylphenidate treatment of cocaine abusers without attention deficit disorder: A negative report. *The American Journal of Drug and Alcohol Abuse*, *11*, 193–197.

Gonzalez, G., Desai, R., Sofuoglu, M., Poling, J., Oliveto, A., Gonsai, K., et al. (2007). Clinical efficacy of gabapentin versus tiagabine for reducing cocaine use among cocaine dependent methadone-treated patients. *Drug and Alcohol Dependence*, *87*, 1–9.

Grabowski, J., Rhoades, H., Elk, R., Schmitz, J., Davis, C., Creson, D., et al. (1995). Fluoxetine is ineffective for treatment of cocaine dependence or concurrent opiate and cocaine dependence: Two placebo-controlled double-blind trials. *Journal of Clinical Psychopharmacology*, *15*, 163–174.

Grabowski, J., Rhoades, H., Stotts, A., Cowan, K., Kopecky, C., Dougherty, A., et al. (2004). Agonist-like or antagonist-like treatment for cocaine dependence with methadone for heroin dependence: Two double-blind randomized clinical trials. *Neuropsychopharmacology*, *29*, 969–981.

Grabowski, J., Roache, J. D., Schmitz, J. M., Rhoades, H., Creson, D., & Korszun, A. (1997). Replacement medication for cocaine dependence: Methylphenidate. *Journal of Clinical Psychopharmacology*, *17*, 485–488.

Grassi, M. C., Cioce, A. M., Giudici, F. D., Antonilli, L., & Nencini, P. (2007). Short-term efficacy of Disulfiram or Naltrexone in reducing positive urinalysis for both cocaine and cocaethylene in cocaine abusers: A pilot study. *Pharmacological Research*, *55*, 117–121.

Grinspoon, L., & Hedblom, P. (2005). A historical overview of amphetamines. In N. Harris (Ed.), *Amphetamines* (pp. 19–30). Detroit: Thomson Gale.

Hagen, E. H., Sullivan, R. J., Schmidt, R., Morris, G., Kempter, R., & Hammerstein, P. (2009). Ecology and neurobiology of toxin avoidance and the paradox of drug reward. *Neuroscience*, *160*, 69–84.

Halberstadt, A. L., & Nichols, D. E. (2010). Serotonin and serotonin receptors in hallucinogen action. In C. P. Müller & B. L. Jacobs (Eds.), *Handbook of the behavioral neurobiology of serotonin* (pp. 621–636). London: Academic Press.

Haney, M., Hart, C. L., & Foltin, R. W. (2006). Effects of baclofen on cocaine self-administration: Opioid- and nonopioid-dependent volunteers. *Neuropsychopharmacology*, *31*, 1814–1821.

Hassan, Z., Muzaimi, M., Navaratnam, V., Yusoff, N. H., Suhaimi, F. W., Vadivelu, R., et al. (2013). From Kratom to mitragynine and its derivatives: Physiological and behavioural effects related to use, abuse, and addiction. *Neuroscience and Biobehavioral Reviews*, *37*, 138–151.

Heilig, M., & Koob, G. F. (2007). A key role for corticotropin-releasing factor in alcohol dependence. *Trends in Neurosciences*, *30*, 399–406.

Heinzerling, K. G., Gadzhyan, J., van Oudheusden, H., Rodriguez, F., McCracken, J., & Shoptaw, S. (2013). Pilot randomized trial of bupropion for adolescent methamphetamine abuse/dependence. *The Journal of Adolescent Health*, *52*, 502–505.

Heinzerling, K. G., Shoptaw, S., Peck, J. A., Yang, X., Liu, J., Roll, J., et al. (2006). Randomized, placebo-controlled trial of baclofen and gabapentin for the treatment of methamphetamine dependence. *Drug and Alcohol Dependence*, *85*, 177–184.

Heinzerling, K. G., Swanson, A. N., Hall, T. M., Yi, Y., Wu, Y., & Shoptaw, S. J. (2014). Randomized, placebo-controlled trial of bupropion in methamphetamine-dependent participants with less than daily methamphetamine use. *Addiction*, *109*, 1878–1886.

Heinzerling, K. G., Swanson, A. N., Kim, S., Cederblom, L., Moe, A., Ling, W., et al. (2010). Randomized, double-blind, placebo-controlled trial of modafinil for the treatment of methamphetamine dependence. *Drug and Alcohol Dependence*, *109*, 20–29.

Higgins, S. T., Bickel, W. K., Hughes, J. R., Lynn, M., Capeless, M. A., & Fenwick, J. W. (1990). Effects of intranasal cocaine on human learning, performance and physiology. *Psychopharmacology*, *102*, 451–458.

Hopitt, W., & Laland, K. N. (2013). *Social learning*. Princeton: Princeton University Press.

Howell, L. L., & Cunningham, K. A. (2015). Serotonin 5-HT2 receptor interactions with dopamine function: Implications for therapeutics in cocaine use disorder. *Pharmacological Reviews*, *67*, 176–197.

Huffman, M. A. (2003). Animal self-medication and ethno-medicine: Exploration and exploitation of the medicinal properties of plants. *The Proceedings of the Nutrition Society*, *62*, 371–381.

Hulka, L. M., Eisenegger, C., Preller, K. H., Vonmoos, M., Jenni, D., Bendrick, K., et al. (2014). Altered social and non-social decision-making in recreational and dependent cocaine users. *Psychological Medicine*, *44*, 1015–1028.

Hyytiä, P., Bäckström, P., & Liljequist, S. (1999). Site-specific NMDA receptor antagonists produce differential effects on cocaine self-administration in rats. *European Journal of Pharmacology*, *378*, 9–16.

Javaid, J. I., Fischman, M. W., Schuster, C. R., Dekirmenjian, H., & Davis, J. M. (1978). Cocaine plasma concentration: Relation to physiological and subjective effects in humans. *Science*, *202*, 227–228.

Johnson, B. A., Ait-Daoud, N., Elkashef, A. M., Smith, E. V., Kahn, R., Vocci, F., et al. (2008). A preliminary randomized, double-blind, placebo-controlled study of the safety and efficacy of ondansetron in the treatment of methamphetamine dependence. *The International Journal of Neuropsychopharmacology*, *11*, 1–14.

Jones, C. A., & McCreary, A. C. (2008). Serotonergic approaches in the development of novel antipsychotics. *Neuropharmacology*, *55*, 1056–1065.

Kahn, R., Biswas, K., Childress, A. R., Shoptaw, S., Fudala, P. J., Gorgon, L., et al. (2009). Multi-center trial of baclofen for abstinence initiation in severe cocaine-dependent individuals. *Drug and Alcohol Dependence*, *103*, 59–64.

Kalivas, P. W. (2004). Recent understanding in the mechanisms of addiction. *Current Psychiatry Reports*, *6*, 347–351.

Kalix, P., & Braenden, O. (1985). Pharmacological aspects of the chewing of khat leaves. *Pharmacological Reviews*, *37*, 149–164.

Kampman, K. M., Dackis, C., Pettinati, H. M., Lynch, K. G., Sparkman, T., & O'Brien, C. P. (2011). A double-blind, placebo-controlled pilot trial of acamprosate for the treatment of cocaine dependence. *Addictive Behaviors*, *36*, 217–221.

Kelley, A. E., Cador, M., & Stinus, L. (1990). Exploration and its measurement. A psychopharmacological perspective. In A. A. Boulton, G. B. Baker, & A. J. Greenshaw (Eds.), *Neuromethods 13—Psychopharmacology* (pp. 95–143). Clifton, New Jersey: Humana Press.

Kerrigan, S., Mott, A., Jatzlau, B., Ortiz, F., Perrella, L., Martin, S., et al. (2014). Designer psychostimulants in urine by liquid chromatography-tandem mass spectrometry. *Journal of Forensic Sciences*, *59*, 175–183.

King, A. J., Johnson, D. D., & Van Vugt, M. (2009). The origins and evolution of leadership. *Current Biology*, *19*, R911–R916.

Kirkham, T. C., Williams, C. M., Fezza, F., & Di Marzo, V. (2002). Endocannabinoid levels in rat limbic forebrain and hypothalamus in relation to fasting, feeding and satiation: Stimulation of eating by 2-arachidonoyl glycerol. *British Journal of Pharmacology*, *136*, 550–557.

Kishi, T., Matsuda, Y., Iwata, N., & Correll, C. U. (2013). Antipsychotics for cocaine or psychostimulant dependence: Systematic review and meta-analysis of randomized, placebo-controlled trials. *The Journal of Clinical Psychiatry*, *74*, e1169–e1180.

Koob, G. F., & Le Moal, M. (1997). Drug abuse: Hedonic homeostatic dysregulation. *Science*, *278*, 52–58.

Kotlińska, J., & Biała, G. (2000). Memantine and ACPC affect conditioned place preference induced by cocaine in rats. *Polish Journal of Pharmacology*, *52*, 179–185.

Landry, M. J. (2002). MDMA: A review of epidemiologic data. *Journal of Psychoactive Drugs*, *34*, 163–169.

LaRowe, S. D., Myrick, H., Hedden, S., Mardikian, P., Saladin, M., McRae, A., et al. (2007). Is cocaine desire reduced by *N*-acetylcysteine? *The American Journal of Psychiatry*, *164*, 1115–1117.

Lende, D. H., & Smith, E. O. (2002). Evolution meets biopsychosociality: An analysis of addictive behavior. *Addiction*, *97*, 447–458.

Levin, F. R., Evans, S. M., Brooks, D. J., & Garawi, F. (2007). Treatment of cocaine dependent treatment seekers with adult ADHD: Double-blind comparison of methylphenidate and placebo. *Drug and Alcohol Dependence*, *87*, 20–29.

Li, Y., White, F. J., & Wolf, M. E. (2000). Pharmacological reversal of behavioral and cellular indices of cocaine sensitization in the rat. *Psychopharmacology*, *151*, 175–183.

Lile, J. A., Stoops, W. W., Allen, T. S., Glaser, P. E., Hays, L. R., & Rush, C. R. (2004). Baclofen does not alter the reinforcing, subject-rated or cardiovascular effects of intranasal cocaine in humans. *Psychopharmacology*, *171*, 441–449.

Lile, J. A., Stoops, W. W., Glaser, P. E., Hays, L. R., & Rush, C. R. (2004). Acute administration of the GABA reuptake inhibitor tiagabine does not alter the effects of oral cocaine in humans. *Drug and Alcohol Dependence*, *76*, 81–91.

Liu, S., Lane, S. D., Schmitz, J. M., Cunningham, K. A., John, V. P., & Moeller, F. G. (2013). Effects of escitalopram on attentional bias to cocaine-related stimuli and inhibitory control in cocaine-dependent subjects. *Journal of Psychopharmacology*, *27*, 801–807.

Longo, M., Wickes, W., Smout, M., Harrison, S., Cahill, S., & White, J. M. (2010). Randomized controlled trial of dexamphetamine maintenance for the treatment of methamphetamine dependence. *Addiction*, *105*, 146–154.

Marcuse, L. (1984). *Philosophie des Gluecks* (2nd ed.). Zürich: Diogenes.

Maremmani, A. G., Pacini, M., Rovai, L., Rugani, F., Dell'osso, L., & Maremmani, I. (2011). Can ropinirole modulate reinforcing subjective effects of cocaine in humans? *Frontiers in Psychology*, *2*, 50.

Margolin, A., Kosten, T. R., Avants, S. K., Wilkins, J., Ling, W., Beckson, M., et al. (1995). A multicenter trial of bupropion for cocaine dependence in methadone-maintained patients. *Drug and Alcohol Dependence*, *40*, 125–131.

Martell, B. A., Mitchell, E., Poling, J., Gonsai, K., & Kosten, T. R. (2005). Vaccine pharmacotherapy for the treatment of cocaine dependence. *Biological Psychiatry*, *58*, 158–164.

Martell, B. A., Orson, F. M., Poling, J., Mitchell, E., Rossen, R. D., Gardner, T., et al. (2009). Cocaine vaccine for the treatment of cocaine dependence in methadone-maintained patients: A randomized, double-blind, placebo-controlled efficacy trial. *Archives of General Psychiatry*, *66*, 1116–1123.

Martinez-Raga, J., Knecht, C., & Cepeda, S. (2008). Modafinil: A useful medication for cocaine addiction? Review of the evidence from neuropharmacological, experimental and clinical studies. *Current Drug Abuse Reviews*, *1*, 213–221.

McCabe, S. E., Knight, J. R., Teter, C. J., & Wechsler, H. (2005). Non-medical use of prescription stimulants among US college students: Prevalence and correlates from a national survey. *Addiction*, *100*, 96–106.

McClure, E. A., Gipson, C. D., Malcolm, R. J., Kalivas, P. W., & Gray, K. M. (2014). Potential role of *N*-acetylcysteine in the management of substance use disorders. *CNS Drugs*, *28*, 95–106.

McCreary, A. C., & Jones, C. A. (2010). Antipsychotic medication: The potential role of 5-HT(1A) receptor agonism. *Current Pharmaceutical Design*, *16*, 516–521.

McElhiney, M. C., Rabkin, J. G., Rabkin, R., & Nunes, E. V. (2009). Provigil (modafinil) plus cognitive behavioral therapy for methamphetamine use in HIV+ gay men: A pilot study. *The American Journal of Drug and Alcohol Abuse*, *35*, 34–37.

Meini, M., Moncini, M., Cecconi, D., Cellesi, V., Biasci, L., Simoni, G., et al. (2012). Aripiprazole and ropinirole treatment for cocaine dependence: Evidence from a pilot study. *Current Pharmaceutical Design*, *17*, 1376–1383.

Miles, S. W., Sheridan, J., Russell, B., Kydd, R., Wheeler, A., Walters, C., et al. (2013). Extended-release methylphenidate for treatment of amphetamine/methamphetamine dependence: A randomized, double-blind, placebo-controlled trial. *Addiction, 108*, 1279–1286.

Mitchell, E. S., & Neumaier, J. F. (2005). 5-HT6 receptors: A novel target for cognitive enhancement. *Pharmacology & Therapeutics, 108*, 320–333.

Moeller, F. G., Schmitz, J. M., Steinberg, J. L., Green, C. M., Reist, C., Lai, L. Y., et al. (2007). Citalopram combined with behavioral therapy reduces cocaine use: A double-blind, placebo-controlled trial. *The American Journal of Drug and Alcohol Abuse, 33*, 367–378.

Morgan, C. J., Noronha, L. A., Muetzelfeldt, M., Fielding, A., & Curran, H. V. (2013). Harms and benefits associated with psychoactive drugs: Findings of an international survey of active drug users. *Journal of Psychopharmacology, 27*, 497–506.

Müller, C. P. (2015). Eyes on the price: Human culture and its teaching. *The Behavioral and Brain Sciences*. (in press).

Müller, C. P., & Homberg, J. R. (2015). The role of serotonin in drug use and addiction. *Behavioural Brain Research, 277*, 146–192.

Müller, C. P., & Jacobs, B. L. (2010). *Handbook of the behavioral neurobiology of serotonin*. London: Academic Press.

Müller, C. P., Lenz, B., & Kornhuber, J. (2012). Gene-independent heritability of behavioural traits: Don't we also need to rethink the "environment"? *The Behavioral and Brain Sciences, 35*, 374–375.

Müller, C. P., Pum, M. E., Amato, D., Schuttler, J., Huston, J. P., & Silva, M. A. (2011). The in vivo neurochemistry of the brain during general anesthesia. *Journal of Neurochemistry, 119*, 419–446.

Müller, C. P., & Schumann, G. (2011a). Drugs as instruments: A new framework for non-addictive psychoactive drug use. *The Behavioral and Brain Sciences, 34*, 293–310.

Müller, C. P., & Schumann, G. (2011b). To use or not to use: Expanding the view on non-addictive psychoactive drug consumption and its implications. *The Behavioral and Brain Sciences, 34*, 328–347.

Nich, C., McCance-Katz, E. F., Petrakis, I. L., Cubells, J. F., Rounsaville, B. J., & Carroll, K. M. (2004). Sex differences in cocaine-dependent individuals' response to disulfiram treatment. *Addictive Behaviors, 29*, 1123–1128.

Nichols, D. E. (2004). Hallucinogens. *Pharmacology & Therapeutics, 101*, 131–181.

O'Malley, P. M., & Johnston, L. D. (2002). Epidemiology of alcohol and other drug use among American college students. *Journal of Studies on Alcohol. Supplement, 14*, 23–39.

Oliveto, A., McCance-Katz, F. E., Singha, A., Petrakis, I., Hameedi, F., & Kosten, T. R. (2001). Effects of cocaine prior to and during bupropion maintenance in cocaine-abusing volunteers. *Drug and Alcohol Dependence, 63*, 155–167.

Oliveto, A., Poling, J., Mancino, M. J., Feldman, Z., Cubells, J. F., Pruzinsky, R., et al. (2011). Randomized, double blind, placebo-controlled trial of disulfiram for the treatment of cocaine dependence in methadone-stabilized patients. *Drug and Alcohol Dependence, 113*, 184–191.

Oliveto, A., Poling, J., Mancino, M. J., Williams, D. K., Thostenson, J., Pruzinsky, R., et al. (2012). Sertraline delays relapse in recently abstinent cocaine-dependent patients with depressive symptoms. *Addiction, 107*, 131–141.

Orson, F. M., Wang, R., Brimijoin, S., Kinsey, B. M., Singh, R. A., Ramakrishnan, M., et al. (2014). The future potential for cocaine vaccines. *Expert Opinion on Biological Therapy, 14*, 1271–1283.

Padwa, H., Ni, Y. M., Barth-Rogers, Y., Arangua, L., Andersen, R., & Gelberg, L. (2014). Barriers to drug use behavior change among primary care patients in urban United States community health centers. *Substance Use & Misuse, 49*, 743–751.

Parran, T. V., Jr., & Jasinski, D. R. (1991). Intravenous methylphenidate abuse. Prototype for prescription drug abuse. *Archives of Internal Medicine, 151*, 781–783.

Patil, S. T., Zhang, L., Martenyi, F., Lowe, S. L., Jackson, K. A., Andreev, B. V., et al. (2007). Activation of mGlu2/3 receptors as a new approach to treat schizophrenia: A randomized Phase 2 clinical trial. *Nature Medicine, 13*, 1102–1107.

Patrick, M. E., & Maggs, J. L. (2008). Short-term changes in plans to drink and importance of positive and negative alcohol consequences. *Journal of Adolescence, 31*, 307–321.

Perez-Mana, C., Castells, X., Torrens, M., Capella, D., & Farre, M. (2013). Efficacy of psychostimulant drugs for amphetamine abuse or dependence. *Cochrane Database of Systematic Reviews, 9,* CD009695.

Perez-Mana, C., Castells, X., Vidal, X., Casas, M., & Capella, D. (2011). Efficacy of indirect dopamine agonists for psychostimulant dependence: A systematic review and meta-analysis of randomized controlled trials. *Journal of Substance Abuse Treatment, 40*, 109–122.

Peroutka, S. J., Newman, H., & Harris, H. (1988). Subjective effects of 3,4-methylenedioxymethamphetamine in recreational users. *Neuropsychopharmacology, 1*, 273–277.

Petrakis, I. L., Carroll, K. M., Nich, C., Gordon, L. T., McCance-Katz, E. F., Frankforter, T., et al. (2000). Disulfiram treatment for cocaine dependence in methadone-maintained opioid addicts. *Addiction, 95*, 219–228.

Pettinati, H. M., Kampman, K. M., Lynch, K. G., Xie, H., Dackis, C., Rabinowitz, A. R., et al. (2008). A double blind, placebo-controlled trial that combines disulfiram and naltrexone for treating co-occurring cocaine and alcohol dependence. *Addictive Behaviors, 33*, 651–667.

Plebani, J. G., Lynch, K. G., Yu, Q., Pettinati, H. M., O'Brien, C. P., & Kampman, K. M. (2012). Results of an initial clinical trial of varenicline for the treatment of cocaine dependence. *Drug and Alcohol Dependence, 121*, 163–166.

Poling, J., Oliveto, A., Petry, N., Sofuoglu, M., Gonsai, K., Gonzalez, G., et al. (2006). Six-month trial of bupropion with contingency management for cocaine dependence in a methadone-maintained population. *Archives of General Psychiatry, 63*, 219–228.

Poling, J., Rounsaville, B., Gonsai, K., Severino, K., & Sofuoglu, M. (2010). The safety and efficacy of varenicline in cocaine using smokers maintained on methadone: A pilot study. *The American Journal on Addictions, 19*, 401–408.

Pomierny-Chamioło, L., Rup, K., Pomierny, B., Niedzielska, E., Kalivas, P. W., & Filip, M. (2014). Metabotropic glutamatergic receptors and their ligands in drug addiction. *Pharmacology & Therapeutics, 142*, 281–305.

Potenza, M. N., Sofuoglu, M., Carroll, K. M., & Rounsaville, B. J. (2011). Neuroscience of behavioral and pharmacological treatments for addictions. *Neuron, 69*, 695–712.

Preller, K. H., Hulka, L. M., Vonmoos, M., Jenni, D., Baumgartner, M. R., Seifritz, E., et al. (2014). Impaired emotional empathy and related social network deficits in cocaine users. *Addiction Biology, 19*, 452–466.

Ramo, D. E., Grov, C., Delucchi, K. L., Kelly, B. C., & Parsons, J. T. (2011). Cocaine use trajectories of club drug-using young adults recruited using time-space sampling. *Addictive Behaviors, 36*, 1292–1300.

Ramsay, R. R., & Hunter, D. J. (2002). Inhibitors alter the spectrum and redox properties of monoamine oxidase A. *Biochimica et Biophysica Acta, 1601*, 178–184.

Resnick, R. B., Kestenbaum, R. S., & Schwartz, L. K. (1977). Acute systemic effects of cocaine in man: A controlled study by intranasal and intravenous routes. *Science, 195*, 696–698.

Riddle, E. L., Topham, M. K., Haycock, J. W., Hanson, G. R., & Fleckenstein, A. E. (2002). Differential trafficking of the vesicular monoamine transporter-2 by methamphetamine and cocaine. *European Journal of Pharmacology, 449*, 71–74.

Rodriguez, E., & Wrangham, R. (1993). Zoopharmacognosy: The use of medicinal plants by animals. *Recent Advances in Phytochemistry*, *27*, 89–105.
Rothman, R. B. (1990). High affinity dopamine reuptake inhibitors as potential cocaine antagonists: A strategy for drug development. *Life Sciences*, *46*, L17–L21.
Sabioni, P., Ramos, A. C., & Galduroz, J. C. (2013). The effectiveness of treatments for cocaine dependence in schizophrenic patients: A systematic review. *Current Neuropharmacology*, *11*, 484–490.
SAMHSA (2011) National survey on drug use and health, Substance Abuse and Mental Health Services Administration, Rockville. http://www.samhsa.gov/data/NSDUH/2011SummNatFindDetTables/Index.aspx.
Sarter, M., Hasselmo, M. E., Bruno, J. P., & Givens, B. (2005). Unraveling the attentional functions of cortical cholinergic inputs: Interactions between signal-driven and cognitive modulation of signal detection. *Brain Research Reviews*, *48*, 98–111.
Satel, S. L., Krystal, J. H., Delgado, P. L., Kosten, T. R., & Charney, D. S. (1995). Tryptophan depletion and attenuation of cue-induced craving for cocaine. *The American Journal of Psychiatry*, *152*, 778–783.
Schmitz, J. M., Green, C. E., Stotts, A. L., Lindsay, J. A., Rathnayaka, N. S., Grabowski, J., et al. (2014). A two-phased screening paradigm for evaluating candidate medications for cocaine cessation or relapse prevention: Modafinil, levodopa-carbidopa, naltrexone. *Drug and Alcohol Dependence*, *136*, 100–107.
Schmitz, J. M., Mooney, M. E., Moeller, F. G., Stotts, A. L., Green, C., & Grabowski, J. (2008). Levodopa pharmacotherapy for cocaine dependence: Choosing the optimal behavioral therapy platform. *Drug and Alcohol Dependence*, *94*, 142–150.
Schmitz, J. M., Stotts, A. L., Sayre, S. L., DeLaune, K. A., & Grabowski, J. (2004). Treatment of cocaine-alcohol dependence with naltrexone and relapse prevention therapy. *The American Journal on Addictions*, *13*, 333–341.
Schoffelmeer, A. N., Vanderschuren, L. J., De Vries, T. J., Hogenboom, F., Wardeh, G., & Mulder, A. H. (2000). Synergistically interacting dopamine. D1 and NMDA receptors mediate nonvesicular transporter-dependent GABA release from rat striatal medium spiny neurons. *The Journal of Neuroscience*, *20*, 3496–3503.
Schubiner, H., Saules, K. K., Arfken, C. L., Johanson, C. E., Schuster, C. R., Lockhart, N., et al. (2002). Double-blind placebo-controlled trial of methylphenidate in the treatment of adult ADHD patients with comorbid cocaine dependence. *Experimental and Clinical Psychopharmacology*, *10*, 286–291.
See, R. E. (2005). Neural substrates of cocaine-cue associations that trigger relapse. *European Journal of Pharmacology*, *526*, 140–146.
Sesack, S. R., & Pickel, V. M. (1990). In the rat medial nucleus accumbens, hippocampal and catecholaminergic terminals converge on spiny neurons and are in apposition to each other. *Brain Research*, *527*, 266–279.
Shearer, J., Darke, S., Rodgers, C., Slade, T., van Beek, I., Lewis, J., et al. (2009). A double-blind, placebo-controlled trial of modafinil (200 mg/day) for methamphetamine dependence. *Addiction*, *104*, 224–233.
Shearer, J., Wodak, A., Mattick, R. P., van Beek, I., Lewis, J., Hall, W., et al. (2001). Pilot randomized controlled study of dexamphetamine substitution for amphetamine dependence. *Addiction*, *96*, 1289–1296.
Shearer, J., Wodak, A., van Beek, I., Mattick, R. P., & Lewis, J. (2003). Pilot randomized double blind placebo-controlled study of dexamphetamine for cocaine dependence. *Addiction*, *98*, 1137–1141.
Shippenberg, T. S., & Koob, G. F. (2002). Recent advances in animal models of drug addiction and alcoholism. In K. L. Davis, D. Charney, J. T. Coyle, & C. Nemeroff (Eds.), *Neuropsychopharmacology: The fifth generation of progress* (pp. 1381–1397). Philadelphia, PA: Lippincott Williams and Wilkins.

Shoptaw, S., Heinzerling, K. G., Rotheram-Fuller, E., Steward, T., Wang, J., Swanson, A. N., et al. (2008). Randomized, placebo-controlled trial of bupropion for the treatment of methamphetamine dependence. *Drug and Alcohol Dependence, 96*, 222–232.

Shoptaw, S., Huber, A., Peck, J., Yang, X., Liu, J., Jeff, D., et al. (2006). Randomized, placebo-controlled trial of sertraline and contingency management for the treatment of methamphetamine dependence. *Drug and Alcohol Dependence, 85*, 12–18.

Shoptaw, S., Yang, X., Rotheram-Fuller, E. J., Hsieh, Y. C., Kintaudi, P. C., Charuvastra, V. C., et al. (2003). Randomized placebo-controlled trial of baclofen for cocaine dependence: Preliminary effects for individuals with chronic patterns of cocaine use. *The Journal of Clinical Psychiatry, 64*, 1440–1448.

Singh, D., Müller, C. P., & Vicknasingam, B. K. (2014). Kratom (Mitragyna speciosa) dependence, withdrawal symptoms and craving in regular users. *Drug and Alcohol Dependence, 139*, 132–137.

Sitte, H. H., Huck, S., Reither, H., Boehm, S., Singer, E. A., & Pifl, C. (1998). Carrier-mediated release, transport rates, and charge transfer induced by amphetamine, tyramine, and dopamine in mammalian cells transfected with the human dopamine transporter. *Journal of Neurochemistry, 71*, 1289–1297.

Skogen, J. C., Harvey, S. B., Henderson, M., Stordal, E., & Mykletun, A. (2009). Anxiety and depression among abstainers and low-level alcohol consumers. The Nord-Trondelag Health Study. *Addiction, 104*, 1519–1529.

Skrinska, V. A., & Gock, S. B. (2005). Measurement of 3,4-MDMA and related amines in diagnostic and forensic laboratories. *Clinical Laboratory Science, 18*, 119–123.

Smirnov, A., Najman, J. M., Hayatbakhsh, R., Plotnikova, M., Wells, H., Legosz, M., et al. (2013). Young adults' trajectories of Ecstasy use: A population based study. *Addictive Behaviors, 38*, 2667–2674.

Sofuoglu, M., & Carroll, K. M. (2011). Effects of galantamine on cocaine use in chronic cocaine users. *The American Journal on Addictions, 20*, 302–303.

Sofuoglu, M., Waters, A. J., Poling, J., & Carroll, K. M. (2011). Galantamine improves sustained attention in chronic cocaine users. *Experimental and Clinical Psychopharmacology, 19*, 11–19.

Spanagel, R., & Kiefer, F. (2008). Drugs for relapse prevention of alcoholism: Ten years of progress. *Trends in Pharmacological Sciences, 29*, 109–115.

Spanagel, R., Vengeliene, V., Jandeleit, B., Fischer, W. N., Grindstaff, K., Zhang, X., et al. (2014). Acamprosate produces its anti-relapse effects via calcium. *Neuropsychopharmacology, 39*, 783–791.

Stillman, R., Jones, R. T., Moore, D., Walker, J., & Welm, S. (1993). Improved performance 4 hours after cocaine. *Psychopharmacology, 110*, 415–420.

Stolerman, I. (1992). Drugs of abuse: Behavioural principles, methods and terms. *Trends in Pharmacological Sciences, 13*, 170–176.

Sulzer, D. (2011). How addictive drugs disrupt presynaptic dopamine neurotransmission. *Neuron, 69*, 628–649.

Swendsen, J., Burstein, M., Case, B., Conway, K. P., Dierker, L., He, J., et al. (2012). Use and abuse of alcohol and illicit drugs in US adolescents: Results of the National Comorbidity Survey-Adolescent Supplement. *Archives of General Psychiatry, 69*, 390–398.

Tatarkiewicz, W. (1976). *Analysis of happiness* (p. 356). The Hague, Martinus Nijhoff.

Thiel, C. M., Müller, C. P., Huston, J. P., & Schwarting, R. K. (1999). High versus low reactivity to a novel environment: Behavioural, pharmacological and neurochemical assessments. *Neuroscience, 93*, 243–251.

Tiihonen, J., Krupitsky, E., Verbitskaya, E., Blokhina, E., Mamontova, O., Fohr, J., et al. (2012). Naltrexone implant for the treatment of polydrug dependence: A randomized controlled trial. *The American Journal of Psychiatry, 169*, 531–536.

Tiihonen, J., Kuoppasalmi, K., Fohr, J., Tuomola, P., Kuikanmaki, O., Vorma, H., et al. (2007). A comparison of aripiprazole, methylphenidate, and placebo for amphetamine dependence. *The American Journal of Psychiatry, 164*, 160–162.

Tzschentke, T. M., & Schmidt, W. J. (2003). Glutamatergic mechanisms in addiction. *Molecular Psychiatry, 8*, 373–382.

Uosukainen, H., Tacke, U., & Winstock, A. R. (2014). Self-reported prevalence of dependence of MDMA compared to cocaine, mephedrone and ketamine among a sample of recreational poly-drug users. *International Journal of Drug Policy, 26*, 78–83.

van Gaalen, M. M., Schetters, D., Schoffelmeer, A. N., & De Vries, T. J. (2010). 5-HT6 antagonism attenuates cue-induced relapse to cocaine seeking without affecting cocaine reinforcement. *The International Journal of Neuropsychopharmacology, 13*, 961–965.

Volkow, N. D., Fowler, J. S., & Wang, G. J. (2003). Positron emission tomography and single-photon emission computed tomography in substance abuse research. *Seminars in Nuclear Medicine, 33*, 114–128.

Wagner, F. A., & Anthony, J. C. (2002). From first drug use to drug dependence; developmental periods of risk for dependence upon marijuana, cocaine, and alcohol. *Neuropsychopharmacology, 26*, 479–488.

Waldorf, D., Reinarman, C., & Murphy, S. (1991). *Cocaine changes: The experience of using and quitting*. Philadelphia: Temple University Press.

Weil, A. (1998). *The natural mind: A new way of looking at drugs and the higher consciousness*. Boston, MA, USA: Houghton Mifflin.

Weintraub, D., Masek, M., & Billingham, M. E. (1985). The lymphocyte subpopulations in cyclosporine-treated human heart rejection. *The Journal of Heart Transplantation, 4*, 213–216.

Westfall, T. C. (2006). Neuropeptide Y and sympathetic control of vascular tone in hypertension. *EXS, 95*, 89–103.

White, N. M. (1996). Addictive drugs as reinforcers: Multiple partial actions on memory systems. *Addiction, 91*, 921–949.

Winhusen, T. M., Kropp, F., Lindblad, R., Douaihy, A., Haynes, L., Hodgkins, C., et al. (2014). Multisite, randomized, double-blind, placebo-controlled pilot clinical trial to evaluate the efficacy of buspirone as a relapse-prevention treatment for cocaine dependence. *The Journal of Clinical Psychiatry, 75*, 757–764.

Winhusen, T., Somoza, E., Singal, B. M., Harrer, J., Apparaju, S., Mezinskis, J., et al. (2006). Methylphenidate and cocaine: A placebo controlled drug interaction study. *Pharmacol ogy, Biochemistry, and Behavior, 85*, 29–38.

Winstanley, E. L., Bigelow, G. E., Silverman, K., Johnson, R. E., & Strain, E. C. (2011). A randomized controlled trial of fluoxetine in the treatment of cocaine dependence among methadone-maintained patients. *Journal of Substance Abuse Treatment, 40*, 255–264.

Zinberg, N. E. (1984). *Drug, set, and setting: The basis for controlled intoxicant use*. New Haven: Yale University Press.

Zinberg, N. E., & Jacobson, R. C. (1976). The natural history of "chipping" *The American Journal of Psychiatry, 133*, 37–40.

Zorick, T., Sugar, C. A., Hellemann, G., Shoptaw, S., & London, E. D. (2011). Poor response to sertraline in methamphetamine dependence is associated with sustained craving for methamphetamine. *Drug and Alcohol Dependence, 118*, 500–503.

Zuckerman, M. (1990). The psychophysiology of sensation seeking. *Journal of Personality, 58*, 313–345.

CHAPTER FIVE

Epigenetic Mechanisms of Psychostimulant-Induced Addiction

Anti Kalda[1], Alexander Zharkovsky
Department of Pharmacology, Institute of Biomedicine and Translational Medicine, University of Tartu, Tartu, Estonia
[1]Corresponding author: e-mail address: anti.kalda@ut.ee

Contents

Abstract

Psychostimulant-induced addiction involves potentially life-long behavioral abnormalities that are caused by repeated exposure to a drug of abuse in vulnerable individuals. The persistence of these behavioral changes suggests that long-lasting alterations in gene expression, particularly within the brain's reward regions, may contribute significantly to the addiction phenotype. An increasing number of works over the past decade have demonstrated the important role of epigenetic regulatory events in mediating the lasting effects of drugs of abuse (including psychostimulants, such as cocaine and amphetamine) in animal models of drug addiction. In this review, we have introduced the importance of epigenetic processes in regulating gene expression and have described the role that dynamic epigenetic changes may play in psychostimulant-induced addiction via long-lasting transcriptional changes following repeated drug exposure. We overviewed the evidence showing that repeated exposure to psychostimulants induces three major modes of epigenetic regulation within the brain's reward regions—histone modification, DNA methylation, and noncoding RNAs.

International Review of Neurobiology, Volume 120
ISSN 0074-7742
http://dx.doi.org/10.1016/bs.irn.2015.02.010

In several instances, it has been possible to demonstrate directly the contribution of these epigenetic changes to psychostimulant-related behavioral abnormalities. Studies of epigenetics may also help to determine the role environmental factors play in an individual's vulnerability to addiction. Further studies are required to validate these epigenetic changes in human addiction and to evaluate the possibility of developing new diagnostic tests and more effective treatments for addiction syndromes.

1. INTRODUCTION

Drug addiction is a multifactorial and polygenic disorder that does not conform to a simple Mendelian transmission pattern (Goldman, Oroszi, & Ducci, 2005; Wong, Mill, & Fernandes, 2011). Extensive epidemiological studies show that roughly half of an individual's risk for drug addiction is genetic; however, the specific genes that confer risk for addiction are unknown (Goldman et al., 2005; Hyman, Malenka, & Nestler, 2006; Nestler, 2001). Individuals are differentially vulnerable to substance abuse and not everyone who uses an addictive substance becomes addicted. Entry into the addicted state results from the interplay between an inherited predisposition (e.g., via genetic variants mediating the personality traits associated with drug-seeking behavior and dependence) and the environment (e.g., actual exposure to drugs of abuse) (Goldman et al., 2005; Nestler, 2001; Wong et al., 2011). In recent years, epigenetic modifications in addition to other risk factors have come into focus. The aim of this review is to introduce the potential role that epigenetic mechanisms play in the pathogenesis of psychostimulant-induced addiction and in mediating addictive behaviors via the triggering of long-lasting changes in gene expression in response to addictive substances.

2. EPIGENETIC PROCESSES

Every cell in our body contains the same DNA sequence but has its own unique phenotype characterized by a specific pattern of gene expression that is in a constant state of flux. In the context of determining the phenotype of a cell, the degree to which specific genes are functionally active at any particular time in development is also important (Smith & Mill, 2011; Wong et al., 2011). Accumulating evidence indicates that above the DNA sequence is a second layer of information—the epigenetic modifications (epigenome) that regulate several genomic functions including when and where genes are turned on or off. Historically, the term epigenetics (literally meaning "above genetics") was coined by Conrad Hal Waddington in 1942 (Haig, 2004; McQuown & Wood, 2010). Currently, epigenetics is defined as a series of biochemical processes through which changes in gene expression are achieved throughout the lifecycle of an organism without changing the DNA sequence itself (Jaenisch & Bird, 2003).

Epigenetic processes are important for normal cellular development and differentiation and allow the long-term regulation of gene function through nonmutagenic mechanisms (Smith & Mill, 2011). Increasingly, studies suggest that alterations of epigenetic mechanisms affect the vast majority of nuclear processes (including gene transcription and silencing), DNA replication and repair, cell cycle and telomere, and centromere function and structure.

Epigenetics can also be viewed as the vehicle through which different environmental factors interacts with an individual's genome to determine all aspects of function during health and disease. Subsets of epigenetic changes are very stable, which makes them ideal mediators of both the vulnerability to addiction and the drug-induced brain maladaptations that underlie an addiction syndrome (Nestler, 2013).

3. CHROMATIN STRUCTURE

Chromatin, the fundamental unit that accomplishes epigenetic modifications on a molecular level, is the complex of DNA, histones, and nonhistone proteins in the cell nucleus. The basic repeating structural unit of chromatin is the nucleosome (Fig. 1), which consists of ~147 base pairs of DNA wrapped around a core nucleosome (Strahl & Allis, 2000). Nucleosomes are composed of octamers that contain four histone homodimers, one each of histones H2A, H2B, H3, and H4, with H1 binding to spans of non-nucleosomal DNA (Robison & Nestler, 2011; Strahl & Allis, 2000). The histone and DNA configuration is maintained by electrostatic bonds between positively charged histones and negatively charged DNA (Grunstein, 1997). This highly condensed histone protein–DNA complex structure means that control over gene expression occurs partly by gating the access of transcriptional activators to the DNA (Felsenfeld & Groudine, 2003; Li, Carey, & Workman, 2007).

The structure of chromatin and access to the DNA sequence wrapped around it is regulated by posttranslational modifications of histones and the DNA itself (Kouzarides, 2007). Numerous types of posttranslational

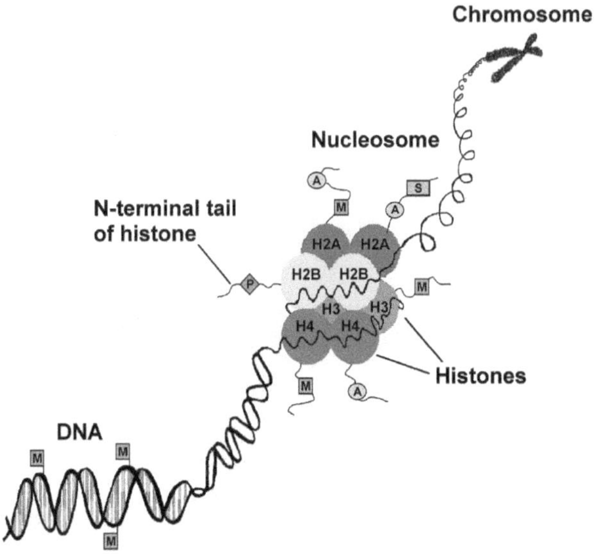

Figure 1 DNA is wrapped around a cluster of histone proteins to form nucleosomes. In posttranslational modifications of histones, a combination of different molecules can attach to the histone N-terminal tails, which consequently change the state of the chromatin around the DNA. When the chromatin becomes opened, the transcription of associated genes is activated and opposite when chromatin becomes closed. In DNA methylation, methyl marks added in promoter region generally repress gene transcription. A, acetylation; M, methylation; P, phosphorylation; S, sumoylation. *Adapted from Wong et al. (2011).*

modifications, such as acetylation, methylation, phosphorylation, ubiquitination, and sumoylation of the amino N-terminal tails of histones, alter chromatin compaction to create more open states (euchromatin, transcriptionally active) versus closed states (heterochromatin, transcriptionally inactive; Berger, 2007; Cheung, Allis, & Sassone-Corsi, 2000; Kouzarides, 2007). In reality, chromatin exists in many states between these two extremes.

4. HISTONE MODIFICATIONS

Each histone protein is composed of a central globular domain and an N-terminal tail that contains multiple sites for posttranslational, covalent modifications including acetylation, ubiquitination, or sumoylation at lysine residues, methylation at lysine or arginine residues, phosphorylation at serine or threonine residues, and ADP ribosylation at glutamate or arginine residues (Jenuwein & Allis, 2001; Okazaki & Moss, 1999).

Acetylation generally promotes decondensation of chromatin and increases gene activity by negating the positive charge of lysine residues in histone tails and by increasing spacing between nucleosomes. In contrast, histone methylation can either promote or repress gene activity depending on the residue undergoing methylation. Histone phosphorylation is also associated with chromatin inhibition or activation. The roles of histone ubiquitylation, sumoylation, and ADP ribosylation are less well understood (Nestler, 2013).

Most histone posttranslational modifications are dynamic (Allis et al., 2007; Berger, 2007; Kouzarides, 2007) and are regulated by a large number of histone-modifying enzymes, such as acetyltransferases, deacetylases, methyltransferases, demethylases, kinases, etc. (Gibney & Nolan, 2010). For example, the enzymes that regulate histone acetylation levels are histone acetyltransferases. The primary function of histone acetyltransferases is to neutralize the charges on histones to relax chromatin structure, enabling greater access of transcription factors to the DNA and thereby increasing transcription (Barrett & Wood, 2008; Norton, Imai, Yau, & Bradbury, 1989). In contrast, histone deacetylases (HDACs) deacetylate histone tails and histone deacetylation has been linked to transcriptional repression (Jenuwein & Allis, 2001; Kuo & Allis, 1998; Narlikar, Fan, & Kingston, 2002). The HDAC family comprises a number of proteins that have a catalytic deacetylase domain, and they are divided into four classes. Class I HDACs (HDAC 1, 2, 3, and 8) are expressed ubiquitously and likely mediate the majority of deacetylase activity within cells. Class II HDACs (HDAC 4–7 and 9–10) are larger proteins containing deacetylase domains and N-terminal regulatory domains that enable them to be shuttled in and out of the nucleus in a neural activity-dependent manner, and they are enriched in specific tissues, such as the brain and heart (Chawla, Vanhoutte, Arnold, Huang, & Bading, 2003; Renthal & Nestler, 2008). Class III HDACs are homologs of Sir2 and sirtuins, and HDAC11 is a class IV HDAC that shares homology with class I and II enzymes. Therefore, balance between the opposing activities of histone acetyltransferases and HDACs determines gene expression levels.

Another group of important enzymes are the histone methyltransferases (such as G9a, SET, MLL, SUV39, etc.), which methylate at lysine or arginine residues, and the histone demethylases that remove these modifications (Hake, Xiao, & Allis, 2004; Shi et al., 2004; Tachibana, Sugimoto, Fukushima, & Shinkai, 2001). Lysine side chains may be mono-, di-, or trimethylated whereas arginine side chains may be mono- or dimethylated.

There are 24 known methylation sites on histones—17 are lysine and 7 are arginine residues (Bannister & Kouzarides, 2005). Trimethylation of histone H3 lysines 4 (H3K4me3) and 36 (H3K36me3) has been observed to be highly associated with transcriptional initiation and often correlates with increased levels of transcriptional activity, whereas di- and trimethylation of histone H3 lysines 9 (H3K9me2/3) and 27 (H3K27me2/3) is associated with transcriptional repression (Maze & Nestler, 2011; Rice & Allis, 2001).

Histone phosphorylation has been shown to be involved in a variety of cellular processes including transcriptional regulation, apoptosis, cell cycle progression, DNA repair, and chromosome condensation (Banerjee & Chakravarti, 2011). The most described histone phosphorylation site is serine 10 on histone H3 (H3S10). This modification has been observed to stabilize a histone acetyltransferase (Gcn5) on gene promoters and to antagonize the methylation of lysine 9 on histone H3 (H3K9) and the recruitment of heterochromatin protein 1 (Kouzarides, 2007; Renthal & Nestler, 2008). Phosphorylation of serine or threonine residues on histone tails may be accomplished by nuclear kinases, such has mitogen- and stress-activated protein kinase (MSK-1), with protein phosphatases (such as protein phosphatase 1, PP1) dephosphorylating the residues (Brami-Cherrier, Roze, Girault, Betuing, & Caboche, 2009; Day & Sweatt, 2011). The exact mechanism by which phosphorylation contributes to transcriptional activation is not well understood; however, it has been hypothesized that the addition of negatively charged phosphate groups to histone tails neutralizes the basic charge of histone tails and reduces their affinity for DNA (Grant, 2001).

The functional consequences of histone modifications are mediated in part via proteins that bind to specific modified residues and affect transcriptional change (Jaenisch & Bird, 2003; Jenuwein & Allis, 2001). For example, different families of chromatin remodeling proteins, which use ATP-derived energy to alter nucleosome spacing and condensation, recognize specific forms of modified histones and enhance or repress the activity of nearby genes.

4.1 Histone Code

Histone modifications are capable of being both gene-specific within the genome and site-specific within a given chromatin particle, meaning that they are in an ideal position to selectively influence gene expression. Whereas the gene-specific modifications change the transcription of a specific gene, the site-specific modifications are known to directly alter chromatin state and transcription via a number of mechanisms. For example, histone acetylation, phosphorylation, and ubiquitination are generally associated with transcriptional activation, whereas histone methylation and other modifications (sumoylation, deimination, and proline isomerization) are more closely correlated with transcriptional repression. Given that histone proteins may be modified at a number of sites, it is possible that specific modifications could work together as a "code" with some codes inducing transcription of a specific gene whereas others repress transcription. This "histone code" hypothesis suggests that the sum of modifications at a particular gene defines epigenetically whether the gene is activated or silenced (Jenuwein & Allis, 2001).

5. DNA METHYLATION AND DEMETHYLATION

DNA methylation is the second-most important epigenetic modification. Methylation of one of the four DNA bases, cytosine, is a stable epigenetic modification that regulates the transcriptional plasticity of mammalian genomes. During DNA methylation, a methyl group is added to the 5′ position on the cytosine pyrimidine ring (5-mC); this occurs primarily where a cytosine (C) is adjacent to a guanine (G) in the DNA sequence (C-phosphate link-G, or cytosine–guanine dinucleotides, CpG) (Holliday & Pugh, 1975; Klose & Bird, 2006). The CpG sequences are not evenly dispersed throughout the genome but are instead clustered in "CpG" islands—short lengths of 0.5–4 kb with rich (60–70%) cytosine–guanine content. Compared with the rest of the genome where the CpG content is ≤20% (Bird, 2002). Approximately 50% of CpG islands are located in promoter regions and around transcription start sites and are unmethylated in normal cells. Normal DNA methylation plays a pivotal role in cell differentiation, genetic imprinting, and X-chromosome inactivation (Chahrour & Zoghbi, 2007; Suzuki & Bird, 2008).

DNA methylation is generally considered to suppress gene transcription. It can either prevent the association of DNA-binding factors to their target sequence or recruit corepressor complexes (e.g., HDACs and histone methyltransferases) that can modify nucleosome structure (Robison & Nestler, 2011). These complexes involve several DNA methyl-CpG-binding domain proteins (MBD; in mammals, they are MeCP2, MBD1–4) (Chahrour & Zoghbi, 2007; Kim, Samaranayake, & Pradhan, 2009; Robertson & Wolffe, 2000). Compared with histone tail modifications, most of which are considered readily reversible, DNA methylation is viewed as a more stable epigenetic change.

DNA methylation is catalyzed by a family of enzymes called DNA methyltransferases (DNMTs). In mammalian genomes, DNMTs are the only enzymes that have been shown to mediate the transfer of a methyl group from *S*-adenosylmethionine (SAM or AdoMet) to cytosine (Goll & Bestor, 2005). There are two main enzyme groups: the DNMT1 and DNMT3 families. DNMT1, the first-identified eukaryotic DNMT, is essential for maintaining DNA methylation patterns in proliferating cells and is involved in establishing new DNA methylation patterns (*de novo* methylation) (Bestor, 2000; Goll & Bestor, 2005; Siedlecki & Zielenkiewicz, 2006). The DNMT3 family includes two active *de novo* DNMTs, DNMT3A and DNMT3B, which are necessary for establishing new DNA methylation patterns (Okano, Bell, Haber, & Li, 1999). In the postnatal brain, DNMT3A is the primary DNMT expressed (Moore, Le, & Fan, 2013).

In contrast to DNA methylation, the enzymatic basis of demethylation is still largely an unresolved area of research (Kapoor, Agius, & Zhu, 2005; Wu et al., 2010). Accumulating evidence indicates that DNA demethylation occurs via a series of chemical reactions that modify 5-mC at two sites, the amino group and the methyl group. One model for DNA demethylation involves the conversion of 5-mC to thymine via deamination or the loss of the amine group following conventional base and nucleotide excision repair processes, thus resynthesizing a nonmethylated cytosine (Day & Sweatt, 2010; Ma, Guo, Ming, & Song, 2009). It is assumed that a growth arrest and DNA damage-inducible protein 45 (GADD45) participates in each step of this process and thereby catalyses DNA demethylation (Ma, Jang, et al., 2009). Furthermore, it appears that DNMTs may also participate in the deamination of methylated cytosine in a strand-specific manner (Métivier et al., 2008); thus, they play a role in both DNA methylation and demethylation.

Another active DNA demethylation mechanism is mediated by the ten-eleven translocation (TET) enzymes TET1–3, which add a hydroxyl group onto the 5-mC to form 5-hydroxymethylcytosine (5-hmC) (Ito et al., 2010; Kriaucionis & Heintz, 2009; Tahiliani et al., 2009). In mammals, once 5-hmC is formed, two separate mechanisms then convert 5-hmC back to cytosine. First, iterative oxidation by TET enzymes continues to oxidize 5-hmC to 5-formylcytosine and then to 5-carboxycytosine (Ito et al., 2011). Second, 5-hmC is deaminated by AID/APOBEC (activation-induced cytidine deaminase/apolipoprotein B mRNA editing enzyme complex) to form 5-hydroxymethyluracil (5-hmU) (Guo, Su, Zhong, Ming, & Song, 2011; Moore et al., 2013). Interestingly, the highest expression of 5-hmC oxidation derivatives is found in neurons. In contrast to the repressive effect of 5-mC on gene expression, 5-hmC is associated more with transactivation (Szulwach et al., 2011). These data indicate that 5-hmC is also an important epigenetic marker that may play a role in active DNA demethylation processes.

6. NONCODING RNA

Another level of epigenetic regulation via small noncoding RNAs (termed microRNAs) has also been discovered (Bergmann & Lane, 2003). MicroRNAs, which are generally 22 base pairs long, are posttranslational regulators that bind to complementary sequences on target mRNAs and regulate gene expression at different levels, e.g., silencing of chromatin (affecting histone modifications), degradation of mRNA, and translation blockade (Dunham et al., 2012; Li & van der Vaart, 2011; Rinn & Chang, 2012; Szyf, McGowan, & Meaney, 2008; Taft, Pang, Mercer, Dinger, & Mattick, 2010). Recently, long noncoding RNAs (lncRNAs), defined as being >200 base pairs in length, have emerged as key regulators of gene transcription. They modulate chromatin-modifying complexes by interacting directly with transcription factors and other nuclear proteins (Nestler, 2013). Thus, like histone modifications and DNA methylation, microRNAs are also important players in the epigenetic control of gene expression.

7. EPIGENETIC MECHANISMS IN PSYCHOSTIMULANT-INDUCED ADDICTION

Addiction is a chronic condition; thus, even after extended periods of abstinence, addicted individuals have a high rate of relapse (Koob & LeMoal, 2005). Drugs of abuse are known to affect neuronal morphology and function in specific brain regions (ventral tegmental area, nucleus accumbens, dorsal striatum, amygdala, hippocampus, prefrontal cortex) resulting in stable and persistent changes from the cellular to behavioral level (Hyman et al., 2006; Nestler, 2001). Therefore, drug addiction can be viewed as maladaptive neural plasticity in response to repeated exposures to a drug of abuse. These features of addiction suggest that epigenetic mechanisms of chromatin regulation may be involved in initiating and establishing these stable changes at the cellular level, which then manifest as long-term behavioral changes.

There are two general roles that epigenetic mechanisms likely play in addiction. (1) Repeated exposures to a drug of abuse (including psychostimulants) in adolescence or adulthood causes addiction in vulnerable individuals by inducing stable changes in gene expression via epigenetic regulation of those specific genes (Nestler, 2013). This epigenetic regulation involves alterations in the steady-state expression levels of one set of genes and also sensitization (priming) or desensitization of other genes without changing their steady-state expression levels. (2) Epigenetic regulation mediates changes in the steady-state gene expression or the induction of genes throughout an individual's lifetime in response to a host of environmental agents, which helps determine that individual's vulnerability to drug exposure and addiction later in life (Hiroi & Agatsuma, 2005; Nestler, 2013).

7.1 Role of Histone Modifications in Psychostimulant-Induced Addiction

7.1.1 Histone Acetylation

Psychostimulants induce changes in histone modifications in the brain, and evidence has begun to accumulate that these modifications underlie some of the functional abnormalities noted in psychostimulant-induced models of addiction (e.g., Kalda, Heidmets, Shen, Zharkovsky, & Chen, 2007; Kumar et al., 2005; Robison & Nestler, 2011). For example, global levels of histone H3 and H4 acetylation (as detected by Western blotting or immunocytochemistry) are increased in the rodent nucleus accumbens (NAc) after acute or chronic exposure to cocaine or other stimulants (Kalda et al., 2007; Kumar et al., 2005; Schroeder et al., 2008; Shen et al., 2008). However, little is known of the intracellular signaling pathways that lead to stimulant-induced global changes in histone acetylation or the histone acetyltransferases and HDACs that modify the various lysine residues that display regulation. Some reports have indicated that CREB-binding protein (a major histone acetyltransferase in brain) and Class II HDACs are implicated (Levine et al., 2005; Malvaez, Mhillaj, Matheos, Palmery, & Wood, 2011; Renthal et al., 2007).

Further experiments have demonstrated that modifications of histone acetyltransferase and HDAC activity in the NAc are important regulators of the rewarding properties of cocaine (Kalda et al., 2007; Kim, Kim, & Kim, 2008; Kumar et al., 2005; Levine et al., 2005, 2011; Malvaez et al.,

2013; Renthal et al., 2007; Romieu et al., 2008; Schroeder et al., 2008; Sun et al., 2008; Wang et al., 2010). For example, it has been demonstrated that mutant mice with decreased expression of CREB-binding protein exhibit reduced sensitivity to chronic cocaine exposure (Levine et al., 2005; Malvaez et al., 2011). Homozygous HDAC5 knockout mice show hypersensitivity (Renthal et al., 2007), and overexpression of HDAC4 or 5 in the NAc attenuates the response to cocaine (Kumar et al., 2005; Renthal et al., 2007; Wang et al., 2010). In contrast, mice with NAc-selective HDAC1 deletions display attenuated behavioral responses to cocaine (Kennedy et al., 2013), and NAc-specific deletion of HDAC3 facilitates the extinction of cocaine-induced place conditioning (Malvaez et al., 2013). Chronic cocaine treatment also induces NAc expression of the two sirtuins SIRT1 and SIRT2, which are Class III HDACs that also deacetylate numerous nonhistone proteins (Renthal et al., 2009). This induction of SIRT (based on experiments that overexpress SIRT in NAc) promotes behavioral responses to cocaine including cocaine self-administration (Renthal et al., 2009). Currently, the protein targets of SIRTs that mediate these behavioral effects are unknown. Based on NAc-specific deletion of HDACs or the actions of systemic or intra-NAc administration of HDAC inhibitors, these accumulating reports suggest that short-term increases in histone acetylation generally promote behavioral responses to psychostimulants, whereas sustained increases instead oppose the effects of stimulants.

At the gene level, it has been demonstrated that acute cocaine treatment is associated with histone H4 hyperacetylation at the promoters of immediate early genes, such as *c-fos* and *fosB*, whereas repeated cocaine treatment is associated with histone H3 hyperacetylation at the promoters of *Cdk5* (cyclin-dependent kinase-5) and *Bdnf* (brain-derived neurotrophic factor) and that these hyperacetylations correlate with changes in their expression (Kumar et al., 2005; Renthal et al., 2008). Induction of CaMKIIa (Ca^{2+}/calmodulin-dependent protein kinase IIa) in the NAc by cocaine is also associated with histone H3 acetylation of the *CaMKIIa* gene (Robison et al., 2013; Wang et al., 2010). Although the majority of studies have focused on the NAc, some others have studied other brain reward regions, e.g., the initial reports of cocaine-induced changes in acetylation of specific genes (Sadri-Vakili et al., 2010; Schmidt et al., 2012).

A genome-wide study using the ChIP-chip method (chromatin immunoprecipitation with antibodies against pan-acetylated histone H3 or H4 followed by promoter microarrays) has provided a more complete map of genes in the NAc that show changes in histone acetylation following chronic cocaine exposure (Renthal et al., 2009). Numerous gene promoters were found to be hyper- or hypoacetylated, with a minimal overlap between genes showing histone H3 versus H4 modifications. However, the majority of genes did not follow this pattern. These data suggest that alterations in histone acetylation are very complex and that these changes contribute to only a fraction of all epigenetic control of the activity of a particular gene.

7.1.2 Histone Methylation

There is evidence that histone methylation is also directly regulated by psychostimulants. A genome-wide study by Renthal et al. (2009) revealed that cocaine-induced alterations in the binding of histone H3 lysine 9 dimethylation (H3K9me2) on numerous gene promoter regions in the NAc. This finding is supported by the report of Maze et al. (2010) who demonstrated that global levels of H3K9me2 are decreased in the mouse NAc following chronic cocaine exposure, which was mediated by the repression of histone methyl transferase G9a. Cocaine-induced downregulation of G9a also increased dentritic arborization of NAc neurons suggesting that G9a affects addiction-associated synaptic plasticity. Further studies have highlighted the possible interaction between histone H3 methylation and transcription factor activity, for exampe, acute cocaine exposure enhanced G9a binding to the *fosB* promoter region and therefore rapidly suppressed cocaine-induced increases in expression of the long-lasting transcription factor ΔFosB (Robison & Nestler, 2011). Following repeated exposure to cocaine, ΔFosB accumulation in the NAc results in G9a repression and a decrease in global levels of H3K9me2, thereby preventing the ability of G9a to maintain normal levels of gene expression and leading to enhanced behavioral responses to the drug (Maze et al., 2010). Consequently, G9a appears to be a critical control point for epigenetic regulation in the NAc, and genetic or pharmacological blockade of G9a in the NAc potentiates behavioral responses to cocaine, whereas increasing G9a function exerts the opposite effect.

Interestingly, Damez-Werno et al. (2012) demonstrated that reduced H3K9me2 binding at the *fosB* gene may be associated with priming—enhanced induction of the *fosB* gene in response to a cocaine challenge in sensitized rats. This priming is not associated with changes in the upstream signaling pathways that control *fosB* expression but is related to reduced H3K9me2 binding at the *fosB* gene and an enrichment of the phosphorylated form of RNA polymerase II. Therefore, *fosB* priming represents an important example of latent regulation that is mediated via chromatin mechanisms.

Recently, cross talk has been demonstrated between the regulation of histone acetylation and methylation in the NAc. Kennedy et al. (2013) demonstrated that G9a is induced in the NAc upon prolonged HDAC inhibition. This report demonstrated that the combination of cocaine and HDAC inhibition resulted in excessive hyperacetylation, which causes (via a negative feedback mechanism) the induction of G9a to counteract the transcriptional-activating effects of increased acetylation.

A major limitation in the field is the difficulty in relating chromatin modifications at a given gene to a functional outcome (Nestler, 2013). Studies to date have relied on overexpressing, knocking out, or pharmacologically inhibiting a chromatin-modifying enzyme (e.g., a HDAC or DNMT) within a given brain region, such as the NAc, and studying the behavioral consequences. However, these manipulations affect hundreds or thousands of genes. A recent report, using a synthetic zinc finger protein and a sequence-specific transcription activator-like effector, which selectively modify chromatin at specific genes *in vivo*, demonstrated that H3K9me2 truly regulates *fosB* transcription in the mouse NAc *in vivo* and consequently blunts the behavioral effects of cocaine (Heller et al., 2014). This approach enabled epigenetic modifications at a given gene to be directly correlated with the regulation of its expression and subsequent effects on reward behavior.

7.1.3 Histone Phosphorylation

Histone phosphorylation is an important component of the epigenetic response to psychostimulants. Brami-Cherrier et al. (2009) reported that cocaine induces the robust phosphorylation of histone H3 within the NAc at the *c-fos* and *c-Jun* promoters, and histone H3 phosphorylation is positively regulated by the MAPK/extracellular-signal-regulated kinase (ERK) cascade including ERK phosphorylation and MSK-1-induced phosphorylation of histone H3 (Bertran-Gonzalez et al., 2008; Brami-Cherrier et al., 2009). Nuclear accumulation of 32 kDa dopamine and cAMP-regulated phosphoprotein (DARPP-32) inhibits protein phosphatase 1 thereby preventing histone dephosphorylation (Stipanovich et al., 2008). These pathways control behavioral responses to cocaine by inhibiting dopamine D1 receptors, ERK, DARPP-32, and MSK-1, all of which diminish drug-induced locomotor responses and conditioned place preference (Brami-Cherrier et al., 2009; Stipanovich et al., 2008).

7.2 Role of DNA Methylation in Psychostimulant-Induced Addiction

Although the majority of studies have focused on histone modifications, DNA methylation is also a critical component of the epigenetic response to psychostimulant-related behaviors. An increasing number of reports have provided crucial evidence of the role of DNA methylation in cocaine-induced neuronal plasticity in the NAc (Anier, Malinovskaja, Aonurm-Helm, Zharkovsky, & Kalda, 2010; Barros et al., 2013; Han et al., 2010; LaPlant et al., 2010). Several studies have demonstrated that expression levels of DNMT3A in the NAc are differentially altered by acute versus chronic cocaine exposure and during extended withdrawal, suggesting that psychostimulants are capable of dynamic control of DNA methylation (Anier et al., 2010; LaPlant et al., 2010). Local knockout of DNMT3A in the NAc or local infusion of the DNMT inhibitor RG108 potentiated cocaine reward, whereas NAc-specific DNMT3A upregulation attenuated cocaine reward and also increased dendritic arborizations of NAc neurons (LaPlant et al., 2010).

There is a growing acceptance that the overall epigenetic status of a cell can be modulated by a variety of environmental factors including nutrients, chemicals, and the early-life environment (Roth, Lubin, Funk, & Sweatt, 2009; Waterland, 2006; Weaver et al., 2005). Some early studies suggested that different environmental factors may also affect DNA methylation in the brain. For example, repeated SAM (donor of methyl groups) pre-treatment significantly potentiated cocaine-induced locomotor sensitization, and the modulating effect of SAM are due in part to decreased methyltransferase activity via the downregulation of DNMT3A (Anier, Zharkovsky, & Kalda, 2013). This study supports the hypothesis that environmental factors that affect the epigenetic status of NAc cells may alter the development of psychostimulant-induced addiction. Moreover, these results may explain, at least in part, why some individuals are more vulnerable to drug addiction.

In addition to DNMT activity, the nuclear proteins capable of binding specifically to methylated DNA (such as methyl-CpG-binding protein-2 or MeCP2) play a role in the epigenetic response. For example, NAc-specific knockout of MeCP2 enhances amphetamine reward (Deng et al., 2010). However, Im, Hollander, Bali, and Kenny (2010) demonstrated that chronic cocaine increased MeCP2 expression in the dorsal striatum, whereas local knockdown of the protein attenuated cocaine self-administration.

A small number of studies have investigated DNA methylation changes at particular genes of interest (Anier et al., 2010; Anier et al., 2013; Nielsen et al., 2009; Ponomarev et al., 2012); however, no genome-wide map of this regulation has been conducted. Recent reports indicate that epigenetic changes in brain regions outside the NAc are also important regulators of drug memories. It has been observed that DNA methylation within the hippocampus and prelimbic cortex is necessary for the establishment and maintenance of cocaine-induced conditioned place preference (Day & Sweatt, 2010; Han et al., 2010).

An initial report showed that chronic cocaine administration decreased DNA demethylase TET1 expression in the NAc thereby potentiating behavioral responses to cocaine (Nestler, 2013). Using genome-wide mapping of 5-hmc in the NAc after cocaine exposure, this study also demonstrated that changes in 5-hmc generally correlated with increased gene expression. These findings further underscore the importance of obtaining genome-wide maps of several forms of DNA methylation in models of drug abuse.

7.3 Role of Noncoding RNAs in Addiction

Several studies have demonstrated that microRNAs are important in addiction-related behaviors. For example, overexpression of miR-124 and let-7d in the NAc of rats reduced cocaine-induced place conditioning, whereas overexpression of miR-181 resulted in the opposite effect (Chandrasekar & Dreyer, 2009, 2011; Sartor, St Laurent, & Wahlestedt, 2012; Schaefer et al., 2010). These data indicate that microRNAs may play an essential role in drug tolerance and escalation of intake. Hollander et al. (2010) noted that cocaine self-administration upregulated microRNA miR-212 expression in the rat striatum and this associated with decreased cocaine reward. These data suggest that the actions of miR-212 depend upon upregulation of CREB, which is known to decrease the rewarding effects of cocaine (Robison & Nestler, 2011). Im et al. (2010) demonstrated that MeCP2 may interact homeostatically with miR-212 to control BDNF expression and cocaine intake. Therefore, it has been suggested that the CREB–miR-212–MeCP2–BDNF pathway is partly responsible for cocaine tolerance and escalation of intake (Im et al., 2010; Robison & Nestler, 2011). Further work is required to identify the definitive mRNA targets of each regulated microRNA and to explore remaining unannotated, novel microRNAs altered by psychostimulants.

8. CONCLUSIONS

In this review, we have introduced the importance of epigenetic processes in regulating gene expression and have described the role that dynamic epigenetic changes may play in psychostimulant-induced addiction via long-lasting transcriptional changes following repeated drug exposure. Epigenetic studies are also important for understanding how an individual's life experiences—exposure to environmental factors—establish stable changes at genomic loci, which then help determine that individual's vulnerability to the addiction-causing effects of subsequent drug exposure.

Because epigenetic mechanisms are dynamic and reversible, chemical agents that alter the modification of histones or the methylation of DNA may prove potent candidates as therapeutic interventions. Moreover, the identification of specific epigenetic patterns associated with specific disease phenotypes may be useful biomarkers for early disease diagnosis and preventative interventions. Future studies should clarify whether drug effects on epigenetic endpoints in peripheral tissues (e.g., blood) may serve as useful biomarkers for clinical features of addiction.

Accumulating reports on drugs of abuse not only demonstrate the imperative role of epigenetic modifications in regulating behavioral responses to drug exposure but also shed light on the complex mechanisms of drug addiction. However, it is worth noting that only a small number of epigenetic studies on addiction have been performed in humans. Further studies must evaluate the possible role of epigenetic mechanism in addicted individuals.

REFERENCES

Allis, C. D., Berger, S. L., Cote, J., Dent, S., Jenuwien, T., Kouzarides, T., et al. (2007). New nomenclature for chromatin-modifying enzymes. *Cell, 131*, 633–636.

Anier, K., Malinovskaja, K., Aonurm-Helm, A., Zharkovsky, A., & Kalda, A. (2010). DNA methylation regulates cocaine-induced behavioral sensitization in mice. *Neuropsychopharmacology, 35*, 2450–2461.

Anier, K., Zharkovsky, A., & Kalda, A. (2013). S-adenosylmethionine modifies cocaine-induced DNA methylation and increases locomotor sensitization in mice. *International Journal of Neuropsychopharmacology, 16*, 2053–2066.

Banerjee, T., & Chakravarti, D. (2011). A peek into the complex realm of histone phosphorylation. *Molecular Cell. Biology, 31*, 4858–4873.

Bannister, A. J., & Kouzarides, T. (2005). Reversing histone methylation. *Nature, 436*, 1103–1106.

Barrett, R. M., & Wood, M. A. (2008). Beyond transcription factors: the role of chromatin modifying enzymes in regulating transcription required for memory. *Learning & Memory, 15*, 460–467.

Barros, M., Dempster, E. L., Illott, N., Chabrawi, S., Maior, R. S., Tomaz, C., et al. (2013). Decreased methylation of the NK3 receptor coding gene (TACR3) after cocaine-induced place preference in marmoset monkeys. *Addiction Biology*, *18*, 452–454.
Berger, S. L. (2007). The complex language of chromatin regulation during transcription. *Nature*, *447*, 407–412.
Bergmann, A., & Lane, M. E. (2003). Hidden targets of microRNAs for growth control. *Trends in Biochemical Sciences*, *28*, 461–463.
Bertran-Gonzalez, J., Bosch, C., Maroteaux, M., Matamales, M., Hervé, D., Valjent, E., et al. (2008). Opposing patterns of signaling activation in dopamine D1 and D2 receptor-expressing striatal neurons in response to cocaine and haloperidol. *Journal of Neuroscience*, *28*, 5671–5685.
Bestor, T. H. (2000). The DNA methyltransferases of mammals. *Human Molecular Genetics*, *9*, 2395–2402.
Bird, A. (2002). DNA methylation patterns and epigenetic memory. *Genes and Development*, *16*, 6–21.
Brami-Cherrier, K., Roze, E., Girault, J. A., Betuing, S., & Caboche, J. (2009). Role of the ERK/MSK1 signalling pathway in chromatin remodelling and brain responses to drugs of abuse. *Journal of Neurochemistry*, *108*, 1323–1335.
Chahrour, M., & Zoghbi, H. Y. (2007). The story of Rett syndrome: From clinic to neurobiology. *Neuron*, *56*, 422–437.
Chandrasekar, V., & Dreyer, J. L. (2009). MicroRNAs miR-124, let-7d and miR-181a regulate cocaine-induced plasticity. *Molecular and Cellular Neuroscience*, *42*, 350–362.
Chandrasekar, V., & Dreyer, J. L. (2011). Regulation of MiR-124, Let-7d, and MiR-181a in the accumbens affects the expression, extinction, and reinstatement of cocaineinduced conditioned place preference. *Neuropsychopharmacology*, *36*, 1149–1164.
Chawla, S., Vanhoutte, P., Arnold, F. J., Huang, C. L., & Bading, H. (2003). Neuronal activity-dependent nucleocytoplasmic shuttling of HDAC4 and HDAC5. *Journal of Neurochemistry*, *85*, 151–159.
Cheung, P., Allis, C. D., & Sassone-Corsi, P. (2000). Signaling to chromatin through histone modifications. *Cell*, *103*, 263–271.
Damez-Werno, D., LaPlant, Q., Dietz, D. M., Sun, S. H., Scobie, K. N., Walker, I., et al. (2012). Drug experience epigenetically primes fosB gene inducibility in rat nucleus accumbens and caudate putamen. *Journal of Neuroscience*, *32*, 10267–10272.
Day, J. J., & Sweatt, J. D. (2010). DNA methylation and memory formation. *Nature Neuroscience*, *13*, 1319–1323.
Day, J. J., & Sweatt, J. D. (2011). Epigenetic mechanisms in cognition. *Neuron*, *70*, 813–829.
Deng, J. V., Rodriguiz, R. M., Hutchinson, A. N., Kim, I. H., Wetsel, W. C., & West, A. E. (2010). MeCP2 in the nucleus accumbens contributes to neural and behavioral responses to psychostimulants. *Nature Neuroscience*, *13*, 1128–1136.
Dunham, I., Kundaje, A., Aldred, S. F., Collins, P. J., Davis, C. A., Doyle, F., et al. (2012). An integrated encyclopedia of DNA elements in the human genome. *Nature*, *489*, 57–74.
Felsenfeld, G., & Groudine, M. (2003). Controlling the double helix. *Nature*, *421*, 448–453.
Gibney, E. R., & Nolan, C. M. (2010). Epigenetics and gene expression. *Heredity*, *105*, 4–13.
Goldman, D., Oroszi, G., & Ducci, F. (2005). The genetics of addictions: Uncovering the genes. *Nature Reviews Genetics*, *6*, 521–532.
Goll, M. G., & Bestor, T. H. (2005). Eukaryotic cytosine methyltransferases. *Annual Review of Biochemistry*, *74*, 481–514.
Grant, P. A. (2001). A tale of histone modifications. *Genome Biology*, *2*, 1–6.
Grunstein, M. (1997). Histone acetylation in chromatin structure and transcription. *Nature*, *389*, 349–352.

Guo, J. U., Su, Y., Zhong, C., Ming, G. L., & Song, H. (2011). Hydroxylation of 5-methylcytosine by TET1 promotes active DNA demethylation in the adult brain. *Cell*, *145*, 423–434.

Haig, D. (2004). The (dual) origin of epigenetics. *Cold Spring Harbor Symposia on Quantitative Biology*, *69*, 67–70.

Hake, S. B., Xiao, A., & Allis, C. D. (2004). Linking the epigenetic 'language' of covalent histone modifications to cancer. *British Journal of Cancer*, *90*, 761–769.

Han, J., Li, Y., Wang, D., Wei, C., Yang, X., & Sui, N. (2010). Effect of 5-aza-2-deoxycytidine microinjecting into hippocampus and prelimbic cortex on acquisition and retrieval of cocaine-induced place preference in C57BL/6 mice. *European Journal of Pharmacology*, *642*, 93–98.

Heller, E. A., Cates, H. M., Peña, C. J., Sun, H., Shao, N., Feng, J., et al. (2014). Locus-specific epigenetic remodeling controls addiction- and depression-related behaviors. *Nature Neuroscience*, *17*, 1720–1727.

Hiroi, N., & Agatsuma, S. (2005). Genetic susceptibility to substance dependence. *Molecular Psychiatry*, *10*, 336–344.

Hollander, J. A., Im, H. I., Amelio, A. L., Kocerha, J., Bali, P., Lu, Q., et al. (2010). Striatal microRNA controls cocaine intake through CREB signalling. *Nature*, *466*, 197–202.

Holliday, R., & Pugh, J. E. (1975). DNA modification mechanisms and gene activity during development. *Science*, *187*, 226–232.

Hyman, S. E., Malenka, R. C., & Nestler, E. J. (2006). Neural mechanisms of addiction: The role of reward-related learning and memory. *Annual Review of Neuroscience*, *29*, 565–598.

Im, H. I., Hollander, J. A., Bali, P., & Kenny, P. J. (2010). MeCP2 controls BDNF expression and cocaine intake through homeostatic interactions with microRNA-212. *Nature Neuroscience*, *13*, 1120–1127.

Ito, S., D'Alessio, A. C., Taranova, O. V., Hong, K., Sowers, L. C., & Zhang, Y. (2010). Role of Tet proteins in 5mC to 5hmC conversion, ES-cell self-renewal and inner cell mass specification. *Nature*, *466*, 1129–1133.

Ito, S., Shen, L., Dai, Q., Wu, S. C., Collins, L. B., Swenberg, J. A., et al. (2011). Tet proteins can convert 5-methylcytosine to 5-formylcytosine and 5-carboxylcytosine. *Science*, *333*, 1300–1303.

Jaenisch, R., & Bird, A. (2003). Epigenetic regulation of gene expression: How the genome integrates intrinsic and environmental signals. *Nature Genetics*, *33*(Suppl.), 245–254.

Jenuwein, T., & Allis, C. D. (2001). Translating the histone code. *Science*, *293*, 1074–1080.

Kalda, A., Heidmets, L. T., Shen, H. Y., Zharkovsky, A., & Chen, J.-F. (2007). Histone deacetylase inhibitors modulates the induction and expression of amphetamine-induced behavioral sensitization partially through an associated learning of the environment in mice. *Behavioural Brain Research*, *181*, 76–84.

Kapoor, A., Agius, F., & Zhu, J. K. (2005). Preventing transcriptional gene silencing by active DNA demethylation. *FEBS Letters*, *579*, 5889–5898.

Kennedy, P. J., Robison, A. J., Maze, I., Feng, J., Badimon, A., Bassel-Duby, R., et al. (2013). HDAC1 inhibition blocks cocaine-induced plasticity through targeted changes in histone methylation. *Nature Neuroscience*, *16*, 434–440.

Kim, W. Y., Kim, S., & Kim, J. H. (2008). Chronic microinjection of valproic acid into the nucleus accumbens attenuates amphetamine-induced locomotor activity. *Neuroscience Letters*, *432*, 54–57.

Kim, J. K., Samaranayake, M., & Pradhan, S. (2009). Epigenetic mechanisms in mammals. *Cellular and Molecular Life Sciences*, *66*, 596–612.

Klose, R. J., & Bird, A. P. (2006). Genomic DNA methylation: The mark and its mediators. *Trends in Biochemical Sciences*, *31*, 89–97.

Koob, G. F., & LeMoal, M. (2005). Plasticity of reward neurocircuitry and the 'dark side' of drug addiction. *Nature Neuroscience*, *8*, 1442–1444.

Kouzarides, T. (2007). Chromatin modifications and their function. *Cell, 128*, 693–705.

Kriaucionis, S., & Heintz, N. (2009). The nuclear DNA base 5-hydroxymethylcytosine is present in Purkinje neurons and the brain. *Science, 324*, 929–930.

Kumar, A., Choi, K. H., Renthal, W., Tsankova, N. M., Theobald, D. E., Truong, H. T., et al. (2005). Chromatin remodeling is a key mechanism underlying cocaine-induced plasticity in striatum. *Neuron, 48*, 303–314.

Kuo, M. H., & Allis, C. D. (1998). Roles of histone acetyltransferases and deacetylases in gene regulation. *Bioessays, 20*, 615–626.

LaPlant, Q., Vialou, V., Covington, H. E., 3rd., Dumitriu, D., Feng, J., Warren, B. L., et al. (2010). Dnmt3a regulates emotional behavior and spine plasticity in the nucleus accumbens. *Nature Neuroscience, 13*, 1137–1143.

Levine, A. A., Guan, Z., Barco, A., Xu, S., Kandel, E. R., & Schwartz, J. H. (2005). CREBbinding protein controls response to cocaine by acetylating histones at the fosB promoter in the mouse striatum. *Proceedings of the National Academy of Sciences of the United States of America, 102*, 19186–19191.

Levine, A., Huang, Y., Drisaldi, B., Griffin, E. A., Jr., Pollak, D. D., Xu, S., et al. (2011). Molecular mechanism for a gateway drug: Epigenetic changes initiated by nicotine prime gene expression by cocaine. *Science Translational Medicine, 3*, 107–109.

Li, B., Carey, M., & Workman, J. L. (2007). The role of chromatin during transcription. *Cell, 128*, 707–719.

Li, M. D., & van der Vaart, A. D. (2011). MicroRNAs in addiction: Adaptation's middlemen? *Molecular Psychiatry, 16*, 1159–1168.

Ma, D. K., Guo, J. U., Ming, G. L., & Song, H. (2009). DNA excision repair proteins and Gadd45 as molecular players for active DNA demethylation. *Cell Cycle, 8*, 1526–1531.

Ma, D. K., Jang, M. H., Guo, J. U., Kitabatake, Y., Chang, M. L., Pow-Anpongkul, N., et al. (2009). Neuronal activity-induced Gadd45b promotes epigenetic DNA demethylation and adult neurogenesis. *Science, 323*, 1074–1077.

Malvaez, M., McQuown, S. C., Rogge, G. A., Astarabadi, M., Jacques, V., Carreiro, S., et al. (2013). HDAC3-selective inhibitor enhances extinction of cocaine-seeking behavior in a persistent manner. *Proceedings of the National Academy of Sciences of the United States of America, 110*, 2647–2652.

Malvaez, M., Mhillaj, E., Matheos, D. P., Palmery, M., & Wood, M. A. (2011). CBP in the nucleus accumbens regulates cocaine-induced histone acetylation and is critical for cocaine-associated behaviors. *Journal of Neuroscience, 31*, 16941–16948.

Maze, I., Covington, H. E., III, Dietz, D. M., LaPlant, Q., Renthal, W., Russo, S. J., et al. (2010). Essential role of the histone methyltransferase G9a in cocaine-induced plasticity. *Science, 327*, 213–216.

Maze, I., & Nestler, E. J. (2011). The epigenetic landscape of addiction. *Annals of the New York Academy of Sciences, 1216*, 99–113.

McQuown, S. C., & Wood, M. A. (2010). Epigenetic regulation in substance use disorders. *Current Psychiatry Reports, 12*, 145–153.

Métivier, R., Huet, G., Gallais, R., Finot, L., Petit, F., Tiffoche, C., et al. (2008). Dynamics of estrogen receptor-mediated transcriptional activation of responsive genes in vivo: Apprehending transcription in four dimensions. *Advances in Experimental Medicine and Biology, 617*, 129–138.

Moore, L. D., Le, T., & Fan, G. (2013). DNA methylation and its basic function. *Neuropsychopharmacology, 38*, 23–38.

Narlikar, G. J., Fan, H. Y., & Kingston, R. E. (2002). Cooperation between complexes that regulate chromatin structure and transcription. *Cell, 108*, 475–487.

Nestler, E. J. (2001). Molecular basis of long-term plasticity underlying addiction. *Nature Reviews Neuroscience, 2*, 119–128.

Nestler, E. J. (2013). Epigenetic mechanisms of drug addiction. *Neuropharmacology, 76*, 259–268.

Nielsen, D. A., Yuferov, V., Hamon, S., Jackson, C., Ho, A., Ott, J., et al. (2009). Increased OPRM1 DNA methylation in lymphocytes of methadone-maintained former heroin addicts. *Neuropsychopharmacology, 34*, 867–873.

Norton, V. G., Imai, B. S., Yau, P., & Bradbury, E. M. (1989). Histone acetylation reduces nucleosome core particle linking number change. *Cell, 57*, 449–457.

Okano, M., Bell, D. W., Haber, D. A., & Li, E. (1999). DNA methyltransferases Dnmt3a and Dnmt3b are essential for de novo methylation and mammalian development. *Cell, 99*, 247–257.

Okazaki, I. J., & Moss, J. (1999). Characterization of glycosylphosphatidylinositiol-anchored, secreted, and intracellular vertebrate mono-ADP-ribosyltransferases. *Annual Review of Nutrition, 19*, 485–509.

Renthal, W., Carle, T. L., Maze, I., Covington, H. E., III, Truong, H.-T., Alibhai, I., et al. (2008). DeltaFosB mediates epigenetic desensitization of the c-fos gene after chronic amphetamine exposure. *Journal of Neuroscience, 28*, 7344–7349.

Renthal, W., Kumar, A., Xiao, G. H., Wilkinson, M., Convington, H. E., III, Maze, I., et al. (2009). Genome wide analysis of chromatin regulation by cocaine reveals a novel role for sirtuins. *Neuron, 62*, 335–348.

Renthal, W., Maze, I., Krishnan, V., Covington, H. E., Xiao, G. H., Kumar, A., et al. (2007). Histone deacetylase 5 epigenetically controls behavioral adaptations to chronic emotional stimuli. *Neuron, 56*, 517–529.

Renthal, W., & Nestler, E. J. (2008). Epigenetic mechanisms in drug addiction. *Trends in Molecular Medicines, 14*, 341–350.

Rice, J. C., & Allis, C. D. (2001). Histone methylation versus histone acetylation: New insights into epigenetic regulation. *Current Opinion in Cell Biology, 13*, 263–273.

Rinn, J. L., & Chang, H. Y. (2012). Genome regulation by long noncoding RNAs. *Annual Review of Biochemistry, 81*, 145–166.

Robertson, K. D., & Wolffe, A. P. (2000). DNA methylation in health and disease. *Nature Reviews Genetics, 1*, 11–19.

Robison, A. J., & Nestler, E. J. (2011). Transcriptional and epigenetic mechanisms of addiction. *Nature Review Neuroscience, 12*, 623–637.

Robison, A. J., Vialou, V., Mazei-Robison, M., Feng, J., Kourrich, S., Collins, M., et al. (2013). Behavioral and structural responses to chronic cocaine require a feed-forward loop involving DeltaFosB and CaMKII in the nucleus accumbens shell. *Journal of Neuroscience, 33*, 4295–4307.

Romieu, P., Host, L., Gobaille, S., Sandner, G., Aunis, D., & Zwiller, J. (2008). Histone deacetylase inhibitors decrease cocaine but not sucrose self-administration in rats. *Journal of Neuroscience, 28*, 9342–9348.

Roth, T. L., Lubin, F. D., Funk, A. J., & Sweatt, J. D. (2009). Lasting epigenetic influence of early-life adversity on the BDNF gene. *Biological Psychiatry, 65*, 760–769.

Sadri-Vakili, G., Kumaresan, V., Schmidt, H. G., Famous, K. R., Chawla, P., Vassoler, F. M., et al. (2010). Cocaine-induced chromatin remodeling increases brain derived neurotrophic factor transcription in the rat medial prefrontal cortex, which alters the reinforcing efficacy of cocaine. *Journal of Neuroscience, 30*, 11735–11744.

Sartor, G. C., St Laurent, G., 3rd., & Wahlestedt, C. (2012). The emerging role of noncoding RNAs in drug addiction. *Frontiers in Genetics, 3*, 106.

Schaefer, A., Im, H. I., Veno, M. T., Fowler, C. D., Min, A., Intrator, A., et al. (2010). Argonaute 2 in dopamine 2 receptor-expressing neurons regulates cocaine addiction. *Journal of Experimental Medicine, 207*, 1843–1851.

Schmidt, H. D., Sangrey, G. R., Darnell, S. B., Schassburger, R. L., Cha, J. H., Pierce, R. C., et al. (2012). Increased brain-derived neurotrophic factor (BDNF) expression in the ventral tegmental area during cocaine abstinence is associated with increased histone acetylation at BDNF exon I-containing promoters. *Journal of Neurochemistry, 120*, 202–209.

Schroeder, F. A., Penta, K. L., Matevossian, A., Jones, S. R., Konradi, C., Tapper, A. R., et al. (2008). Drug-induced activation of dopamine D(1) receptor signaling and inhibition of class I/II histone deacetylase induce chromatin remodeling in reward circuitry and modulate cocaine-related behaviors. *Neuropsychopharmacology, 33*, 2981–2992.

Shen, H. Y., Kalda, A., Yu, L., Ferrara, J., Zhu, J., & Chen, J.-F. (2008). Additive effects of histone deacetylase inhibitors and amphetamine on histone H4 acetylation, cAMP responsive element binding protein phosphorylation and DeltaFosB expression in the striatum and locomotor sensitization in mice. *Neuroscience, 157*, 644–655.

Shi, Y., Lan, F., Matson, C., Mulligan, P., Whetstine, J. R., Cole, P. A., et al. (2004). Histone demethylation mediated by the nuclear amine oxidase homolog LSD1. *Cell, 119*, 941–953.

Siedlecki, P., & Zielenkiewicz, P. (2006). Mammalian DNA methyltransferases. *Acta Biochimica Polonica, 53*, 245–256.

Smith, R., & Mill, J. (2011). Epigenetics and chronic diseases: An overview. In H. I. Roach, F. Bronner, & R. O. C. Oreffo (Eds.), *Epigenetic aspects of chronic diseases* (pp. 1–20). London: Springer-Verlag London Ltd.

Stipanovich, A., Valjent, E., Mata, M., Nishi, A., Ahn, J. H., Maroteaux, M., et al. (2008). A phosphatase cascade by which rewarding stimuli control nucleosomal response. *Nature, 453*, 879–884.

Strahl, B. D., & Allis, C. D. (2000). The language of covalent histone modifications. *Nature, 403*, 41–45.

Sun, J., Wang, L., Jiang, B., Hui, B., Lv, Z., & Ma, L. (2008). The effects of sodium butyrate, an inhibitor of histone deacetylase, on the cocaine- and sucrose-maintained self administration in rats. *Neuroscience Letters, 441*, 72–76.

Suzuki, M. M., & Bird, A. (2008). DNA methylation landscapes: Provocative insights from epigenomics. *Nature Reviews Genetics, 9*, 465–476.

Szulwach, K. E., Li, X., Li, Y., Song, C. X., Wu, H., Dai, Q., et al. (2011). 5-hmC-mediated epigenetic dynamics during postnatal neurodevelopment and aging. *Nature Neuroscience, 14*, 1607–1616.

Szyf, M., McGowan, P., & Meaney, M. J. (2008). The social environment and the epigenome. *Environmental and Molecular Mutagenesis, 49*, 46–60.

Tachibana, M., Sugimoto, K., Fukushima, T., & Shinkai, Y. (2001). Set domain-containing protein, G9a, is a novel lysine preferring mammalian histone methyltransferase with hyperactivity and specific selectivity to lysines9 and 27 of histone H3. *Journal of Biological Chemistry, 276*, 25309–25317.

Taft, R. J., Pang, K. C., Mercer, T. R., Dinger, M., & Mattick, J. S. (2010). Non-coding RNAs: Regulators of disease. *Journal of Pathology, 220*, 126–139.

Tahiliani, M., Koh, K. P., Shen, Y., Pastor, W. A., Bandukwala, H., Brudno, Y., et al. (2009). Conversion of 5-methylcytosine to 5-hydroxymethylcytosine in mammalian DNA by MLL partner TET1. *Science, 324*, 930–935.

Wang, L., Lv, Z., Hu, Z., Sheng, J., Hui, B., Sun, J., et al. (2010). Chronic cocaine-induced H3 acetylation and transcriptional activation of CaMKIIalpha in the nucleus accumbens is critical for motivation for drug reinforcement. *Neuropsychopharmacology, 35*, 913–928.

Waterland, R. A. (2006). Assessing the effects of high methionine intake on DNA methylation. *Journal of Nutrition, 136*, 1706S–1710S.

Weaver, I. C., Champagne, F. A., Brown, S. E., Dymov, S., Sharma, S., Meaney, M. J., et al. (2005). Reversal of maternal programming of stress responses in adult offspring through methyl supplementation: Altering epigenetic marking later in life. *Journal of Neuroscience, 25*, 11045–11054.

Wong, C. C., Mill, J., & Fernandes, C. (2011). Drugs and addiction: An introduction to epigenetics. *Addiction, 106*, 480–489.

Wu, H., Coskun, V., Tao, J., Xie, W., Ge, W., Yoshikawa, K., et al. (2010). Dnmt3a dependent nonpromoter DNA methylation facilitates transcription of neurogenic genes. *Science, 329*, 444–448.

CHAPTER SIX

Experimental Models on Effects of Psychostimulants

Sulev Kõks[1]
Department of Pathophysiology, University of Tartu, Tartu, Estonia
[1]Corresponding author: e-mail address: sulev.koks@ut.ee

Contents

Abstract

Psychostimulants are a diverse group of substances that cause an increase in psychomotor activity at least in part through their actions on catecholaminergic systems including the dopaminergic mesolimbic pathways. Animal models used to study addiction are based on the psychomotor stimulant theory of addiction. The basics of this theory are that the reinforcing effects and the addition liabilities of the drugs can be predicted from their ability to induce psychomotor activation. This approach focuses on the ability of the drugs to directly control the animal's behavior and to induce psychomotor stimulation, and is consistent with the behavioral definition of addiction and behavioral sensitization. Animal experiments have the advantage over clinical studies of lower variation and fewer confounding effects.

International Review of Neurobiology, Volume 120
ISSN 0074-7742
http://dx.doi.org/10.1016/bs.irn.2015.03.002

1. INTRODUCTION

Drug addiction can be understood as an altered behavioral response induced by repetitive drug intake (Nestler, 2005; Vezina, 2004). These changes can persist for weeks or even years and are difficult to correct. Chronic administration of psychostimulants induces adaptive alterations in the brain cytoarchitecture and biochemistry that are necessary for the long-lasting behavioral effects characteristic for drug abuse. Animal models that simulate this behavioral phenotype by repeated administration of the drug usually result in an enhanced behavioral response to further later drug exposure. This phenomenon is referred to as behavioral sensitization and is associated with structural changes in the brain. Understanding behavioral sensitization and its molecular mechanisms better could potentially help us to develop intervention programs against drug addition.

2. CHANGES IN THE BRAIN IN RESPONSE TO PSYCHOSTIMULANTS

The neuroanatomical substrate for sensitization is believed to be the mesocorticolimbic dopaminergic pathway (Kalivas & Stewart, 1991; Pierce & Kalivas, 1997) that originates in the ventral tegmental area (VTA) and projects to the nucleus accumbens (NAc), amygdala, prefrontal cortex, and other forebrain regions (Robinson & Becker, 1986). The VTA-NAc pathway is the most important target for the rewarding effects of all drugs of abuse. The early action of psychostimulants in the VTA is considered a critical cellular event for initiation of behavioral sensitization. During repetitive drug exposure, the neural circuitry in the ventral striatum is recruited for behavioral expression. It has been shown that prior repeated doses of amphetamine to the VTA can sensitize rats, to subsequent parenteral administration of amphetamine leading to a potentiated locomotor responses (Perugini & Vezina, 1994), suggesting that neurons in the VTA are crucial for the induction of psychostimulant sensitization, while the NAc is essential for its behavioral expression (Di Chiara et al., 2004). Enhanced dopamine neuronal activity in VTA also seems essential for the initiation of subsequent behavioral changes. Receptors that can modulate VTA dopamine activity may also affect the severity of behavioral sensitization. For example, antagonists of dopamine D1 or glutamate NMDA receptors or agonists of $GABA_B$ receptors administered to the VTA were able to prevent the induction of amphetamine sensitization (Kalivas & Alesdatter, 1993; Perugini & Vezina, 1994; Vezina, 1996). Peripheral administration of a D1 antagonist completely inhibits the development of sensitization induced by amphetamine (Vezina, 1996).

The enhanced dopamine release in the NAc contributes to behavioral augmentation (Wolf, White, Nassar, Brooderson, & Khansa, 1993). Dopamine release activates the endogenous opioid and cannabinoid systems within the VTA-NAc pathway which is also believed to be important for the development of behavioral sensitization.

Chronic administration of psychostimulants induces chronic functional changes in the dopaminergic VTA-NAc pathway (Hyman, Malenka, & Nestler, 2006; Robinson & Becker, 1986). Numerous adaptations to chronic exposure have been described and these can be split into circuitry-level adaptations and cellular (molecular) adaptations (Di Chiara et al., 2004). Chronic exposure to psychostimulant drugs causes an impaired dopamine system, which can be viewed as a homeostatic response to repeated drug-induced activation system (Di Chiara et al., 1999; Everitt & Wolf, 2002). This impairment involves decreased baseline levels of dopamine function leading to a reduced efficiency of natural rewarding stimuli. These changes contribute to the dysphoria caused by drug withdrawal. In addition, chronic exposure induces sensitization of dopamine system what eventually causes an augmented dopaminergic response to psychostimulants (Everitt & Wolf, 2002; Wise, 2004) that can last long after the drug discontinuation and is related to the drug-seeking behavior. Chronic drug administration also induces adaptations at the cellular and molecular level (Dong et al., 2004; Saal, Dong, Bonci, & Malenka, 2003). Sensitization is caused by the long-term potentiation-like state in VTA dopaminergic neurons (Borgland, Malenka, & Bonci, 2004; Dong et al., 2004; Thomas, Kalivas, & Shaham, 2008; Thomas & Malenka, 2003) that is produced by increased AMPA glutamate receptor responsiveness that in turn occurs through the activation of the GluR1 receptor subunit (Carlezon & Nestler, 2002; Thomas & Malenka, 2003). The glutamatergic adaptations are directly related to the observed behavioral sensitization. One of the most dramatic biochemical changes induced by drugs of abuse is induction of the transcription factor DeltaFosB that accumulates in the NAc after chronic exposure to psychostimulants and is considered to be a molecular switch for addiction (McClung et al., 2004; Nestler, Barrot, & Self, 2001).

3. ANIMAL MODELS

Animal models have been extremely useful in understanding the pathophysiology of addiction and abuse of psychostimulants. In contrast to clinical studies, the subject population can be controlled for virtually all variables (Lynch, Nicholson, Dance, Morgan, & Foley, 2010), thereby permitting study design with much lower variations and fewer confounding effects.

Animal studies have demonstrated that the rewarding effect is not dependent on preexisting conditions, and exposure to the drug alone is sufficient to motivate drug-taking behavior. The notion of reinforcement has been integral to most of the leading theories proposed to explain drug addiction (Bozarth, 1990; Calabrese, 2008). A reinforcer (Table 1 for the terms) is defined as "any event that increases the probability of a response" and is used interchangeably with "reward" (National Institute on Drug Abuse, 2007).

Table 1 Overview of the Most Common Terms Used in Animal Studies of Addiction (Lynch et al., 2010; National Institute on Drug Abuse, 2007)

Term	Explanation
Acquisition	The process by which new behavior is added to the behavioral repertoire
Addiction	A chronic, relapsing brain disease that is characterized by compulsive drug seeking and use
Choice procedure	The allocation of one of two or more alternative responses
Fixed-ratio schedule	A schedule in which response is reinforced only after the animal has responded a specified number times
Operant behavior	A schedule in which response is reinforced only after the animal has responded a specified number times
Progressive-ratio schedule	A higher-order schedule that requires the animal to emit an increasing number of responses for each successive reinforcer
Reinforcement	The process whereby a behavior is strengthened by the event that follows the behavior
Reinforcer	A stimulus event that strengthens the behavior that follows
Reinforcing efficacy	The likelihood that a drug would act as a reinforcer
Reinstatement paradigm	A model of relapse where animal is tested on responding by pressing the lever that was formerly associated with the drug

In general, drugs with rewarding effects function as positive or conditioned reinforcers. Reward is often associated with other attributes such as pleasure that are much more difficult to measure or even define. Self-administration of addictive drugs by animals supports the concept that drugs act as universal reinforcers and that animal models are an accurate reflection of what occurs in the human brain (Bozarth, 1990).

Animal models that address behavioral or neurobiological constructs believed to be responsible for drug abuse have been widely developed and have provided substantial information about the molecular targets of addictive drugs as well as the neurobiological and psychological adaptations resulting from either acute or chronic drug exposure (Geyer & Markou, 1995; Swerdlow & Geyer, 1998). Models that focus on specific features of drug addiction provide a powerful framework for determining brain mechanisms underlying the pathology. However, they rarely address other clinical dimensions of the disorder such as behavioral predictive factors or interactions between different symptoms. Another type of animal model has tried to incorporate several symptoms of pathology in humans (Geyer & Markou, 1995; Geyer & Moghaddam, 2002; Young, Zhou, & Geyer, 2010) and has been particularly valuable for longitudinal studies or testing pharmacological treatments. The behavioral complexity of these models limits their value in studying causative mechanisms (Koob & Le Moal, 2005; Koob & Weiss, 1992).

Reliability refers to the consistency and stability with which the independent and the dependent variables are measured. Thus, a reliable model of drug addiction allows a precise and reproducible manipulation of an independent variable and an objective and reproducible measure of a dependent variable in standard conditions. A further key criterion for the validation of an animal model is its predictive validity (Belzung & Lemoine, 2011). A valid animal model should predict either the pharmacological potential of a compound in humans or a predicting variable that may influence both the dependent variable of the model and the process under investigation in humans (Belzung & Lemoine, 2011).

Additional criteria which are sometimes used to evaluate the reliability of animal models in drug addiction include face validity and construct validity (Belzung & Lemoine, 2011; Geyer & Markou, 1995). Face validity refers to the similarities between the dependent variable of the model (behavior during the drug addiction) and symptoms of disease (Belzung & Lemoine, 2011; Edwards & Koob, 2012). It is almost impossible to provide good criteria to evaluate similarities between the behavioral responses in an animal model and therefore the validity and drug addiction in humans because the behavioral repertoire is so different (Mead, 2014; Peck & Ranaldi, 2014). Construct validity (Edwards & Koob, 2012; Shippenberg & Koob, 2002) is the ability of a model to take into account neurobiological processes that characterize specific human pathological processes. Thus, incentive sensitization, habit formation, or top-down prefrontal executive control failures are examples of constructs investigated by animal models (Barr & Markou, 2005; Epstein, Preston, Stewart, & Shaham, 2006).

4. PSYCHOSTIMULANT ANIMAL MODELS

In animals, two main behavioral effects are associated with psychomotor activation and both result from enhancement of central dopaminergic pathways (Wise & Bozarth, 1987): low doses of psychostimulants enhance "locomotion," and high doses of psychostimulants induce "stereotypies" (Creese & Iversen, 1975; Kelly, Seviour, & Iversen, 1975). Increased locomotor activity is associated with activation of mesolimbic dopaminergic projection from the VTA to the NAc. Stereotypy on the other hand is caused by the activation of adjacent dopaminergic nigrostriatal projection from the *zona compacta* of the *substantia nigra* to the caudate nucleus and putamen (Creese & Iversen, 1975; Kelly et al., 1975). The mesolimbic and nigrostriatal fibers are subdivisions of the same anatomical system, and considerable cross talk is known to occur (Fallon & Moore, 1978).

There are several reasons why increased locomotion or stereotyped behavior should be looked upon as "psychomotor" activation and not simply "motor" activation. Lesions of the central dopaminergic systems cause a form of sensorimotor neglect (Ackil & Frommer, 1984; Carli, Evenden, & Robbins, 1985; Hoyman, Weese, & Frommer, 1979). Similarly, pharmacological blockade of the dopamine system reduces motivation for lever pressing or running an alleyway while their motor abilities remain intact (Fouriezos, Hansson, & Wise, 1978; Fouriezos & Wise, 1976; Wise, Spindler, deWit, & Gerberg, 1978). This motivational deficiency may underlie anhedonia and apathy (Wise et al., 1978). When the lesions are unilateral, animals generally fail to orient to visual, olfactory, or tactile stimuli contralateral to the side of lesion. Animals fail to make contralateral responses to stimuli, while they have perfect contralateral sensory or motor capability supporting a disturbance of sensorimotor integration (Ackil & Frommer, 1984).

In recent studies, we saw clear activation of the locomotor activity and increased stereotypy after administration of methcathinone indicating its psychostimulant activity (Asser et al., 2009, 2010, 2012).

5. ANIMAL MODELS TO ANALYZE REINFORCING PROPERTIES

Drug abuse and dependence are characterized by persistent drug-taking behavior (Stoops, 2008). Drugs of abuse have positive reinforcing abilities and induce repetitive self-administration. This phenomenon has provided the framework for currently used animal models of addiction. It is clear that humans and experimental animals will readily self-administer drugs in the absence of a withdrawal state. Drug reinforcement models use operant paradigms developed in primates and now are successfully utilized in rodents (Gardner, 2000).

5.1 Intravenous Drug Self-Administration

Drugs with high abuse potential are readily self-administered by experimental animals. However, not all drugs abused by humans are self-administered by experimental animals. Furthermore, there are species- and strain-related differences in the degree to which a drug is self-administered (Fattore, Piras, Corda, & Giorgi, 2009; Kuzmin & Johansson, 2000; Mello & Negus, 1996).

During self-administration studies, the subject acquires a drug infusion by performing a particular response. The pattern of responding required for each intravenous (IV) infusion is determined by the schedule of reinforcement imposed by the experimenter. Drug availability is typically signaled by an environmental stimulus. The dependent variables are the number of infusions obtained or the rate of responding during a session. In addition to the IV route of administration, the oral route can also be used.

In fixed-ratio simple schedules, the number of responses required for drug infusion is set at a fixed number. These schedules generally will not maintain a stable response below a certain unit dose in rodents. Within the range of doses that maintain stable responding, animals increase their self-administration rate as the unit dose is decreased. Conversely, animals reduce their rate of self-administration as the unit dose is increased. In a fixed-interval schedule, the frequency of injections is determined by the imposed interval schedule and not the response rate.

A self-administration experiment involves the administration of a compound (drug or placebo) related to a response on a specific schedule of reinforcement (e.g., 1 lever press or the first lever press after 1 min). For example, 0.5 mg/kg IV cocaine was available to drug-naive rats on a one-response fixed-ratio schedule (Pickens & Thompson, 1968). Under this schedule, stable levels of responding were observed when cocaine administration was paired with each response. However, when saline was substituted for cocaine or when only the stimulus light paired with cocaine administration was presented, responding ceased, indicating that administration of cocaine was maintaining responding and functioning as a positive reinforce (Pickens & Thompson, 1968; Roberts, Gabriele, & Zimmer, 2013). Therefore, the use of these schedules can provide information regarding both the motivational effects of a drug and potential nonspecific motor effects that can confound data interpretation (Meisch, 2001; Roberts, Morgan, & Liu, 2007).

Progressive-ratio schedules are used to evaluate the reinforcing efficacy of a self-administered drug. The progressive-ratio schedule was initially used to examine the reinforcing effects of sweetened milk solutions in rats (Hodos, 1961). The schedule begins with one response requirement for the initial presentation of a reinforcer and then requires an escalating number of responses for each subsequent presentation of that reinforcer. The response frequency for each successive drug reinforcement is increased and the breaking point (the point at which the animal will no longer respond) is determined (Stafford, LeSage, & Glowa, 1998). Breaking points are defined either as the largest ratio requirement that the subject completes or as the number of ratios completed by the subject per session. This value represents the maximum effort a subject will perform to receive an infusion of a drug. The progressive-ratio schedule can be used as a measure of the reinforcing efficacy of drugs and is sensitive to numerous manipulations in animals (Stoops, 2008).

Clinical definitions of drug addiction and dependence typically refer to the disruptive effects of addiction on patient's social activities. The use of multiple schedules of reinforcement enables the application of concepts of behavioral economics (e.g., consumption, price, and demand) to operant behavior (Johnson & Bickel, 2003; Petry & Heyman, 1995). This scheme also provides a control for nonselective effects of drug reinforcement. Under this scheme, self-administration of a drug is incorporated into a multiple component schedule with confounding reinforcers. These procedures have shown that the relation of concurrent reinforcers affects behavior asymmetrically (Bickel, DeGrandpre, & Higgins, 1995; Johnson & Bickel, 2003). Moreover, the response requirement for reinforcers can affect drug self-administration (Bickel et al., 1995; Johnson & Bickel, 2003). For instance, the reinforcing effects of nicotine can be difficult to demonstrate in laboratory studies across schedules of reinforcement. This is consistent with the notion that nonpharmacological factors heavily influence cigarette smoking and contribute to the considerable abuse potential of nicotine. Reinforcement procedures using multiple schedules can also provide information for behavioral or pharmacological therapies for the treatment of addiction.

In a second-order schedule, completion of a single component (or part) produces the terminal event (drug infusion) according to another overall schedule. Typically, completion of a unit schedule results in the presentation of a brief stimulus, while completion of the overall schedule results in the delivery of the stimulus and the drug. Second-order schedules have the advantage that they maintain high rates of response and extended sequences of behavior before any drug infusion occurs, thereby minimizing the influence of acute drug effects on response rates. High response rates can be maintained even with diminishing dose rates when several injections are self-administered during a session (Katz, Newman, & Izenwasser, 1997). This schedule also requires extended sequences of behavior attempting to reproduce the rituals of drug taking (e.g., procurement, preparation). Although second-order schedules are more typically used in nonhuman primate studies of addiction, their use in rodents is increasing (Arroyo, Markou, Robbins, & Everitt, 1998; Fattore et al., 2009; Markou, Arroyo, & Everitt, 1999; Ranaldi & Roberts, 1996).

5.2 Oral Self-Administration

Oral self-administration has focused largely on alcohol because of the obvi ous face validity and because IV self-administration of alcohol is difficult to sustain in rodents (Abramov et al., 2006; Hyytia, Schulteis, & Koob, 1996).

The first approach is to analyze the home cage drinking and preference in experimental animals. A simple design to study motivation to consume a drug is to measure the volume consumed from a drinking bottle available in the home cage. These procedures have been particularly useful for characterizing genetic differences in drug preference, most often alcohol preference, and for initial studies on the effects of pharmacologic treatments on drug intake and preference (Crabbe, Belknap, & Buck, 1994; Kuzmin & Johansson, 2000; Li, 2000). Usually, a choice is offered between a drug solution and alternative solutions, one of which is often water, and the proportion of drug intake relative to total intake is calculated as a preference ratio.

For two-bottle choice testing of alcohol in mice or rats, animals are singly housed and a bottle containing 10% alcohol and a bottle containing water are placed in each cage. Most commonly, animals are allowed free choice of these drinking solutions for successive 24-h periods with simultaneous free access to food (Abramov et al., 2006). However, limited access to the drug can induce high drug intakes in a short period of time. Similar studies have also been done with cocaine (Jentsch, Henry, Mason, Merritt, & Ziriax, 1998).

A more "motivational" approach is to use operant conditioning and to have animals work to obtain drugs. These experiments permit the effort to obtain the substance to be separated from the summation response (e.g., drinking). Different schedules of reinforcement can be used to change the baseline parameters and intake easily can be charted over time.

For operant self-administration of alcohol, animals can be trained to lever press using a variety of techniques all designed to overcome the aversive taste and after-effects of initial exposure. One approach involves using a sweetened solution fading procedure (Samson, 1986). Alcohol concentrations are increased to a final concentration of 10% over 20 days, with each concentration being mixed first with saccharin or sucrose and then presented alone. The animals can be trained to lever press for concentrations of alcohol up to 40% and will perform on fixed-ratio schedules and progressive-ratio schedules and obtain significant blood alcohol levels in a 30-min session.

Operant self-administration of oral alcohol has also been validated as a measure of the reinforcing effects of alcohol in primates (Stewart, Bass, Wang, & Meisch, 1996). Similar studies have been published on other drugs of abuse (Meisch, Lemaire, & Cutrell, 1992; Stewart et al., 1996; Stewart, Lemaire, Roache, & Meisch, 1994).

Drug self-administration has both reliability and predictive validity. The dependent variable provides a reliable measure of the motivation to obtain drugs and in demonstrating that drugs function as powerful reinforcers. The responses maintained by drugs as reinforcers are stable across sessions and can be altered predictably by neurotransmitter antagonists. Self-administration also has very good predictive validity. Drugs with high reinforcement potential in experimental animals have reinforcing effects in humans as measured by both operant and subjective reports (Lamb et al., 1991).

6. CONDITIONED PLACE PREFERENCE

Conditioned place preference is a classical conditioning procedure in which an abused drug is paired with a particular environment

(Shippenberg & Koob, 2002). In this model, animals receive a dose of a drug or vehicle and are placed into one of two sides of an experimental chamber, which have different visual (that is, vertical versus horizontal lines on the walls) and tactile (that is, grid versus bars for the floor) cues (Lynch et al., 2010). The animal's choice to spend more time in either environment provides a direct measure of the conditioned reinforcing effect of a drug. Conditioned preference is exhibited for an environment associated with positive reinforcing drugs (e.g., spend more time in the drug-paired compared to placebo-paired environment). Animals avoid the environment that induces aversive states (e.g., conditioned place aversion). This procedure permits assessment of the conditioning of drug reinforcement and can provide indirect information regarding the positive and negative reinforcing effects of drugs. Place conditioning has been used in conjunction with gene transfer and homologous recombination techniques to delineate the neural basis of drug-induced reinforcement (Carlezon et al., 1998; Innos et al., 2013; Risinger, Bormann, & Oakes, 1996; Runkorg, Varv, Matsui, Koks, & Vasar, 2006; Runkorg et al., 2003).

The apparatus used in conditioning experiments consists of two highly distinctive environments that are differentiated from each other on the basis of color, texture, and/or lighting. In the unbiased design, the environments are manipulated so that animals differentiate one from the other but do not exhibit an innate preference for either of the place cues. Pairing of drug with a particular environment is counterbalanced and change in the time spent in the drug-paired environment can be directly attributed to the conditioned reinforcing effects of a drug. Although quality control experiments confirming the unbiased nature of the procedure are conducted periodically, experiments do not require a preconditioning phase to assess pretest preferences, preventing the potential confound of latent inhibition and decreasing the time necessary for a particular experiment (Lynch et al., 2010).

In the biased design, animals exhibit a preference for one of the place cues prior to conditioning. During preconditioning phase, animals are allowed access to both environments and the innate preference of each animal is determined. The drug then is paired with the preferred or nonpreferred environment depending on whether the drug is assumed to produce aversive or positive reinforcing effects, respectively. Although this design is commonly used, data interpretation can be problematic because place preferences may indicate incentive motivational effects of a drug or a decrease in the aversive properties of the least-preferred environment.

The conditioned place preference paradigm is reliable and valid. Drugs that produce conditioned preferences for the drug-associated environment are those that function as positive reinforcers in other paradigms. Conditioned aversions also are observed in response to drugs that are negative reinforcers or produce aversive or dysphoric states in humans (Hand, Koob, Stinus, & Le Moal, 1988; Mucha & Herz, 1985).

7. DRUG DISCRIMINATION AS A TOOL TO MEASURE SUBJECTIVE EFFECTS

The drug-discrimination paradigm is an experimental model frequently used as a component of the overall assessment of the abuse liability of a novel drug. This paradigm is based on two hypotheses (Shippenberg & Koob, 2002). First, similar mechanisms of drug action have discriminative stimulus effects in animals and in humans. Second, discriminative stimulus effects of drugs may contribute to drug taking and to relapse in drug addicts. Therefore, discriminative stimuli help the animal engage in those behaviors that enable consumption of the reinforcing drug. The stimuli that predict drug administration elicit drug-seeking behavior and can reestablish extinguished cocaine-seeking behavior (Weiss et al., 2000). These data suggest that the discriminative stimulus effects of a drug contribute to drug-seeking behaviors (Falk & Lau, 1995; See, Grimm, Kruzich, & Rustay, 1999; Weiss et al., 2000).

In a typical experiment, animals are trained to carry out a particular response following administration of a fixed drug dose (depression of one lever designated the drug-associated lever) and to carry out another response (depression of saline designated lever) following administration of saline. Most commonly, an appetitively motivated operant procedure is used in which animals are food or water deprived. Responding on the training condition, appropriate lever results in the delivery of food or water. Training is continued until the animal reliably selects the appropriate lever after drug or saline administration. Once discrimination between drug and vehicle conditions has been acquired, novel compounds can be substituted for the training drug.

As with other operant paradigms, various reinforcement schedules (fixed-ratio, fixed-interval, differential reinforcement of low response rate) and response measures (nose poking, maze running) can be used. Dose 1 versus dose 2 and drug 1 versus drug 2 versus saline discriminations also can be employed (Bowen, Gatto, & Grant, 1997; Gauvin & Holloway, 1991; Picker & Cook, 1997).

8. ANIMAL MODELS FOR DRUG WITHDRAWAL

Drug administration withdrawal is characterized by responses opposite to the acute initial actions of the drug. Several physical signs associated with withdrawal from drugs can be quantified and measured. In addition, motivational aspects of abstinence are very sensitive measures of drug withdrawal.

8.1 Conditioned Place Aversion Model

The conditioned place preference paradigm can be used to characterize the conditioned aversive effects of drug withdrawal (Shippenberg & Koob, 2002). Rodents are exposed to one environment while undergoing drug withdrawal and to another in the absence of a withdrawal state. During tests of conditioning, animals are allowed access to both environments, and the time spent in each is determined. This procedure has been used to study withdrawal from opiate drugs (Runkorg et al., 2003). Administration of opioid receptor antagonists to animals physically dependent on opiates produces dose-dependent conditioned place aversions, an effect that can be observed only after a single-conditioning session with the antagonist (Funada & Shippenberg, 1996; Hand et al., 1988). Interestingly, the administration of the same doses of antagonist to opiate-naive animals fails to produce a conditioned response. The minimum effective dose of an antagonist that produces conditioned place aversions in animals physically dependent on morphine is less than that producing quantifiable somatic withdrawal signs. This suggests that this technique is a sensitive model for evaluating the affective component of drug withdrawal. Place aversion conditioning can be used also for studies of spontaneous withdrawal (Bechara, Nader, & van der Kooy, 1995).

9. TOXICITY OF PSYCHOSTIMULANTS

Amphetamine-type psychostimulants possess remarkable toxicity potential and their abuse is related to the increased incidence of different health problems. Their difference in neurotoxicity comes from their respective mechanism of action. In addition to the blocking of synaptic reuptake that is common with other psychostimulants (like methylphenidate), amphetamines enter the synaptic terminal and they interact with the vesicular transporters what are responsible for the intracellular storage of dopamine (Schiffer et al., 2006). Amphetamines displace dopamine from the vesicles and induce profound release of dopamine from intracellular depots. This difference produces rapid and greater increase in synaptic monoamines compared with other psychostimulants and accounts for their greater toxicity (Fone & Nutt, 2005).

Hyperthermia is the most life-threatening acute physiological consequence of amphetamine intoxication. Case reports indicate that the incidence of hyperthermia differs from drug to drug (Green, O'Shea, & Colado, 2004; Jaehne, Salem, & Irvine, 2007). Hyperthermia is most frequent with methamphetamine, MDMA, 3,4-methylenedioxyethamphetamine, and *p*-methoxyamphetamine (Green et al., 2004). In case of MDMA, the body temperature has been reported to rise up to 43 °C (Green, Mechan, Elliott, O'Shea, & Colado, 2003; Green et al., 2004). Hyperthermia can lead to fatal complications, such as rhabdomyolysis, acute renal failure, disseminated intravascular coagulation, multiple organ failure, and acidosis (Henry, 1992; Kalant, 2001). The MDMA-induced hyperthermia seems to be caused by the activation of the skeletal muscle thermogenic protein, UCP3 (Mills, Banks, Sprague, & Finkel, 2003). Mice deficient in a mitochondrial protein (UCP3 −/−) are protected against MDMA toxic effect and do not express thermogenic response (Mills, Rusyniak, & Sprague, 2004).

There is still much debate relating to the neurotoxic effects of amphetamines on catecholaminergic neurons. Amphetamines act as substance-releasers. They bind to monoamine transporters and stimulate the release of different monoamines, including dopamine (Kahlig et al., 2005). Amphetamine-type psychostimulants present different affinities toward the monoamine transporters, DAT, NET, and 5-HTT. Amphetamines are recognized by these transporters and internalized to the monoaminergic neurons (Carvalho et al., 2012). Once in the cytoplasm, the rapid enhancement of monoamine release from the storage vesicles by amphetamines occurs via a carrier-mediated exchange mechanism. Amphetamine-type psychostimulants are substrates for vesicular monoamine transporter (VMAT) and may be incorporated into the vesicles through active competition with the transporter. This leads to depletion of vesicular neurotransmitter storage by reversal of transporter activity (Baumann, Partilla, & Lehner, 2013; Partilla et al., 2006). This explains why all amphetamines are potent monoamine releasers. An increase in the cytoplasmic pool of monoamines triggers oxidative stress inside the nerve terminal by the autoxidation properties of dopamine and norepinephrine and by oxidative stress induced by catabolic by-products (Carvalho et al., 2012). It is conceivable, therefore, that these effects could lead to nerve terminal damage. In our recent study, we showed that both acute and chronic administration of methcathinone could induce loss of neurons in mice (Fig. 1). Three times a day chronic administration of methcathinone in 100 mg/kg for a month induced loss of D2 binding in mice comparable to that seen with manganese.

Clinical relevance of preclinical toxicity in rodents is regarded uncertain and their utility is commonly questioned in scientific literature. However, toxicity of amphetamines has also clearly been described in mammals. Single dose of MDMA induces long-term (2 weeks) depletions of brain 5-HT, its major metabolites, and its vesicular transporter, VMAT2 (Green et al., 2003; Steele, McCann, & Ricaurte, 1994). Morphologic examinations have identified fragmented 5-HT-positive axons within days of MDMA treatment, followed by marked reductions in 5-HT axon density weeks later (Ricaurte et al., 1988; Wilson, Mamounas, Fasman, Axt, & Molliver, 1993). Numerous studies have concluded that MDMA has the potential to damage brain 5-HT axons. High-dose studies with methamphetamine have resulted in conclusive evidence that its use causes severe toxicity symptoms (Harvey, Lacan, & Melegan, 2000; Melega et al., 1997). Moreover,

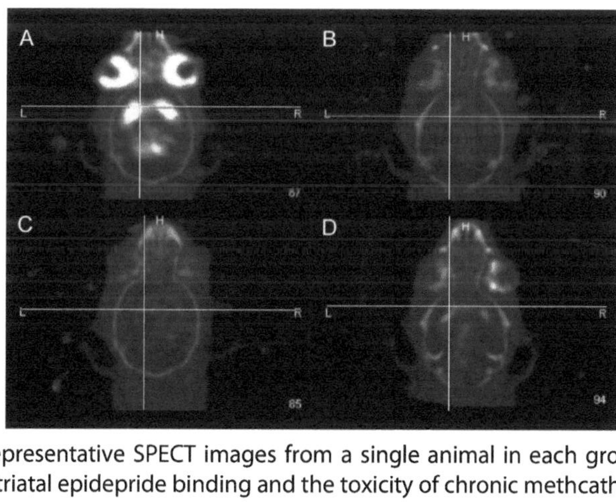

Figure 1 Representative SPECT images from a single animal in each group show the decreased striatal epidepride binding and the toxicity of chronic methcathinone abuse. The white crosshair marks the striatal area selected for binding ratio calculations and for quantitative analysis. The treatment groups were as follows: (A) control animals; (B) 100 mg/kg methcathinone; (C) 30 mg/kg manganese chloride 2; and (D) home-made psychostimulant mixture (contains 100 mg/kg methcathinone) made of Sudafed used by drug addicts. Drugs were injected three times a day for 4 weeks. It is clearly seen that methcathinone has neurotoxicity comparable to the manganese (author's unpublished data).

even in the range of doses used recreationally by humans, methamphetamine is able to produce significant decrements in brain dopaminergic neurons in baboons (Villemagne et al., 1998). Therefore, abuse of psychostimulants and amphetamines has significant deleterious effect on the health of user. Most remarkable effects are related to their neurotoxic effects, but other systems are damaged as well.

10. CONCLUSIONS

In this chapter, we gave a systematic overview about the models that can be used for drug addiction studies. Drug addiction is a complex phenomenon and its modeling in animals is time consuming. However, most of the models have been available for decades and they are validated on a high level. The procedures for different models and neurochemical changes induced by different study designs are described in different textbooks and can easily be implemented. As the models are validated and reliable, their utility is wide. On the other hand, as drug addiction is a behavior with diverse aspects, no single model is perfect. Therefore, depending on the aims of the study, an appropriate model should be chosen.

REFERENCES

Abramov, U., Raud, S., Innos, J., Koks, S., Matsui, T., & Vasar, E. (2006). Gender specific effects of ethanol in mice, lacking CCK2 receptors. *Behavioural Brain Research*, *175*(1), 149–156. http://dx.doi.org/10.1016/j.bbr.2006.08.015.

Ackil, J. E., & Frommer, G. P. (1984). Deficits in visual discrimination performance following neglect-producing unilateral lateral hypothalamic lesions in the albino rat. *Physiology & Behavior*, *32*(6), 915–922.

Arroyo, M., Markou, A., Robbins, T. W., & Everitt, B. J. (1998). Acquisition, maintenance and reinstatement of intravenous cocaine self-administration under a second-order schedule of reinforcement in rats: Effects of conditioned cues and continuous access to cocaine. *Psychopharmacology*, *140*(3), 331–344.

Asser, A., Kõks, S., Haaparanta-Solin, M., Grönroos, T., Pakkanen, A., Nairismägi, J., et al. (2009). The effects of chronic administration of ephedrone (methcathinone) and manganese in mice. *Movement Disorders*, *24*, S48–S49.

Asser, A., Kõks, S., Soomets, U., Terasmaa, A., Sauk, M., Eltermaa, M., et al. (2010). Acute effects of methcathinone and manganese in mice: A dose response study. *Movement Disorders*, *25*, S226.

Asser, A., Raki, M. J. J., Krispin, V., Muldmaa, M., Põldsepp, S., Rätsep, H., et al. (2012). Methcathinone (ephedrone) and manganese both reduce D2-receptor function: An animal SPECT study. *Movement Disorders*, *27*, S430.

Barr, A. M., & Markou, A. (2005). Psychostimulant withdrawal as an inducing condition in animal models of depression. *Neuroscience and Biobehavioral Reviews*, *29*(4–5), 675–706. http://dx.doi.org/10.1016/j.neubiorev.2005.03.012.

Baumann, M. H., Partilla, J. S., & Lehner, K. R. (2013). Psychoactive "bath salts": Not so soothing. *European Journal of Pharmacology*, *698*(1–3), 1–5. http://dx.doi.org/10.1016/j.ejphar.2012.11.020.

Bechara, A., Nader, K., & van der Kooy, D. (1995). Neurobiology of withdrawal motivation: Evidence for two separate aversive effects produced in morphine-naive versus morphine-dependent rats by both naloxone and spontaneous withdrawal. *Behavioral Neuroscience*, *109*(1), 91–105.

Belzung, C., & Lemoine, M. (2011). Criteria of validity for animal models of psychiatric disorders: Focus on anxiety disorders and depression. *Biology of Mood & Anxiety Disorders*, *1*(1), 9. http://dx.doi.org/10.1186/2045-5380-1-9.

Bickel, W. K., DeGrandpre, R. J., & Higgins, S. T. (1995). The behavioral economics of concurrent drug reinforcers: A review and reanalysis of drug self-administration research. *Psychopharmacology*, *118*(3), 250–259.

Borgland, S. L., Malenka, R. C., & Bonci, A. (2004). Acute and chronic cocaine-induced potentiation of synaptic strength in the ventral tegmental area: Electrophysiological and behavioral correlates in individual rats. *The Journal of Neuroscience*, *24*(34), 7482–7490. http://dx.doi.org/10.1523/jneurosci.1312-04.2004.

Bowen, C. A., Gatto, G. J., & Grant, K. A. (1997). Assessment of the multiple discriminative stimulus effects of ethanol using an ethanol-pentobarbital-water discrimination in rats. *Behavioural Pharmacology*, *8*(4), 339–352.

Bozarth, M. (1990). Drug addiction as a psychobiological process. In D. M. Warburton (Ed.), *Addiction controversies* (pp. 112–134). London: Harwood Academic Publishers.

Calabrese, E. J. (2008). Addiction and dose response: The psychomotor stimulant theory of addiction reveals that hormetic dose responses are dominant. *Critical Reviews in Toxicology*, *38*(7), 599–617. http://dx.doi.org/10.1080/10408440802026315.

Carlezon, W. A., Jr., & Nestler, E. J. (2002). Elevated levels of GluR1 in the midbrain: A trigger for sensitization to drugs of abuse? *Trends in Neurosciences*, *25*(12), 610–615.

Carlezon, W. A., Jr., Thome, J., Olson, V. G., Lane-Ladd, S. B., Brodkin, E. S., Hiroi, N., et al. (1998). Regulation of cocaine reward by CREB. *Science*, *282*(5397), 2272–2275.

Carli, M., Evenden, J. L., & Robbins, T. W. (1985). Depletion of unilateral striatal dopamine impairs initiation of contralateral actions and not sensory attention. *Nature*, *313*(6004), 679–682.

Carvalho, M., Carmo, H., Costa, V. M., Capela, J. P., Pontes, H., Remiao, F., et al. (2012). Toxicity of amphetamines: An update. *Archives of Toxicology*, *86*(8), 1167–1231. http://dx.doi.org/10.1007/s00204-012-0815-5.

Crabbe, J. C., Belknap, J. K., & Buck, K. J. (1994). Genetic animal models of alcohol and drug abuse. *Science*, *264*(5166), 1715–1723.

Creese, I., & Iversen, S. D. (1975). The pharmacological and anatomical substrates of the amphetamine response in the rat. *Brain Research*, *83*(3), 419–436.

Di Chiara, G., Bassareo, V., Fenu, S., De Luca, M. A., Spina, L., Cadoni, C., et al. (2004). Dopamine and drug addiction: The nucleus accumbens shell connection. *Neuropharmacology*, *47*(Suppl. 1), 227–241. http://dx.doi.org/10.1016/j.neuropharm.2004.06.032.

Di Chiara, G., Tanda, G., Bassareo, V., Pontieri, F., Acquas, E., Fenu, S., et al. (1999). Drug addiction as a disorder of associative learning. Role of nucleus accumbens shell/extended amygdala dopamine. *Annals of the New York Academy of Sciences*, *877*, 461–485.

Dong, Y., Saal, D., Thomas, M., Faust, R., Bonci, A., Robinson, T., et al. (2004). Cocaine-induced potentiation of synaptic strength in dopamine neurons: Behavioral correlates in GluRA(-/-) mice. *Proceedings of the National Academy of Sciences of the United States of America*, *101*(39), 14282–14287. http://dx.doi.org/10.1073/pnas.0401553101.

Edwards, S., & Koob, G. F. (2012). Experimental psychiatric illness and drug abuse models: From human to animal, an overview. *Methods in Molecular Biology*, *829*, 31–48. http://dx.doi.org/10.1007/978-1-61779-458-2_2.

Epstein, D. H., Preston, K. L., Stewart, J., & Shaham, Y. (2006). Toward a model of drug relapse: An assessment of the validity of the reinstatement procedure. *Psychopharmacology, 189*(1), 1–16. http://dx.doi.org/10.1007/s00213-006-0529-6.

Everitt, B. J., & Wolf, M. E. (2002). Psychomotor stimulant addiction: A neural systems perspective. *The Journal of Neuroscience, 22*(9), 3312–3320.

Falk, J. L., & Lau, C. E. (1995). Stimulus control of addictive behavior: Persistence in the presence and absence of a drug. *Pharmacology, Biochemistry, and Behavior, 50*(1), 71–75.

Fallon, J. H., & Moore, R. Y. (1978). Catecholamine innervation of the basal forebrain. IV. Topography of the dopamine projection to the basal forebrain and neostriatum. *The Journal of Comparative Neurology, 180*(3), 545–580. http://dx.doi.org/10.1002/cne.901800310.

Fattore, L., Piras, G., Corda, M. G., & Giorgi, O. (2009). The Roman high- and low-avoidance rat lines differ in the acquisition, maintenance, extinction, and reinstatement of intravenous cocaine self-administration. *Neuropsychopharmacology, 34*(5), 1091–1101. http://dx.doi.org/10.1038/npp.2008.43.

Fone, K. C., & Nutt, D. J. (2005). Stimulants: Use and abuse in the treatment of attention deficit hyperactivity disorder. *Current Opinion in Pharmacology, 5*(1), 87–93. http://dx.doi.org/10.1016/j.coph.2004.10.001.

Fouriezos, G., Hansson, P., & Wise, R. A. (1978). Neuroleptic-induced attenuation of brain stimulation reward in rats. *Journal of Comparative and Physiological Psychology, 92*(4), 661–671.

Fouriezos, G., & Wise, R. A. (1976). Pimozide-induced extinction of intracranial self-stimulation: Response patterns rule out motor or performance deficits. *Brain Research, 103*(2), 377–380.

Funada, M., & Shippenberg, T. S. (1996). Differential involvement of D1 and D2 dopamine receptors in the expression of morphine withdrawal signs in rats. *Behavioural Pharmacology, 7*(5), 448–453.

Gardner, E. L. (2000). What we have learned about addiction from animal models of drug self-administration. *The American Journal on Addictions, 9*(4), 285–313.

Gauvin, D. V., & Holloway, F. A. (1991). Cue dimensionality in the three-choice pentylenetetrazole-saline-chlordiazepoxide discrimination task. *Behavioural Pharmacology, 2*(4 and 5), 417–428.

Geyer, M. A., & Markou, A. (1995). Animal models of psychiatric disorders. In F. E. Bloom, & D. J. Kupfer (Eds.), *Neuropsychopharmacology: The fourth generation of progress* (pp. 787–798). New York: Raven Press.

Geyer, M. A., & Moghaddam, B. (2002). Animal models relevant to schizophrenia disorders. In K. L. Davis, D. Charney, J. T. Coyle, & C. Nemeroff (Eds.), *Neuropsychopharmacology: The fifth generation of progress* (pp. 689–701). Pennsylvania: Lippincott, Williams & Wilkins.

Green, A. R., Mechan, A. O., Elliott, J. M., O'Shea, E., & Colado, M. I. (2003). The pharmacology and clinical pharmacology of 3,4-methylenedioxymethamphetamine (MDMA, "ecstasy"). *Pharmacological Reviews, 55*(3), 463–508. http://dx.doi.org/10.1124/pr.55.3.3.

Green, A. R., O'Shea, E., & Colado, M. I. (2004). A review of the mechanisms involved in the acute MDMA (ecstasy)-induced hyperthermic response. *European Journal of Pharmacology, 500*(1–3), 3–13. http://dx.doi.org/10.1016/j.ejphar.2004.07.006.

Hand, T. H., Koob, G. F., Stinus, L., & Le Moal, M. (1988). Aversive properties of opiate receptor blockade: Evidence for exclusively central mediation in naive and morphine-dependent rats. *Brain Research, 474*(2), 364–368.

Harvey, D. C., Lacan, G., & Melegan, W. P. (2000). Regional heterogeneity of dopaminergic deficits in vervet monkey striatum and substantia nigra after methamphetamine exposure. *Experimental Brain Research, 133*(3), 349–358.

Henry, J. A. (1992). Ecstasy and the dance of death. *BMJ*, *305*(6844), 5–6.
Hodos, W. (1961). Progressive ratio as a measure of reward strength. *Science*, *134*(3483), 943–944.
Hoyman, L., Weese, G. D., & Frommer, G. P. (1979). Tactile discrimination performance deficits following neglect-producing unilateral lateral hypothalamic lesions in the rat. *Physiology & Behavior*, *22*(1), 139–147.
Hyman, S. E., Malenka, R. C., & Nestler, E. J. (2006). Neural mechanisms of addiction: The role of reward-related learning and memory. *Annual Review of Neuroscience*, *29*, 565–598. http://dx.doi.org/10.1146/annurev.neuro.29.051605.113009.
Hyytia, P., Schulteis, G., & Koob, G. F. (1996). Intravenous heroin and ethanol self-administration by alcohol-preferring AA and alcohol-avoiding ANA rats. *Psychopharmacology*, *125*(3), 248–254.
Innos, J., Leidmaa, E., Philips, M. A., Sutt, S., Alttoa, A., Harro, J., et al. (2013). Lsamp(-)/(-) mice display lower sensitivity to amphetamine and have elevated 5-HT turnover. *Biochemical and Biophysical Research Communications*, *430*(1), 413–418. http://dx.doi.org/10.1016/j.bbrc.2012.11.077.
Jaehne, E. J., Salem, A., & Irvine, R. J. (2007). Pharmacological and behavioral determinants of cocaine, methamphetamine, 3,4-methylenedioxymethamphetamine, and para-methoxyamphetamine-induced hyperthermia. *Psychopharmacology*, *194*(1), 41–52. http://dx.doi.org/10.1007/s00213-007-0825-9.
Jentsch, J. D., Henry, P. J., Mason, P. A., Merritt, J. H., & Ziriax, J. M. (1998). Establishing orally self-administered cocaine as a reinforcer in rats using home-cage pre-exposure. *Progress in Neuro-Psychopharmacology & Biological Psychiatry*, *22*(1), 229–239.
Johnson, M. W., & Bickel, W. K. (2003). The behavioral economics of cigarette smoking: The concurrent presence of a substitute and an independent reinforcer. *Behavioural Pharmacology*, *14*(2), 137–144. http://dx.doi.org/10.1097/01.fbp.0000063266.43827.42.
Kahlig, K. M., Binda, F., Khoshbouei, H., Blakely, R. D., McMahon, D. G., Javitch, J. A., et al. (2005). Amphetamine induces dopamine efflux through a dopamine transporter channel. *Proceedings of the National Academy of Sciences of the United States of America*, *102*(9), 3495–3500. http://dx.doi.org/10.1073/pnas.0407737102.
Kalant, H. (2001). The pharmacology and toxicology of "ecstasy" (MDMA) and related drugs. *CMAJ: Canadian Medical Association Journal*, *165*(7), 917–928.
Kalivas, P. W., & Alesdatter, J. E. (1993). Involvement of N-methyl-D-aspartate receptor stimulation in the ventral tegmental area and amygdala in behavioral sensitization to cocaine. *The Journal of Pharmacology and Experimental Therapeutics*, *267*(1), 486–495.
Kalivas, P. W., & Stewart, J. (1991). Dopamine transmission in the initiation and expression of drug- and stress-induced sensitization of motor activity. *Brain Research. Brain Research Reviews*, *16*(3), 223–244.
Katz, J. L., Newman, A. H., & Izenwasser, S. (1997). Relations between heterogeneity of dopamine transporter binding and function and the behavioral pharmacology of cocaine. *Pharmacology, Biochemistry, and Behavior*, *57*(3), 505–512.
Kelly, P. H., Seviour, P. W., & Iversen, S. D. (1975). Amphetamine and apomorphine responses in the rat following 6-OHDA lesions of the nucleus accumbens septi and corpus striatum. *Brain Research*, *94*(3), 507–522.
Koob, G. F., & Le Moal, M. (2005). Plasticity of reward neurocircuitry and the 'dark side' of drug addiction. *Nature Neuroscience*, *8*(11), 1442–1444. http://dx.doi.org/10.1038/nn1105-1442.
Koob, G. F., & Weiss, F. (1992). Neuropharmacology of cocaine and ethanol dependence. *Recent Developments in Alcoholism*, *10*, 201–233.
Kuzmin, A., & Johansson, B. (2000). Reinforcing and neurochemical effects of cocaine: Differences among C57, DBA, and 129 mice. *Pharmacology, Biochemistry, and Behavior*, *65*(3), 399–406.

Lamb, R. J., Preston, K. L., Schindler, C. W., Meisch, R. A., Davis, F., Katz, J. L., et al. (1991). The reinforcing and subjective effects of morphine in post-addicts: A dose-response study. *The Journal of Pharmacology and Experimental Therapeutics, 259*(3), 1165–1173.

Li, T. K. (2000). Pharmacogenetics of responses to alcohol and genes that influence alcohol drinking. *Journal of Studies on Alcohol, 61*(1), 5–12.

Lynch, W. J., Nicholson, K. L., Dance, M. E., Morgan, R. W., & Foley, P. L. (2010). Animal models of substance abuse and addiction: Implications for science, animal welfare, and society. *Comparative Medicine, 60*(3), 177–188.

Markou, A., Arroyo, M., & Everitt, B. J. (1999). Effects of contingent and non-contingent cocaine on drug-seeking behavior measured using a second-order schedule of cocaine reinforcement in rats. *Neuropsychopharmacology, 20*(6), 542–555. http://dx.doi.org/10.1016/S0893-133X(98)00080-3.

McClung, C. A., Ulery, P. G., Perrotti, L. I., Zachariou, V., Berton, O., & Nestler, E. J. (2004). DeltaFosB: A molecular switch for long-term adaptation in the brain. *Brain Research. Molecular Brain Research, 132*(2), 146–154. http://dx.doi.org/10.1016/j.molbrainres.2004.05.014.

Mead, A. N. (2014). Appropriate experimental approaches for predicting abuse potential and addictive qualities in preclinical drug discovery. *Expert Opinion on Drug Discovery, 9*(11), 1281–1291. http://dx.doi.org/10.1517/17460441.2014.956077.

Meisch, R. A. (2001). Oral drug self-administration: An overview of laboratory animal studies. *Alcohol, 24*(2), 117–128.

Meisch, R. A., Lemaire, G. A., & Cutrell, E. B. (1992). Oral self-administration of pentobarbital by rhesus monkeys: Relative reinforcing effects under concurrent signalled differential-reinforcement-of-low-rates schedules. *Drug and Alcohol Dependence, 30*(3), 215–225.

Melega, W. P., Raleigh, M. J., Stout, D. B., Lacan, G., Huang, S. C., & Phelps, M. E. (1997). Recovery of striatal dopamine function after acute amphetamine- and methamphetamine-induced neurotoxicity in the vervet monkey. *Brain Research, 766*(1–2), 113–120.

Mello, N. K., & Negus, S. S. (1996). Preclinical evaluation of pharmacotherapies for treatment of cocaine and opioid abuse using drug self-administration procedures. *Neuropsychopharmacology, 14*(6), 375–424. http://dx.doi.org/10.1016/0893-133x(95)00274-h.

Mills, E. M., Banks, M. L., Sprague, J. E., & Finkel, T. (2003). Pharmacology: Uncoupling the agony from ecstasy. *Nature, 426*(6965), 403–404. http://dx.doi.org/10.1038/426403a.

Mills, E. M., Rusyniak, D. E., & Sprague, J. E. (2004). The role of the sympathetic nervous system and uncoupling proteins in the thermogenesis induced by 3,4-methylenedioxymethamphetamine. *Journal of Molecular Medicine (Berlin, Germany), 82*(12), 787–799. http://dx.doi.org/10.1007/s00109-004-0591-7.

Mucha, R. F., & Herz, A. (1985). Motivational properties of kappa and mu opioid receptor agonists studied with place and taste preference conditioning. *Psychopharmacology, 86*(3), 274–280.

National Institute on Drug Abuse. (2007). *Drugs, brains and behavior: The science of addiction.* Retrieved from, http://www.drugabuse.gov/scienceofaddiction/sciofaddiction.pdf.

Nestler, E. J. (2005). Is there a common molecular pathway for addiction? *Nature Neuroscience, 8*(11), 1445–1449. http://dx.doi.org/10.1038/nn1578.

Nestler, E. J., Barrot, M., & Self, D. W. (2001). DeltaFosB: A sustained molecular switch for addiction. *Proceedings of the National Academy of Sciences of the United States of America, 98*(20), 11042–11046. http://dx.doi.org/10.1073/pnas.191352698.

Partilla, J. S., Dempsey, A. G., Nagpal, A. S., Blough, B. E., Baumann, M. H., & Rothman, R. B. (2006). Interaction of amphetamines and related compounds at the vesicular monoamine transporter. *The Journal of Pharmacology and Experimental Therapeutics, 319*(1), 237–246. http://dx.doi.org/10.1124/jpet.106.103622.

Peck, J. A., & Ranaldi, R. (2014). Drug abstinence: Exploring animal models and behavioral treatment strategies. *Psychopharmacology, 231*(10), 2045–2058. http://dx.doi.org/10.1007/s00213-014-3517-2.

Perugini, M., & Vezina, P. (1994). Amphetamine administered to the ventral tegmental area sensitizes rats to the locomotor effects of nucleus accumbens amphetamine. *The Journal of Pharmacology and Experimental Therapeutics, 270*(2), 690–696.

Petry, N. M., & Heyman, G. M. (1995). Behavioral economics of concurrent ethanol-sucrose and sucrose reinforcement in the rat: Effects of altering variable-ratio requirements. *Journal of the Experimental Analysis of Behavior, 64*(3), 331–359. http://dx.doi.org/10.1901/jeab.1995.64-331.

Pickens, R., & Thompson, T. (1968). Cocaine-reinforced behavior in rats: Effects of reinforcement magnitude and fixed-ratio size. *The Journal of Pharmacology and Experimental Therapeutics, 161*(1), 122–129.

Picker, M. J., & Cook, C. D. (1997). Discriminative stimulus effects of opioids in pigeons trained to discriminate fentanyl, bremazocine and water: Evidence of pharmacological selectivity. *Behavioural Pharmacology, 8*(2–3), 160–173.

Pierce, R. C., & Kalivas, P. W. (1997). A circuitry model of the expression of behavioral sensitization to amphetamine-like psychostimulants. *Brain Research. Brain Research Reviews, 25*(2), 192–216.

Ranaldi, R., & Roberts, D. C. (1996). Initiation, maintenance and extinction of cocaine self-administration with and without conditioned reward. *Psychopharmacology, 128*(1), 89–96.

Ricaurte, G. A., Forno, L. S., Wilson, M. A., DeLanney, L. E., Irwin, I., Molliver, M. E., et al. (1988). (+/-)3,4-Methylenedioxymethamphetamine selectively damages central serotonergic neurons in nonhuman primates. *JAMA, 260*(1), 51–55.

Risinger, F. O., Bormann, N. M., & Oakes, R. A. (1996). Reduced sensitivity to ethanol reward, but not ethanol aversion, in mice lacking 5-HT1B receptors. *Alcoholism, Clinical and Experimental Research, 20*(8), 1401–1405.

Roberts, D. C., Gabriele, A., & Zimmer, B. A. (2013). Conflation of cocaine seeking and cocaine taking responses in IV self-administration experiments in rats: Methodological and interpretational considerations. *Neuroscience and Biobehavioral Reviews, 37*(9 Pt. A), 2026–2036. http://dx.doi.org/10.1016/j.neubiorev.2013.04.017.

Roberts, D. C., Morgan, D., & Liu, Y. (2007). How to make a rat addicted to cocaine. *Progress in Neuro-Psychopharmacology & Biological Psychiatry, 31*(8), 1614–1624. http://dx.doi.org/10.1016/j.pnpbp.2007.08.028.

Robinson, T. E., & Becker, J. B. (1986). Enduring changes in brain and behavior produced by chronic amphetamine administration: A review and evaluation of animal models of amphetamine psychosis. *Brain Research, 396*(2), 157–198.

Runkorg, K., Varv, S., Matsui, T., Koks, S., & Vasar, E. (2006). Differences in behavioural effects of amphetamine and dopamine-related gene expression in wild-type and homozygous CCK2 receptor deficient mice. *Neuroscience Letters, 406*(1–2), 17–22. http://dx.doi.org/10.1016/j.neulet.2006.07.016.

Runkorg, K., Veraksits, A., Kurrikoff, K., Luuk, H., Raud, S., Abramov, U., et al. (2003). Distinct changes in the behavioural effects of morphine and naloxone in CCK2 receptor-deficient mice. *Behavioural Brain Research, 144*(1–2), 125–135.

Saal, D., Dong, Y., Bonci, A., & Malenka, R. C. (2003). Drugs of abuse and stress trigger a common synaptic adaptation in dopamine neurons. *Neuron, 37*(4), 577–582.

Samson, H. H. (1986). Initiation of ethanol reinforcement using a sucrose-substitution procedure in food- and water-sated rats. *Alcoholism, Clinical and Experimental Research, 10*(4), 436–442.

Schiffer, W. K., Volkow, N. D., Fowler, J. S., Alexoff, D. L., Logan, J., & Dewey, S. L. (2006). Therapeutic doses of amphetamine or methylphenidate differentially increase synaptic and extracellular dopamine. *Synapse, 59*(4), 243–251. http://dx.doi.org/10.1002/syn.20235.

See, R. E., Grimm, J. W., Kruzich, P. J., & Rustay, N. (1999). The importance of a compound stimulus in conditioned drug-seeking behavior following one week of extinction from self-administered cocaine in rats. *Drug and Alcohol Dependence, 57*(1), 41–49.

Shippenberg, T. S., & Koob, G. F. (2002). Recent advances in animal models of drug addiction. In K. L. Davis, D. Charney, J. T. Coyle, & C. Nemeroff (Eds.), *Neuropsychopharmacology: The fifth generation of progress* (pp. 1381–1397). Pennsylvania: Lippincott, Williams & Wilkins.

Stafford, D., LeSage, M. G., & Glowa, J. R. (1998). Progressive-ratio schedules of drug delivery in the analysis of drug self-administration: A review. *Psychopharmacology, 139*(3), 169–184.

Steele, T. D., McCann, U. D., & Ricaurte, G. A. (1994). 3,4-Methylenedioxymethamphetamine (MDMA, "Ecstasy"): Pharmacology and toxicology in animals and humans. *Addiction, 89*(5), 539–551.

Stewart, R. B., Bass, A. A., Wang, N. S., & Meisch, R. A. (1996). Ethanol as an oral reinforcer in normal weight rhesus monkeys: Dose-response functions. *Alcohol, 13*(4), 341–346.

Stewart, R. B., Lemaire, G. A., Roache, J. D., & Meisch, R. A. (1994). Establishing benzodiazepines as oral reinforcers: Midazolam and diazepam self-administration in rhesus monkeys. *The Journal of Pharmacology and Experimental Therapeutics, 271*(1), 200–211.

Stoops, W. W. (2008). Reinforcing effects of stimulants in humans: Sensitivity of progressive-ratio schedules. *Experimental and Clinical Psychopharmacology, 16*(6), 503–512. http://dx.doi.org/10.1037/a0013657.

Swerdlow, N. R., & Geyer, M. A. (1998). Using an animal model of deficient sensorimotor gating to study the pathophysiology and new treatments of schizophrenia. *Schizophrenia Bulletin, 24*(2), 285–301.

Thomas, M. J., Kalivas, P. W., & Shaham, Y. (2008). Neuroplasticity in the mesolimbic dopamine system and cocaine addiction. *British Journal of Pharmacology, 154*(2), 327–342. http://dx.doi.org/10.1038/bjp.2008.77.

Thomas, M. J., & Malenka, R. C. (2003). Synaptic plasticity in the mesolimbic dopamine system. *Philosophical Transactions of the Royal Society of London. Series B, Biological Sciences, 358*(1432), 815–819. http://dx.doi.org/10.1098/rstb.2002.1236.

Vezina, P. (1996). D1 dopamine receptor activation is necessary for the induction of sensitization by amphetamine in the ventral tegmental area. *The Journal of Neuroscience, 16*(7), 2411–2420.

Vezina, P. (2004). Sensitization of midbrain dopamine neuron reactivity and the self-administration of psychomotor stimulant drugs. *Neuroscience and Biobehavioral Reviews, 27*(8), 827–839. http://dx.doi.org/10.1016/j.neubiorev.2003.11.001.

Villemagne, V., Yuan, J., Wong, D. F., Dannals, R. F., Hatzidimitriou, G., Mathews, W. B., et al. (1998). Brain dopamine neurotoxicity in baboons treated with doses of methamphetamine comparable to those recreationally abused by humans: Evidence from [11C] WIN-35,428 positron emission tomography studies and direct in vitro determinations. *The Journal of Neuroscience, 18*(1), 419–427.

Weiss, F., Maldonado-Vlaar, C. S., Parsons, L. H., Kerr, T. M., Smith, D. L., & Ben-Shahar, O. (2000). Control of cocaine-seeking behavior by drug-associated stimuli in rats: Effects on recovery of extinguished operant-responding and extracellular dopamine levels in amygdala and nucleus accumbens. *Proceedings of the National Academy of Sciences of the United States of America*, *97*(8), 4321–4326.

Wilson, M. A., Mamounas, L. A., Fasman, K. H., Axt, K. J., & Molliver, M. E. (1993). Reactions of 5-HT neurons to drugs of abuse: Neurotoxicity and plasticity. *NIDA Research Monograph*, *136*, 155–178, discussion 178–187.

Wise, R. A. (2004). Dopamine, learning and motivation. *Nature Reviews. Neuroscience*, *5*(6), 483–494. http://dx.doi.org/10.1038/nrn1406.

Wise, R. A., & Bozarth, M. A. (1987). A psychomotor stimulant theory of addiction. *Psychological Review*, *94*(4), 469–492.

Wise, R. A., Spindler, J., deWit, H., & Gerberg, G. J. (1978). Neuroleptic-induced "anhedonia" in rats: Pimozide blocks reward quality of food. *Science*, *201*(4352), 262–264.

Wolf, M. E., White, F. J., Nassar, R., Brooderson, R. J., & Khansa, M. R. (1993). Differential development of autoreceptor subsensitivity and enhanced dopamine release during amphetamine sensitization. *The Journal of Pharmacology and Experimental Therapeutics*, *264*(1), 249–255.

Young, J. W., Zhou, X., & Geyer, M. A. (2010). Animal models of schizophrenia. *Current Topics in Behavioral Neurosciences*, *4*, 391–433.

CHAPTER SEVEN

Neurologic Complications of Psychomotor Stimulant Abuse

Juan Sanchez-Ramos[1]
Ellis Endowed Chair of Neurology, University of South Florida, Tampa, Florida, USA
[1]Corresponding author: e-mail address: jsramos@health.usf.edu

Contents

Abstract

Psychomotor stimulants are drugs that act on the central nervous system (CNS) to increase alertness, elevate mood, and produce a sense of well-being. These drugs also decrease appetite and the need for sleep. Stimulants can enhance stamina and improve performance in tasks that have been impaired by fatigue or boredom. Approved therapeutic applications of stimulants include attention deficit hyperactivity disorder (ADHD), narcolepsy, and obesity. These agents also possess potent reinforcing properties that can result in excessive self-administration and abuse. Chronic use is associated with adverse effects including psychosis, seizures, and cerebrovascular accidents, though these complications usually occur in individuals with preexisting risk factors.

This chapter reviews the adverse neurologic consequences of chronic psychomotor stimulant use and abuse, with a focus on two prototypical stimulants methamphetamine and cocaine.

International Review of Neurobiology, Volume 120
ISSN 0074-7742
http://dx.doi.org/10.1016/bs.irn.2015.02.003

1. HISTORICAL OVERVIEW

Humans have used natural stimulants for at least several thousand years by consuming amphetamine-producing plants such as *Catha edulis* (khat) and plants from the genus *Ephedrae* (family *Ephedraceae*) including má huáng (*Ephedra sinica*) (Carvalho et al., 2012). Khat is an evergreen plant that grows at high altitudes in East Africa and the Arabian Peninsula. Users of khat report increased levels of energy, alertness, and self-esteem, a sensation of elation, enhanced imaginative ability, and a higher capacity to detect patterns of connectivity (Carvalho, 2003). These effects have been attributed to khat's content of cathinone, a potent natural amphetamine. Some other less-potent amphetamines may also be present in khat, namely norpseudoephedrine (cathine) and norephedrine.

One of the oldest medicinal herbs known to mankind is probably *Ephedra*, or má huáng as it is known in Traditional Chinese Medicine. The aerial parts of different *Ephedra* species contain at least six optically active amphetamines (Fig. 1). The amphetamines ephedrine and pseudoephedrine are the main psychoactive constituents of the plant, the others being their optical isomers and N-methylated derivatives (Abourashed, El-Alfy, Khan, & Walker, 2003). Ephedroxane (Fig. 2), a less-known amphetamine, has also been isolated from the aerial parts of *E. intermedia* and has been detected in at least six more species containing ephedrine alkaloids (Konno, Taguchi, Tamada, & Hikino, 1979).

1.1 Amphetamines

Methamphetamine was synthesized from ephedrine (derived from the plant *E. sinica*) in 1893 and eventually a synthetic version became available to the consumer as an over-the-counter (OTC) decongestant and bronchodilator (Rusyniak, 2011). Before the abuse potential of methamphetamine was recognized, its clinical effects were considered to be ideal for warfare. Combat capability was markedly enhanced by a drug-induced state of alertness and aggression, as well as decreased hunger and need to sleep. The United States, Germany, and Japan all issued it to their troops during World War II (WWII) (Anglin, Burke, Perrochet, Stamper, & Dawud-Noursi, 2000). After the war, Japan experienced an epidemic of methamphetamine abuse as army surplus flooded the market. Its usage declined in the 1960s, only for a resurgence to occur in the 1970s and continues to be a problem in Japan today (Suwaki, Fukui, & Konuma, 1997). A 2008 United Nations Office on

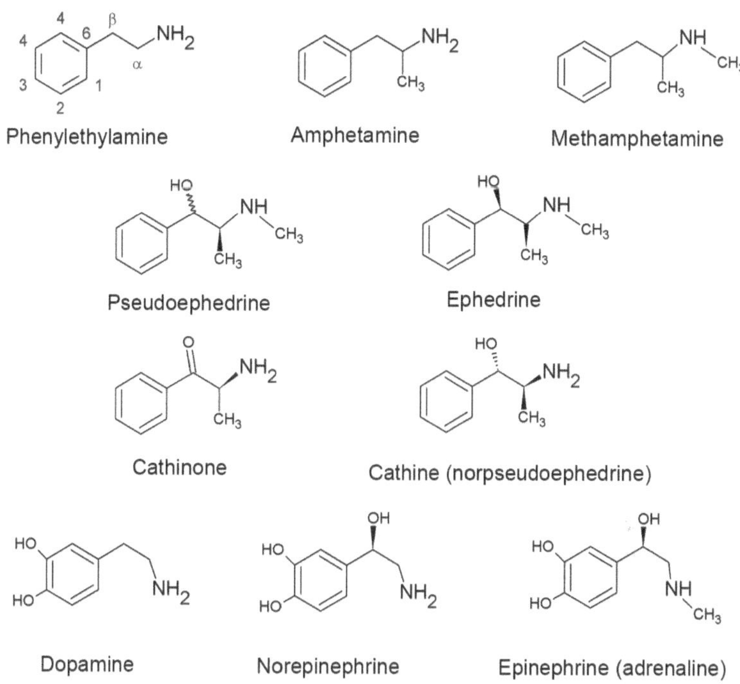

Figure 1 Chemical structures of β-phenylethylamine (numbered), amphetamine, and methamphetamine. Also depicted are the natural amphetamines pseudoephedrine, ephedrine, cathinone, and cathine (norpseudoephedrine). The neurotransmitters dopamine, norepinephrine (noradrenaline), and epinephrine (adrenaline) are based on the same phenylethylamine structure.

Drugs and Crime reported there were 25 million abusers of amphetamines worldwide, exceeding the number of users of both cocaine (14 million) and heroin (11 million) (UNDOC, 2008).

After WWII, many US soldiers and civilians continued to use methamphetamine, which at that time was available by prescription in an injectable form. When pharmaceutical companies terminated their injectable formulations in the early 1960s, methamphetamine manufacturing was taken up in clandestine labs and distributed by west coast motorcycle gangs to meet the demand for the drug (Gonzales, Mooney, & Rawson, 2010). At that time, methamphetamine was produced primarily from the precursors phenyl-2-propanone and methylamine (the P-2-P method) (Anglin et al., 2000). In the 1980s, a crystalline form of methamphetamine that could be smoked, called "ice," began to be imported from Asia to Hawaii (Gonzales et al., 2010). This form of methamphetamine quickly found its way to the US west coast and slowly began working its way east (Office of National Drug

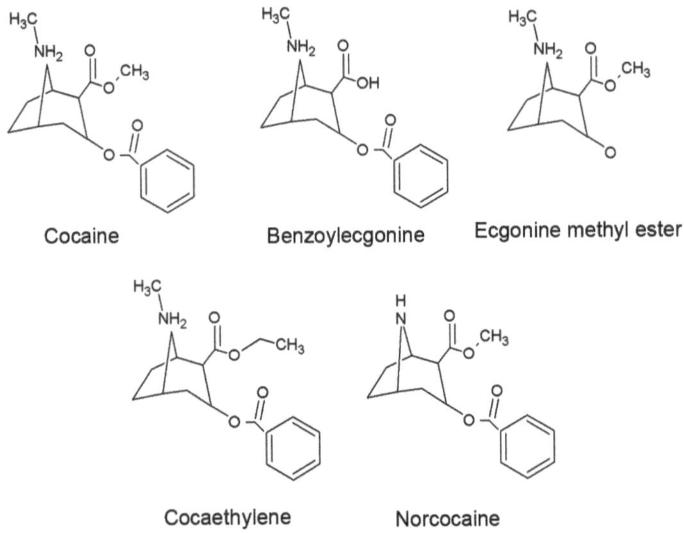

Figure 2 Chemical structure of cocaine (benzoylmethylecgonine) and its metabolic products. Hydrolysis of cocaine yields benzoylecgonine, and the action of serum and liver esterases produces ecgonine methyl ester. Cocaethylene is a product of trans-esterification of cocaine with ethanol. Cocaine is also N-demethylated by the liver cytochrome P450 system into norcocaine.

Control Policy, 2011). By 1990, methamphetamine had replaced cocaine as the stimulant of choice among drug users in many areas of California (Derlet & Heischober, 1990). Methamphetamine abuse was moved to the forefront of the Drug Enforcement Administration's war on drugs, and to a popular topic of mainstream media, primarily because of the ubiquitous rural "meth lab." Methamphetamine manufacture was not limited by geographic location, unlike other drugs of abuse that required cultivation of a plant source (e.g., coca leaf or opium poppy plant). By using "OTC" ephedrine and pseudoephedrine as the main precursors, production of methamphetamine became simpler, more efficient, and available to intrepid, unskilled "kitchen chemists." Despite the relative simplicity of its synthesis (by traditional chemistry standards), "cooking" methamphetamine requires heating volatile hydrocarbons. When done by those without chemistry backgrounds in poorly ventilated areas, fires and explosions were not uncommon. In an attempt to decrease the growing methamphetamine crisis, US Congress passed the 2005 Combat Methamphetamine Epidemic Act which limited access to pseudoephedrine. This led to the closure of large numbers of small and medium-sized clandestine laboratories resulting in a decrease in numbers of methamphetamine abusers in 2006—the first time for 10 years (Gonzales et al., 2010).

Despite the decline in illicit use of amphetamines, they remain important and useful treatments in medicine. Methamphetamine (Desoxyn™) and the combination of amphetamine and dextroamphetamine (Adderall™) are listed as Schedule II drugs and are currently available by prescription for treatment of attention deficit hyperactivity disorder (ADHD), extreme obesity, and narcolepsy.

1.2 Cocaine

Cocaine is a natural alkaloid with a chemical structure (benzoylmethylecgonine) that is distinct from the amphetamines but it shares the properties of central nervous system (CNS) stimulant activity and a high proclivity for abuse. It was first extracted from the plant *Erythroxylum coca* in the mid-nineteenth century. Leaves of the plant were used by the indigenous population of the Andes for centuries before the European conquest and formed an integral part of Inca rites and customs. Coca leaves continue to be chewed by natives of the altiplano to alleviate the diminish fatigue and alleviate altitude sickness. The leaves are sprinkled with lime alkali (or nowadays readily available baking soda—sodium bicarbonate) to facilitate extraction of the base and absorption into the blood stream by the oral mucosa.

Cocaine was extracted from coca in pure form in 1860, but it was not until Sigmund Freud's *Über Coca* was published in 1884 that Europeans became aware of it as a possible therapeutic agent (Byck, 1974). Among many potential applications suggested by Freud (including treatment of alcohol and opiate dependence), its use as a local anesthetic was widely adopted by physicians. Its stimulant effects were also considered to be of potential value as a treatment for neurasthenia and depression by many eminent physicians, and the popular press extolled its use for innumerable ailments from the common cold to impotence. Cocaine was added to many tonics and popular alcohol and nonalcoholic beverages such as Vin Mariani and Coca Cola. Such publicity and widespread use inevitably led to reports of cocaine intoxication and addiction. Opposition by the medical profession then followed, with sensationalized newspaper stories describing the dangers and violence associated with cocaine use by "black dope fiends." By 1914, even before the passage of the Harrison Narcotics Act, the majority of states had passed laws prohibiting the sale and use of cocaine. Despite its criminalization as a recreational drug, its use was resurrected by bohemians and artists and jazz musicians in the 1950s, and its use and abuse gradually spread over the next decade to all echelons of society. Despite the declaration of the "War on Drugs" by the US Federal Government in 1970, cocaine was transformed into a "champagne" drug, obtainable only by those who could afford its inflated price. In 1980s, the drug became available in a smokable form known as "crack," supposedly because of the sound made by popping cocaine crystals during heating. Crack could be synthesized readily from cocaine hydrochloride, and because of its relatively lower price, soon it became the stimulant of choice among the urban American poor.

Cocaine and amphetamines have alternated in abuse prevalence during the past 70 years, with peaks in amphetamine abuse roughly corresponding to troughs of cocaine abuse. The most recent data from 2007 to 2012 indicate methamphetamine use has remained steady, from 530,000 current users in 2007 to 440,000 in 2012. In contrast over the same period, cocaine use has gone down, the number of current users aged 12 or older having dropped from 2.1 to 1.7 million (NIDA, 2014).

2. NEUROPHARMACOLOGY

The primary amphetamine structure permits substitutions at the aromatic ring and at the α and β carbons of the aliphatic chain and the amine terminal, making it possible to synthesize a wide range of compounds (see Fig. 1). Amphetamines without ring substitutions have sympathomimetic, antifatigue, and strong reinforcing effects, those with side-chain substitutions may cause anorexia, while those derivatives with terminal amine substitutions have psychomotor stimulant effects at low doses and hallucinogenic activity at higher doses (Young & Glennon, 1986). Amphetamines with aromatic ring substitutions are usually weak stimulants, but some possess hallucinogenic activity (Kleven & Seiden, 1992). Compounds such as 2,5-dimethoxyphenylisopropylamine, 2,5-dimethoxy-4-methylphenylisopropylamine, and 3,4,5-trimethoxyamphetamine have behavioral effects similar to lysergic acid (LSD). Amphetamines with methylenedioxy substitutions on the phenyl ring such as 3,4-methylenedioxymethamphetamine (MDMA) (Ecstasy) or 3,4-methylenedioxyamphetamine have hallucinogenic and stimulant actions at relatively low doses, but most users of MDMA would deny any resemblance to the classic hallucinogens LSD and psilocybin.

Methamphetamine rapidly crosses the blood–brain barrier, regardless of the route of administration (intranasal insufflation, intravenous injection, or oral consumption). Compared to its parent compound amphetamine, methamphetamine has increased CNS penetration and is more potent because of its increased lipophilicity (Lake & Quirk, 1984). Once in the CNS, it binds to transporter proteins for dopamine, norepinephrine, and, to a lesser extent, serotonin located on neuronal cell bodies and nerve fibers; at higher concentrations, methamphetamine may also cross cell membranes independent of transporter binding. Once bound, the neurotransmitter transporters pump methamphetamine into the neuron where it is taken up by vesicular monoamine transporters (VMATs). The drug then displaces the monoamine from the storage vesicles to the cytoplasm where they are reverse-transported out of the cell through the same transporters that pumped methamphetamine into the cell (Fleckenstein, Volz, Riddle, Gibb, & Hanson, 2007). Methamphetamine also decreases monoamine neurotransmitter reuptake and degradation (Suzuki, Hattori, Asano, Oya, & Katsumata, 1980). The net result is a rapid and sustained increase in the extracellular concentrations of monoamine neurotransmitters. One of the reasons methamphetamine has superseded cocaine in worldwide usage is that it has a longer half-life (12 h compared to 90 min) and therefore a much longer duration of action (Rusyniak, 2013).

While many receptors have been implicated in mediating the complex physiologic responses to amphetamines, the clinical effects associated with methamphetamine and cocaine use are mediated by stimulation of the sympathetic nervous system. It is the rapid and sustained activation of catecholamines that is responsible for the adrenergic toxic syndrome: tachycardia, hypertension, mydriasis, diaphoresis, and psychomotor agitation. In addition, most of the acute neurologic complications associated with methamphetamine use also occur through similar mechanisms (e.g., strokes, seizures, agitation, and hyperthermia) (Halpin, Collins, & Yamamoto, 2014; O'Connor, Rusyniak, & Bruno, 2005; Schep, Slaughter, & Beasley, 2010). With repeated use in both humans and experimental animal models, methamphetamine depletes the brain's stores of dopamine and damages dopamine and serotonin nerve terminals. When chronic users stop taking methamphetamine, they may exhibit an impaired ability to experience pleasure (anhedonia) and slip into a deep depression.

Cocaine is absorbed from mucous membranes and the gastrointestinal mucosa following which it is hydrolyzed rapidly to benzoylecgonine and metabolized to ecgonine and ecgonine methyl ester by serum and liver esterases (Fig. 2).

A small fraction (3–6%) of cocaine is N-demethylated in liver by the cytochrome P450 system (Inaba, Stewart, & Kalow, 1978). Although the plasma half-life of cocaine after oral or nasal administration is 60–90 min, benzoylecgonine, a nonpsychotropic metabolite, has been detected in brain tissue of chronic cocaine users for up to 22 days after last drug use (Madden & Powers, 1990). In the presence of ethanol, a transesterification process leads to the production of cocaethylene, which has similar pharmacological properties to cocaine and prolongs the duration of euphoria (Hearn et al., 1991). Individuals who are genetically deficient in plasma cholinesterase may be acutely sensitive to even small doses of the drug (Ritchie & Greene, 1985). Inducers of the cytochrome P450 system such as alcohol, phenobarbital, and phenytoin may increase metabolic oxidation of cocaine, thereby decreasing its potential toxicity (Shuster, Garhart, Powers, Grunfeld, & Kanel, 1988).

An important therapeutic effect of cocaine is that of local anesthesia, especially when administered to mucosal membranes of the eye or nose. The capacity of cocaine and other similar compounds, e.g., procaine and other local anesthetics, to block nerve conduction is a function of a direct membrane effect that impacts the sodium channel (Ritchie & Greene, 1985). Cocaine prevents the large transient increase in the permeability of the membrane to sodium ions that are produced by a slight depolarization of the membrane.

Cocaine modulates monoaminergic neurotransmission in several different ways, the most studied being its capacity to block the reuptake of monoamines released at the synapse. Unlike amphetamines, cocaine does not inhibit monoamine oxidase. The reinforcing effects of cocaine or those actions that lead to compulsive self-administration of the drug are believed to be mediated by the blockade of the dopamine transporter in the mesolimbic dopaminergic system (Ritz, Lamb, Goldberg, & Kuhar, 1987). With higher doses and with chronic use, other neurotransmitter systems such as serotonin and norepinephrine are involved, directly or indirectly in mediating CNS toxicity. With chronic use, neuroadaptive mechanisms result in development of tolerance, reverse tolerance (behavioral sensitization), and psychological dependence.

3. STIMULANT ABUSE, TOLERANCE, AND DEPENDENCE

Most individuals who have used stimulants in low doses do not progress to higher and more frequent dosing. Of the 30 million Americans who have tried snorting cocaine (intranasal insufflation), 80% did not become regular users and 95% did not become dependent on the drug (Gawin & Ellinwood, 1988). Similarly, when amphetamines were prescribed to millions of individuals in the 1960s to treat obesity or depression, most of them were weaned easily when restrictions were applied. The determinants of compulsive stimulant use have not been identified clearly, but clinical observations indicate that the extent of stimulant exposure may be the most important factor leading to abuse. Stimulant abusers report that controlled use commonly shifts to compulsive use, either when access to the drug increases and dosages escalate markedly or when the user switches to a more rapid route of administration such as the intravenous route or smoking. Large doses and rapid routes of administration result in high plasma concentrations that result in a euphoria so intense that it has been compared to sexual orgasm. Being able to induce a powerful state of euphoria at will tends to shift the pattern of stimulant use to high-dose bouts of repetitive and compulsive use (binges).

Binges are characterized by repeated administration of the drug up to every 10 min, causing rapid and frequent mood changes. Although cocaine binges can last as long as 7 consecutive days, the average length is 12 h (Jaffe, 1985). Amphetamine binges often last more than 24 h, with one to several hours between readministrations.

Tolerance or diminished effects with repeated doses develop to some but not all of the central actions of amphetamines such as its euphoriant, anorectic, and hyperthermic actions (Jaffe, 1985). This may lead to escalation of dose or increased dose frequency in order to obtain the same degree of euphoria. Simultaneously, increased sensitivity to other CNS effects occurs. For example, repeated use of cocaine lowers seizure threshold through a mechanism similar to the pathophysiological phenomenon of "kindling" (Stripling, 1983). Cross-tolerance between the amphetamine-like sympathomimetic drugs has been observed clinically, and cross-tolerance between the anorectic effect of cocaine and amphetamine has been reported in pri mates (Jaffe, 1985). Tolerance does not develop to certain effects of amphetamine, and toxic psychosis can result after continual use for weeks to months.

It was believed for a long time that stimulants did not induce a state of drug dependence. In fact, dependence can develop to stimulants. Acute abstinence (crash) after chronic or binge use of cocaine is not life-threatening and is typically free of gross autonomic nervous system derangements that are seen with opiate, alcohol, and CNS depressant withdrawal. This does not negate the significance of the physiologic and neurochemical alterations that underlie stimulant abstinence, causing disturbance of affect and disruption of sleep cycles during the first hours to days of abstinence (Gawin, 1991; Gawin & Ellinwood, 1988). The subsequent weeks to months of abstinence are associated with anhedonia, anxiety, and high levels of stimulant drug craving that usually result in relapse to former patterns of stimulant use.

3.1 Neuropsychological Consequences of Abuse

The immediate subjective effects of amphetamine closely resemble the effects seen with other psychomotor stimulants when matched for relative potency (Jaffe, 1985). These drugs include dextroamphetamine (Dexedrine™, the dextrorotatory stereo-isomer of amphetamine), methamphetamine, phenmetrazine, methylphenidate, diethylpropion, cocaine, and cathinone. Even experienced drug users cannot distinguish the immediate subjective effects of 16 mg of cocaine from 10 mg of dextroamphetamine, when both are administered intravenously (Fischman et al., 1976). Moreover, the toxic psychosis that may develop with chronic cocaine use is clinically indistinguishable from that induced by chronic amphetamine use. Although the actions and toxicity of amphetamine are emphasized as a prototype, this should not imply that all stimulant drugs have identical mechanisms of action. Even further from the truth would be the assertion that experienced drug abusers cannot distinguish differences between stimulants.

Nevertheless, the similarities in the pharmacology, toxicology, and clinical effects between methamphetamine, amphetamine, and other CNS stimulants (e.g., cocaine and methylphenidate) make the following discussion of neuropsychological effects applicable to CNS stimulants in general.

Chronic methamphetamine use has been associated with deficits in cognition, anxiety, depression, and psychosis. Approximately 40% of regular methamphetamine users have cognitive deficits that can be documented by neuropsychiatric tests (Rippeth et al., 2004). The most frequently reported deficits involved episodic memory, executive function, and motor function (Scott et al., 2007). The greatest impairments were in episodic memory (Tulving, 2002). Some experts have speculated that this memory deficit causes them to forget past errors and hence condemns them to relapse into the same self-destructive pattern of stimulant self-administration. Chronic methamphetamine abuse also impacts executive function, leading to impulsiveness, perseveration, and inability to delay gratification and to carry out long-term goals (Gilbert & Burgess, 2008). Some studies report motor deficits in chronic methamphetamine abusers, especially noted when testing fine motor dexterity (Caligiuri & Buitenhuys, 2005).

Chronic methamphetamine abusers can exhibit a range of mental disturbances including anxiety, depression, and psychosis (Sanchez-Ramos,

1993). The fully developed toxic psychosis from chronic methamphetamine or cocaine use is characterized by vivid visual, auditory, and occasionally tactile hallucinations (Rusyniak, 2013). Delusions of parasitosis and compulsive picking at imaginary bugs under the skin (formication) may develop (Rusyniak, 2013). Interestingly, chronic users with toxic psychosis often display little or no sympathomimetic effects and blood pressure is not elevated unduly (Jaffe, 1985).

The amphetamine-induced paranoid ideation and thought disorder are similar to paranoid schizophrenia. The most frequently reported symptoms are delusions of persecution and auditory hallucinations (Iwanami et al., 1994; Mahoney, Kalechstein, De La Garza, & Newton, 2008; Srisurapanont et al., 2003; Yui, Ikemoto, Ishiguro, & Goto, 2000). Although not as commonly reported, negative symptoms (e.g., poverty of speech and psychomotor retardation) have also been seen with methamphetamine-induced psychosis (Srisurapanont et al., 2003). Both schizophrenia and amphetamine-evoked psychosis can be effectively treated with dopamine antagonists (Angrist, Lee, & Gershon, 1974). The development of psychosis is more readily seen in people using higher methamphetamine concentrations for prolonged periods of time (Chen et al., 2003, 2005). The reported doses required, duration of abuse, and onset of symptoms are highly variable, as is the duration of psychotic symptoms (1 week—indefinitely) (Cruickshank & Dyer, 2009). Even if symptoms abate with abstinence, they can reemerge with repeat usage or under stressful situations (Sato, 1992). One of the debates associated with psychosis and methamphetamine is whether it is the result of methamphetamine-induced neurotoxicity (i.e., altered dopaminergic neurotransmission), or whether the two disorders coexist so that persons with mental illness are more likely to abuse methamphetamine (so-called dual diagnosis). The latter seems to be supported by data showing that persons with predisposition to mental illness, such as strong family histories, are significantly more likely to develop methamphetamine-associated psychosis (Chen et al., 2003, 2005). Furthermore, schizophrenics given low doses of methamphetamine will have exacerbations of their symptoms (Lieberman, Kinon, & Loebel, 1990). Therefore, it has been suggested that in susceptible individuals, methamphetamine abuse may be a trigger which unmasks schizophrenia/psychosis (Bell, 1965). Some experts have suggested that persons with schizophrenia/psychosis seek out illicit drugs as a form of self-treatment (Buckley, 1998) and others claim that neuronal deficits underlying the development of schizophrenia make individuals more prone to develop drug addiction

(Chambers, Krystal, & Self, 2001). Regardless of the perspective, it is clear that methamphetamine abuse can result in the development of acute, and in some cases chronic, psychosis.

4. STIMULANTS AND MOVEMENT DISORDERS

Chronic stimulant abuse can result in a range of movement disorders including stereotypies, tics, chorea, and dystonia. Stereotypy is a drug-triggered behavioral phenomenon that may occur in stimulant users, and should not be confused with stereotypic movement disorders, which typically have onset in childhood and by definition cannot be due to a direct drug effect (APA, 2013). Stereotypic movements involve repetitive, nonfunctional motor behaviors that may be self-injurious (head banging, hand shaking, rocking movements, self-biting, skin picking). Although stereotypic movement disorders are associated with autism, Lesch–Nyhan syndrome, and other neurodevelopmental disorders, methamphetamine can trigger stereotypic movements such as frequent blinking, facial grimacing, lip licking, and grunting in normal individuals. In addition, methamphetamine abuse has been reported to increase the risk for developing Parkinson's disease (PD), but this association is not generally accepted (Moszczynska et al., 2004).

4.1 Stereotypy (Punding)

The word punding, derived from Swedish for "block-head," is often used interchangeably with the term stereotypy (Rusyniak, 2013). Many examples seem to have a compulsive component with rearrangement of furniture, fastidious bathing, and distinctive and repetitive walking patterns (Sanchez-Ramos, 1993). There seems to be a predilection for activities that users tend to do normally. For example, an artist may doodle, draw, or paint excessively to the point that all walls of the house are covered with the art. A housekeeper may repetitively polish silverware or rearrange the furniture for hours. Along this line, there is a gender-related component, with men typically spending hours disassembling watches, locks, or household appliances that are in good working order and women's stereotypy consisting of more commonly involving grooming behaviors like excessive hair brushing and nail polishing (Rusyniak, 2013).

Punding was first reported in amphetamine users where in one study 26% (40 of 150) of heavy users experienced it (Rylander, 1972). Punding has also been reported in cocaine users (Fasano et al., 2008), and more recently in patients with PD receiving dopamine replacement therapy (Fasano & Petrovic, 2010; O'Sullivan, Evans, & Lees, 2009). Like chronic stimulant abusers, patients with PD have dysfunctional dopaminergic neurotransmission and can develop psychosis (O'Sullivan et al., 2009). This suggests a similar pathophysiologic mechanism. While few controlled studies have been done on punding in substance abusers, there are some data available on its incidence. In a study of 50 patients addicted to cocaine, 38% had some form of punding (Fasano & Petrovic, 2010). These patients spent on average 3 h a day engaged in repetitive activities. One patient reported spending up to 14 h a day playing computer games and collecting things (O'Sullivan et al., 2009). It is interesting that the majority of interviewed patients in this study noted their behavior began shortly after their first medication usage. In addition, the duration and amount of drug used did not seem to predict which users would develop punding and which would not (O'Sullivan et al., 2009). As mentioned above, the same abnormal brain circuitry that increases ones risk for becoming psychologically dependent may also be involved in the development of such stereotyped behaviors.

Interestingly, most drug abuse subjects did not describe associated anxiety or distress over their activities, but found them amusing or pleasurable. When drug usage ceases, punding typically decreases or stops.

While the neurobiological mechanisms behind punding are not yet well understood, animal research has provided some insights. Repeated dosing of amphetamines in animals results in stereotypic behaviors such as excessive gnawing, sniffing, and head bobbing (Randrup & Munkvad, 1967). In addition, repeated dosing results in behavioral sensitization: this is manifested as increased locomotor activity and stereotypic behavior with each subsequent dose of amphetamine. This sensitization appears to involve both glutamate and dopamine, and more recently dopamine-mediated decreases in acetylcholine have been implicated (Aliane, Perez, Bohren, Deniau, & Kemel, 2011; O'Sullivan et al., 2009; Pierce & Kalivas, 1997). As concentrations of extracellular dopamine increase with each subsequent dose of amphetamine, one could envision over time this excess dopamine causing neurotoxicity to dopamine receptor-bearing striatal neurons or changing the normal balance between dopamine 1 (D1) and dopamine 2 (D2) receptor activity (Lieberman et al., 1990). The imbalance in the striatal D1 and D2 receptors would impact the "direct" and "indirect" striatal outflow pathways, resulting in abnormal involuntary movements (Albin, Young, & Penney, 1995).

4.2 Tic Disorders

Psychomotor stimulants can elicit tics, which are defined as brief, repetitive, purposeless, nonrhythmic, involuntary movements (motor tics) or sounds (vocal tics, grunts, snorting) that share some, but not all, features of stereotypic movement disorders (APA, 2013). Stimulant-induced tics are similar to the stereotypic movements (excessive sniffing, gnawing, and head bobbing) produced by amphetamines in animals (Randrup & Munkvad, 1967). Tics, like some stereotypies in humans, can be voluntarily suppressed, at least transiently. After volitional suppression of tics, there is usually an outburst of pent-up tics.

Tics can be elicited by stimulant drug therapy in a small proportion of patients with ADHD who previously did not exhibit tics. It is not clear whether or not the patients would have developed tics if stimulants had not been used (Weiner & Sanchez-Ramos, 1992). Certainly, stimulant drugs may exacerbate tics in as many as 50% of patients who already have tics as part of Tourette's syndrome. Symptoms usually revert to the prior baseline level after discontinuation of the stimulant drug.

4.3 Dyskinesias (Chorea, Athetosis, and Dystonia)

A potential complication of chronic methamphetamine abuse is the development of abnormal involuntary movements (dyskinesia) most commonly characterized as a combination of chorea and athetosis. Choreoathetoid movements typically involve the limbs, neck, and face and often have a dance-like quality. Like other dyskinesias, symptoms disappear while patients sleep. There have been numerous reports of choreoathetosis in patients using or abusing amphetamines (Downes & Whyte, 2005; Lundh & Tunving, 1981; Morgan, Winter, & Wooten, 2004; Rhee, Albertson, & Douglas, 1988; Sperling & Horowitz, 1994). In one report, patients with underlying chorea intrinsic to specific diseases (e.g., Sydenham's, Huntington's, and Lupus) were given an intravenous dose of amphetamine to assess its effect on their baseline movements. In all of these patients, amphetamine dramatically worsened the underlying chorea (Klawans & Weiner, 1974). The increases in limb movements provoked by amphetamines could be prevented if patients were pretreated with the D2 receptor antagonist haloperidol (Klawans & Weiner, 1974). Since a group of control patients without chorea given amphetamine did not develop movement disorders, the authors suggested that the development of chorea from amphetamines may require an underlying damage to the striatum (Klawans & Weiner, 1974). This supposition would seem to be supported from several lines of evidence. Several studies have shown that methamphetamine abusers have evidence of dopaminergic deficits in the striatum (Volkow, Chang, Wang, Fowler, Ding, et al., 2001; Wilson et al., 1996; Yamamoto, Moszczynska, & Gudelsky, 2010) and chronic methamphetamine abusers, even without frank chorea, often exhibit movement disorders (Bartzokis et al., 1999). In some patients, movement disorders can last for years even after they have stopped using amphetamines (Lundh & Tunving, 1981; Rylander, 1972). Lastly, patients who have stopped abusing amphetamine, and subsequently recovered from their choreoathetoid movement disorder, will often redevelop symptoms the first time they use amphetamines again suggesting that patients may become permanently susceptible (Lundh & Tunving, 1981). Although in some patients dopamine antagonists and benzodiazepines have been found to relieve symptoms (Downes & Whyte, 2005; Klawans & Weiner, 1974; Rhee et al., 1988), in other studies they have had no benefit (Lundh & Tunving, 1981). Choreoathetoid movements have also been reported with other stimulants including cocaine (known as "crack dancing") (Bartzokis et al., 1999; Daras, Koppel, & Atos-Radzion, 1994; Rylander, 1972; Stork & Cantor, 1997). Although the paucity of literature on this topic suggests that the development of these symptoms is relatively rare, the fact that there are street names for this in English and Spanish would suggest it may occur much more commonly than has been reported in the medical literature (Daras et al., 1994).

Acute dystonic reactions (abnormal sustained posturing of the limbs, trunk, or facial grimacing due to prolonged contracture of skeletal muscles) have been reported in chronic cocaine abusers given haloperidol in a research setting (Kumor, Sherer, & Jaffe, 1986). These patients had been abstinent from cocaine for at least 10 days prior to treatment with haloperidol. Other researchers have reported that a history of cocaine abuse is associated with a threefold increased risk of dystonic reaction to neuroleptic drugs (Choy-Kwong & Lipton, 1989a). Acute dystonic reactions have also been reported in cocaine abusers not exposed to neuroleptic medications. Shortly after cocaine use, one patient developed transient focal dystonic movements that lasted 45 min (Merab, 1988). In another single case report, a 15-year-old girl admitted to a psychiatric service developed acute generalized dystonia 16 h after admission. She had not been treated with neuroleptics and the authors speculated that the dystonia was associated with cocaine withdrawal (Choy-Kwong & Lipton, 1989a). Most experts, however, do not report motor signs as a manifestation of a cocaine withdrawal syndrome. Instead, the cocaine abstinence syndrome is characterized by symptoms of psychological dependence such as drug craving, dysphoria, depression, and anhedonia.

4.4 PD and Methamphetamine Abuse

The animal and human research findings indicate that high-dose methamphetamine abuse causes alterations in striatal dopaminergic neurotransmission. Numerous pathology and imaging studies have shown reductions in striatal dopamine, tyrosine hydroxylase, and dopamine transporters (Guilarte, 2001; McCann et al., 2008; Moszczynska et al., 2004; Truong et al., 2005; Volkow, Chang, Wang, Fowler, Franceschi, et al., 2001; Volkow, Chang, Wang, Fowler, Leonido-Yee, et al., 2001; Wilson et al., 1996). More severe but similar findings are typical in persons with PD, so one might infer that chronic methamphetamine abusers could potentially trigger PD at least in susceptible individuals (Caligiuri & Buitenhuys, 2005; Guilarte, 2001; Moszczynska et al., 2004). PD involves loss of nigral dopaminergic neurons and their innervation of the striatum; methamphetamine abuse affects dopaminergic nerve terminals, but not the nigral cell bodies (Moszczynska et al., 2004). Moreover, reductions in striatal dopamine have a different distribution in methamphetamine abusers than in PD patients. Methamphetamine users have greater dopamine reductions in the caudate compared to the putamen with PD patients showing the inverse, with greater reduction in the putamen (Moszczynska et al., 2004). In addition, damaged dopaminergic nerve terminals in methamphetamine abusers begin to recover during abstinence. For example, the diminution of dopamine transporters in methamphetamine abusers was found to significantly recover with prolonged (>12 months) abstinence (Volkow, Chang, Wang, Fowler, Franceschi, et al., 2001). It is also possible that methamphetamine abusers do not actually damage their dopaminergic nerve terminals, and that the findings of reduced indicators of dopamine innervation (e.g., DA transporter (DAT) or VMAT2) represent compensatory responses to repeated amphetamine-triggered release of monoamines from storage vesicles. Evidence for this has been found in positron emission tomography (PET) studies showing reduction of VMAT2 in patients with PD, but not in abstinent methamphetamine abusers (Johanson et al., 2006; Wilson et al., 1996). A more recent PET scan study of nonabstinent methamphetamine abusers actually found increases in VMAT2 (Boileau et al., 2008). This was thought to be due to reductions in vesicular dopamine, depleted from recent release and resulting in less dopamine being available to compete for binding to VMAT2 (Boileau et al., 2008). Another consideration when comparing methamphetamine abusers to PD patients is the role of nicotinic cholinergic receptors. Activation of nicotinic receptors can influence the behavioral and neurochemical effects of psychomotor stimulant drugs and vice versa (Desai & Bergman, 2010). A significantly greater number of methamphetamine users smoke cigarettes compared to the general population (87–92% vs. 22%) (Weinberger & Sofuoglu, 2009). It is believed that cigarette smoking negatively correlates with development of PD (Hernan, Takkouche, Caamano-Isorna, & Gestal-Otero, 2002), so one can infer that methamphetamine abusers may be protected against PD (Caligiuri & Buitenhuys, 2005).

In contrast, there is some evidence that methamphetamine abuse does increase the risk for developing PD (Callaghan, Cunningham, Sajeev, & Kish, 2010; Christine, Garwood, Schrock, Austin, & McCulloch, 2010; Guilarte, 2001). A retrospective review of hospital admissions over a 10-year period found an increased incidence of PD among patients who had a prior history of being admitted with a methamphetamine-related problem (Callaghan et al., 2010). A phone survey revealed that PD patients were more likely (OR = 8, CI 1.6–41) to have used amphetamines than their unaffected spouses. In addition, the majority of these patients reported their exposures to amphetamines occurred years (~27) before symptom onset (Garwood, Bekele, McCulloch, & Christine, 2006). Compared to Parkinson's patients without a history of exposure, those patients with a history of amphetamine use were significantly younger at age of symptom onset, but not at age of diagnosis (Christine et al., 2010). These reports are subject to recall bias and other limitations inherent in retrospective studies. Much more research, especially prospective longitudinal long-term studies, will be necessary to establish a strong link between amphetamine use and the development of PD.

5. SERIOUS ADVERSE EFFECTS LEADING TO EMERGENCY ROOM VISITS AND HOSPITALIZATIONS

US nationwide estimates on drug-related visits to hospital emergency departments (EDs) are obtained from the Drug Abuse Warning Network (DAWN), a public health surveillance system managed by the Substance Abuse and Mental Health Services Administration (SAMHSA), US Department of Health and Human Services (HHS) (NIDA, 2011). In 2009, cocaine was involved in 422,896 ED visits and stimulants, including amphetamines and methamphetamine, were involved in 93,562 ED visits. According to data from a 2012 National Survey on Drug Use and Health

(NSDUH), over 12 million people (4.7% of the population) have tried methamphetamine at least once. NSDUH also reports that approximately 1.2 million people used methamphetamine in the year leading up to the survey.

5.1 Stimulant Abuse and Stroke

Abuse of either cocaine or amphetamine, or both, is considered a risk factor for stroke and is described as such in many textbooks of medicine and neurology. In addition, the Causative Classification System for Ischemic Stroke (Arsava et al., 2010; Ay et al., 2007) recognizes cocaine as a potential cause of stroke by virtue of exclusion. Recently, a systematic review of the literature was conducted on the relationship between stroke and cocaine use (Sordo et al., 2014). The authors searched all bibliographic databases until January 2014 for articles on the epidemiological association between cocaine use and strokes. Of 996 articles found, 9 were selected for thorough review. Seven were case–control studies (CCSs) and two were cross-sectional studies (CSSs). One CCS and one CSS showed an association between cocaine and hemorrhagic strokes. The latter study also reported a positive relationship with ischemic stroke. Another CCS found the cocaine exposure to be associated with stroke without distinguishing between stroke types. One forensic CCS found that deaths with cocaine-positive toxicology presented a 14.3- and 4.6-fold increased risk of atherosclerosis compared to opioid-related deaths and hanging deaths, respectively. However, the authors pointed out that not all the reviewed epidemiological studies reported an association between stroke and cocaine use. Indeed, three CCSs and one CSS did not find any relationship between cocaine and strokes.

Nevertheless, the biological plausibility for cocaine as a causative factor in stroke is supported by preclinical evidence in animal models. Cocaine administration increases blood pressure, heart rate, and causes diffuse vasoconstriction (Knuepfer, Rowe, Schwartz, & Lomax, 2005; Matsumura, Tsuchihashi, & Abe, 2001; Mo, Arruda, Dunea, & Singh, 1999). These factors lead to reduced supply of cerebral blood (Johnson et al., 1998; Mathew, Wilson, Lowe, & Humphries, 1996) and oxygen (Gollub et al., 1998; Yonetani et al., 1994) and increased vascular resistance in the CNS in both animals and humans (Herning, Better, Nelson, Gorelick, & Cadet, 1999). Cocaine can elicit hypercoagulable states (Heesch et al., 2000; Hobbs, Moore, Penkala, Bolgiano, & Lopez, 2013; Rinder, Ault, Jatlow, Kosten, & Smith, 1994) and can produce cardiac arrhythmias (O'Leary &

Hancox, 2010) that could lead to cardioembolic strokes. Cocaine consumption has also been associated with inflammatory changes in blood vessels and endothelial dysfunction (Ross et al., 2002; Su, Li, Li, Altura, & Altura, 2003), which are considered a possible pathogenesis of CNS vasculitis (Fiala et al., 1998; Gan et al., 1999). The vasculitis is frequently manifested clinically after a stroke, and several cases have been published describing both conditions following cocaine consumption (Merkel, Koroshetz, Irizarry, & Cudkowicz, 1995). Furthermore, cocaine may be implicated in the exacerbation of pathologies like cerebral aneurysm rupture due to sudden increases in blood pressure (Buttner, 2012) or ischemic stroke secondary to atherosclerosis in cerebral vessels (Su et al., 2003), or in large and small vessel (lacunar stroke) disease (Lucena et al., 2010).

Despite some epidemiological data mentioned above showing an association between stroke and cocaine use, inadequate control for confounding factors is not uncommon. The relationship between strokes and cocaine use in humans may be affected by numerous factors such as demographics, lifestyle, patterns of cocaine use, concomitant use of other drugs (European Monitoring Centre for Drugs and Drug Addiction, 2007; Nakamura et al., 2012; Patra et al., 2010), and other health conditions (i.e., diabetes mellitus, hypertension, and cerebral vascular malformations) (Ferro, Massaro, & Mas, 2010; National Institute of Neurological Disorders and Stroke, 2012; O'Donnell, et al., 2010; Rothwell, et al., 2010). Experts have called for more rigorous observational studies, including cohort approaches, to better quantify this risk, and stroke type, hypertension variation, frequency/length of cocaine use, amphetamines co-use, and other factors that also will need to be taken into consideration.

Is amphetamine abuse, with its longer duration of action, more likely to cause stroke than cocaine? Review of a database of Texas hospital discharges from 2000 to 2003 was conducted to determine if young adults who abuse amphetamine or cocaine were at higher risk of stroke (Westover, McBride, & Haley, 2007). During the 3-year interval under review, the rate of increase of amphetamine abuse was greater than that of cocaine abuse. The rate of stroke also increased, especially among amphetamine abusers. Amphetamine abuse was significantly associated with hemorrhagic stroke, but not with ischemic stroke. Cocaine was associated with both hemorrhagic and ischemic stroke. The abuse of amphetamine, but not of cocaine, was associated with a higher risk of death after hemorrhagic stroke. Potential misclassification of drug abuse history is an unavoidable hazard in studies of this sort.

Animal studies also support a causal link between amphetamine abuse and stroke. Intravenous amphetamine administration to rhesus monkey causes microhemorrhages, thrombosis, infarction, poor vascular filling, and fragmentation of small arterioles and capillary beds (Rumbaugh et al., 1971).

5.2 Stimulants and Seizures

The relationship between cocaine use and convulsions in humans has been known for at least 100 years (Pulay, 1922). The mechanism responsible for its convulsive properties is believed to be a combination of cocaine's effects on monoaminergic neurons and its local anesthetic effects (Russell & Stripling, 1987). Repeated use of cocaine may lower seizure threshold, an effect that has pathophysiologic parallels with the kindling phenomenon (Stripling, 1983). Interestingly, cocaine-elicited seizures do not occur as frequently as a primary toxic effect in humans as one might predict from preclinical animal studies. In a review of records of 283 consecutive cocaine abusers admitted to a municipal hospital over a period of 18 months, only 8 patients (2.8%) had seizures (Choy-Kwong & Lipton, 1989b). There was a clear temporal association between seizures and cocaine use in four patients (1.4%). In the remaining four patients, the seizures were secondary to postanoxic encephalopathy, stroke, brain contusion, or alcohol withdrawal. A similar low incidence of seizures was reported based on a review of emergency room visits and hospitalizations (Lowenstein et al., 1987). Generalized seizures occurred in 2.3% of the patients; they occurred in 1.6% of patients within 12 h of cocaine use. A higher seizure frequency of 7.9% was reported in a retrospective study of 474 patients with cocaine-related medical complications (Pascual-Leone, Dhuna, Altafullah, & Anderson, 1990). In this study, cocaine-induced seizures were defined as convulsion occurring within 90 min of cocaine ingestion as per witness report; 32 of 403 (7.9%) patients met this criterion. Of 474 patient records reviewed, 403 patients had no prior history of epilepsy. The majority of seizures were single, generalized, induced by intravenous or smoked crack cocaine, and were not associated with any lasting neurologic deficits. Most of the seizures that were focal, multiple, or induced by intranasal cocaine were associated with an acute intracerebral complication or concurrent use of other drugs. Of 71 patients with a prior history of noncocaine-related seizures, 12 (16.9%) presented with cocaine-induced seizures. Most of these patients had multiple seizures that were of the same type as those recorded in their history. In general, cocaine elicited seizures faster and more frequently following intravenous and crack cocaine administration due to rapid attainment of high serum and brain levels (Pascual-Leone et al., 1990). Snorting of cocaine, however, induced seizures primarily in patients with a history of seizures, with concurrent use of other epileptogenic drugs or with stroke.

In contrast to the low frequency of seizures in hospital-based reviews, analysis of seizures occurring prior to cocaine-related deaths demonstrates a much higher frequency of fits. An autopsy study of 36 fatalities due to cocaine use in Dade County, Florida, revealed that 13 (36%) of the patients experienced seizures prior to death (Mittleman & Wetli, 1984).

5.3 Stimulants, Hyperpyrexia, and Rhabdomyolysis

Methamphetamine use is responsible for an estimated 94,000 ED admissions annually, with elevated body temperature appearing as an invariable presenting symptom (Matsumoto et al., 2014; NIDA, 2011). Hyperthermia can promote rhabdomyolysis, multiorgan failure, release of excitotoxic neurotransmitters, increased reactive oxygen species production, and heightened breakdown of cytoskeletal proteins (Matsumoto et al., 2014). However, rhabdomyolysis is not an inevitable consequence of hyperthermia. In a series of cocaine-related cases of rhabdomyolysis, 33% of the patients presented with hyperpyrexia and 90% with agitation (Roth, Alarcon, Fernandez, Preston, & Bourgoignie, 1988). The mechanism of stimulant-induced rhabdomyolysis has been postulated to be due to exaggeration of normal sympathomimetic actions, e.g., prolonged vasoconstriction of intramuscular vascular beds, combined with agitation, increased muscle activity, and hyperpyrexia. Increased muscle activity or muscle rigidity and hyperpyrexia from a number of causes, including heat stroke and neuroleptic malignant syndrome, have been known causes of rhabdomyolysis (Knochel, 1981). Hyperpyrexia has been observed frequently in cocaine intoxication and has been thought to be due to central sympathomimetic actions in the hypothalamus, combined with increased muscle activity (Ritchie & Greene, 1985).

Other stimulants such as MDMA and drugs, such as phencyclidine, that cause hyperpyrexia and agitation have also been associated with rhabdomyolysis (Cogen, Rigg, Simmons, & Domino, 1978; Kendrick, Hull, & Knochel, 1977). Cocaine has been postulated to exert direct toxicity to skeletal muscle just as it can to cardiac muscle (Peng & Duan, 1989). Another potential explanation for the rhabdomyolysis associated with stimulant abuse is the possibility of contamination of the drug with adulterants such as arsenic, strychnine, and phencyclidine, any of which can cause rhabdomyolysis (Nolte, 1991).

Dantrolene is a recommended treatment for rhabdomyolysis associated with cocaine use, based on its usefulness in treatment of malignant hyperthermia (Gay, 1982; Hard, 1989). It has also been reported anecdotally to be useful in alleviating rigidity in other types of intoxication caused by agents as diverse as neuroleptics, phenelzine, amitriptyline, and carbon monoxide (Fox, 1989). However, there are no reported cases of successful treatment of cocaine-associated rigidity with dantrolene (Fox, 1989).

A recent review of the literature on the hyperthermic effects of amphetamine underscores that no specific pharmacological profile exists for the treatment of stimulant-induced hyperthermia and clinicians must focus on cooling the body (Matsumoto et al., 2014). Cooling, accomplished with external or internal means, remains the primary method for the clinical treatment of hyperthermia (Matsumoto et al., 2014). External cooling measures can include cool water submersion, misting accompanied by fans, or hypothermia blankets. Attention must be paid to ensure skin cooling is not performed too quickly as rapid skin cooling produces shivering and vasoconstriction, which would minimize therapeutic benefit. Endovascular cooling, in which the temperature of the patient's blood is lowered via a cooling catheter, while not generally deemed necessary, is capable of inducing rapid cooling while reducing the impact of shivering and vasoconstriction. While these methods have been shown to be beneficial in the treatment of hyperthermia for other disease states, currently it is unknown if these treatments result in better patient outcomes following stimulant overdoses.

6. SUMMARY

Psychomotor stimulants increase alertness, elevate mood, and decrease appetite and the need for sleep. These agents also possess powerful reinforcing properties, mediated by dopamine release in the mesolimbic system that may lead to excessive self-administration and dependence. Epidemics of stimulant abuse have occurred historically usually related to the introduction of new compounds or new routes of administration. The beneficial actions, as well as toxic effects of stimulants, are related primarily to interaction with monoaminergic neurotransmission in the central and peripheral sympathetic nervous systems. The most common complications of stimulant use that result in visits to emergency rooms and hospital admissions are referable to psychiatric and neurologic symptoms. Neurologic complications most commonly include seizures and stroke, both hemorrhagic and ischemic. Relative to the prevalence of stimulant abuse in most cities, the incidence of stroke and seizures is small. Stimulant-induced stroke can be linked to underlying abnormalities of the cerebrovascular system in almost one half of the cases. Other complications such as movement disorders (punding, tics, choreoathetosis, and dystonia) and rhabdomyolysis are reported in the literature, but are relatively rare.

ACKNOWLEDGMENT

This work was supported by Helen Ellis Endowment. Thanks to Sofia O'Neill-Sanchez for editing the manuscript.

REFERENCES

Abourashed, E. A., El-Alfy, A. T., Khan, I. A., & Walker, L. (2003). Ephedra in perspective—A current review. *Phytotherapy Research*, *17*(7), 703–712. http://dx.doi.org/10.1002/ptr.1337.

Albin, R. L., Young, A. B., & Penney, J. B. (1995). The functional anatomy of disorders of the basal ganglia. *Trends in Neurosciences*, *18*(2), 63–64.

Aliane, V., Perez, S., Bohren, Y., Deniau, J. M., & Kemel, M. L. (2011). Key role of striatal cholinergic interneurons in processes leading to arrest of motor stereotypies. *Brain*, *134*(Pt. 1), 110–118. http://dx.doi.org/10.1093/brain/awq285.

Anglin, M. D., Burke, C., Perrochet, B., Stamper, E., & Dawud-Noursi, S. (2000). History of the methamphetamine problem. *Journal of Psychoactive Drugs*, *32*(2), 137–141. http://dx.doi.org/10.1080/02791072.2000.10400221.

Angrist, B., Lee, H. K., & Gershon, S. (1974). The antagonism of amphetamine-induced symptomatology by a neuroleptic. *The American Journal of Psychiatry*, *131*(7), 817–819.

APA. (2013). *Diagnostic and statistical manual of mental disorders* (5th ed.). Arlington, VA: American Psychiatric Publishing.

Arsava, E. M., Ballabio, E., Benner, T., Cole, J. W., Delgado-Martinez, M. P., Dichgans, M., et al. (2010). The causative classification of stroke system: An international reliability and optimization study. *Neurology*, *75*(14), 1277–1284. http://dx.doi.org/10.1212/WNL.0b013e3181f612ce.

Ay, H., Benner, T., Arsava, E. M., Furie, K. L., Singhal, A. B., Jensen, M. B., et al. (2007). A computerized algorithm for etiologic classification of ischemic stroke: The causative classification of stroke system. *Stroke*, *38*(11), 2979–2984. http://dx.doi.org/10.1161/STROKEAHA.107.490896.

Bartzokis, G., Beckson, M., Wirshing, D. A., Lu, P. H., Foster, J. A., & Mintz, J. (1999). Choreoathetoid movements in cocaine dependence. *Biological Psychiatry*, *45*(12), 1630–1635.

Bell, D. S. (1965). Comparison of amphetamine psychosis and schizophrenia. *The British Journal of Psychiatry*, *111*, 701–707.

Boileau, I., Rusjan, P., Houle, S., Wilkins, D., Tong, J., Selby, P., et al. (2008). Increased vesicular monoamine transporter binding during early abstinence in human methamphetamine users: Is VMAT2 a stable dopamine neuron biomarker? *The Journal of Neuroscience*, *28*(39), 9850–9856. http://dx.doi.org/10.1523/JNEUROSCI.3008-08.2008.

Buckley, P. F. (1998). Substance abuse in schizophrenia: A review. *The Journal of Clinical Psychiatry*, *59*(Suppl. 3), 26–30.

Buttner, A. (2012). Neuropathological alterations in cocaine abuse. *Current Medicinal Chemistry, 19*(33), 5597–5600.

Byck, R. (1974). Introduction. In R. Byck (Ed.), *Cocaine papers* (p. xvii). New York: Stonehill Publishing.

Caligiuri, M. P., & Buitenhuys, C. (2005). Do preclinical findings of methamphetamine-induced motor abnormalities translate to an observable clinical phenotype? *Neuropsychopharmacology, 30*(12), 2125–2134. http://dx.doi.org/10.1038/sj.npp.1300859.

Callaghan, R. C., Cunningham, J. K., Sajeev, G., & Kish, S. J. (2010). Incidence of Parkinson's disease among hospital patients with methamphetamine-use disorders. *Movement Disorders, 25*(14), 2333–2339. http://dx.doi.org/10.1002/mds.23263.

Carvalho, F. (2003). The toxicological potential of khat. *Journal of Ethnopharmacology, 87*(1), 1–2.

Carvalho, M., Carmo, H., Costa, V. M., Capela, J. P., Pontes, H., Remiao, F., et al. (2012). Toxicity of amphetamines: An update. *Archives of Toxicology, 86*(8), 1167–1231. http://dx.doi.org/10.1007/s00204-012-0815-5.

Chambers, R. A., Krystal, J. H., & Self, D. W. (2001). A neurobiological basis for substance abuse comorbidity in schizophrenia. *Biological Psychiatry, 50*(2), 71–83.

Chen, C. K., Lin, S. K., Sham, P. C., Ball, D., Loh el, W., & Murray, R. M. (2005). Morbid risk for psychiatric disorder among the relatives of methamphetamine users with and without psychosis. *American Journal of Medical Genetics. Part B, Neuropsychiatric Genetics, 136B*(1), 87–91. http://dx.doi.org/10.1002/ajmg.b.30187.

Chen, C. K., Lin, S. K., Sham, P. C., Ball, D., Loh, E. W., Hsiao, C. C., et al. (2003). Premorbid characteristics and co-morbidity of methamphetamine users with and without psychosis. *Psychological Medicine, 33*(8), 1407–1414.

Choy-Kwong, M., & Lipton, R. B. (1989a). Dystonia related to cocaine withdrawal: A case report and pathogenic hypothesis. *Neurology, 39*(7), 996–997.

Choy-Kwong, M., & Lipton, R. B. (1989b). Seizures in hospitalized cocaine users. *Neurology, 39*(3), 425–427.

Christine, C. W., Garwood, E. R., Schrock, L. E., Austin, D. E., & McCulloch, C. E. (2010). Parkinsonism in patients with a history of amphetamine exposure. *Movement Disorders, 25*(2), 228–231. http://dx.doi.org/10.1002/mds.22915.

Cogen, F. C., Rigg, G., Simmons, J. L., & Domino, E. F. (1978). Phencyclidine-associated acute rhabdomyolysis. *Annals of Internal Medicine, 88*(2), 210–212.

Cruickshank, C. C., & Dyer, K. R. (2009). A review of the clinical pharmacology of methamphetamine. *Addiction, 104*(7), 1085–1099. http://dx.doi.org/10.1111/j.1360-0443.2009.02564.x.

Daras, M., Koppel, B. S., & Atos-Radzion, E. (1994). Cocaine-induced choreoathetoid movements ('crack dancing'). *Neurology, 44*(4), 751–752.

Derlet, R. W., & Heischober, B. (1990). Methamphetamine. Stimulant of the 1990s? *The Western Journal of Medicine, 153*(6), 625–628.

Desai, R. I., & Bergman, J. (2010). Drug discrimination in methamphetamine-trained rats: Effects of cholinergic nicotinic compounds. *The Journal of Pharmacology and Experimental Therapeutics, 335*(3), 807–816. http://dx.doi.org/10.1124/jpet.110.173773.

Downes, M. A., & Whyte, I. M. (2005). Amphetamine-induced movement disorder. *Emergency Medicine Australasia, 17*(3), 277–280. http://dx.doi.org/10.1111/j.1742-6723.2005.00735.x.

European Monitoring Centre for Drugs and Drug Addiction. (2007). *Cocaine and crack cocaine: A growing public health issue.* Luxembourg. Retrieved from, http://www.emcdda.europa.eu/attachements.cfm/att_44748_EN_TDSI07002ENC.pdf.

Fasano, A., Barra, A., Nicosia, P., Rinaldi, F., Bria, P., Bentivoglio, A. R., et al. (2008). Cocaine addiction: From habits to stereotypical-repetitive behaviors and punding. *Drug and Alcohol Dependence, 96*(1–2), 178–182. http://dx.doi.org/10.1016/j.drugalcdep.2008.02.005.

Fasano, A., & Petrovic, I. (2010). Insights into pathophysiology of punding reveal possible treatment strategies. *Molecular Psychiatry*, *15*(6), 560–573. http://dx.doi.org/10.1038/mp.2009.95.

Ferro, J. M., Massaro, A. R., & Mas, J. L. (2010). Aetiological diagnosis of ischaemic stroke in young adults. *Lancet Neurology*, *9*(11), 1085–1096. http://dx.doi.org/10.1016/S1474-4422(10)70251-9.

Fiala, M., Gan, X. H., Zhang, L., House, S. D., Newton, T., Graves, M. C., et al. (1998). Cocaine enhances monocyte migration across the blood–brain barrier. Cocaine's connection to AIDS dementia and vasculitis? *Advances in Experimental Medicine and Biology*, *437*, 199–205.

Fischman, M. W., Schuster, C. R., Resnekov, L., Shick, J. F., Krasnegor, N. A., Fennell, W., et al. (1976). Cardiovascular and subjective effects of intravenous cocaine administration in humans. *Archives of General Psychiatry*, *33*(8), 983–989.

Fleckenstein, A. E., Volz, T. J., Riddle, E. L., Gibb, J. W., & Hanson, G. R. (2007). New insights into the mechanism of action of amphetamines. *Annual Review of Pharmacology and Toxicology*, *47*, 681–698. http://dx.doi.org/10.1146/annurev.pharmtox.47.120505.105140.

Fox, A. W. (1989). More on rhabdomyolysis associated with cocaine intoxication. *The New England Journal of Medicine*, *321*(18), 1271.

Gan, X., Zhang, L., Berger, O., Stins, M. F., Way, D., Taub, D. D., et al. (1999). Cocaine enhances brain endothelial adhesion molecules and leukocyte migration. *Clinical Immunology*, *91*(1), 68–76. http://dx.doi.org/10.1006/clim.1998.4683.

Garwood, E. R., Bekele, W., McCulloch, C. E., & Christine, C. W. (2006). Amphetamine exposure is elevated in Parkinson's disease. *Neurotoxicology*, *27*(6), 1003–1006. http://dx.doi.org/10.1016/j.neuro.2006.03.015.

Gawin, F. H. (1991). Cocaine addiction: Psychology and neurophysiology. *Science*, *251*(5001), 1580–1586.

Gawin, F. H., & Ellinwood, E. H., Jr. (1988). Cocaine and other stimulants. Actions, abuse, and treatment. *The New England Journal of Medicine*, *318*(18), 1173–1182. http://dx.doi.org/10.1056/NEJM198805053181806.

Gay, G. R. (1982). Clinical management of acute and chronic cocaine poisoning. *Annals of Emergency Medicine*, *11*(10), 562–572.

Gilbert, S. J., & Burgess, P. W. (2008). Executive function. *Current Biology*, *18*(3), R110–R114. http://dx.doi.org/10.1016/j.cub.2007.12.014.

Gollub, R. L., Breiter, H. C., Kantor, H., Kennedy, D., Gastfriend, D., Mathew, R. T., et al. (1998). Cocaine decreases cortical cerebral blood flow but does not obscure regional activation in functional magnetic resonance imaging in human subjects. *Journal of Cerebral Blood Flow and Metabolism*, *18*(7), 724–734. http://dx.doi.org/10.1097/00004647-199807000-00003.

Gonzales, R., Mooney, L., & Rawson, R. A. (2010). The methamphetamine problem in the United States. *Annual Review of Public Health*, *31*, 385–398. http://dx.doi.org/10.1146/annurev.publhealth.012809.103600.

Guilarte, T. R. (2001). Is methamphetamine abuse a risk factor in parkinsonism? *Neurotoxicology*, *22*(6), 725–731.

Halpin, L. E., Collins, S. A., & Yamamoto, B. K. (2014). Neurotoxicity of methamphetamine and 3,4-methylenedioxymethamphetamine. *Life Sciences*, *97*(1), 37–44. http://dx.doi.org/10.1016/j.lfs.2013.07.014.

Hard, C. (1989). Acute rhabdomyolysis associated with cocaine intoxication. *The New England Journal of Medicine*, *320*(10), 667–668. http://dx.doi.org/10.1056/NEJM198903093201011.

Hearn, W. L., Flynn, D. D., Hime, G. W., Rose, S., Cofino, J. C., Mantero-Atienza, E., et al. (1991). Cocaethylene: A unique cocaine metabolite displays high affinity for the dopamine transporter. *Journal of Neurochemistry*, *56*(2), 698–701.

Heesch, C. M., Wilhelm, C. R., Ristich, J., Adnane, J., Bontempo, F. A., & Wagner, W. R. (2000). Cocaine activates platelets and increases the formation of circulating platelet containing microaggregates in humans. *Heart, 83*(6), 688–695.

Hernan, M. A., Takkouche, B., Caamano-Isorna, F., & Gestal-Otero, J. J. (2002). A meta-analysis of coffee drinking, cigarette smoking, and the risk of Parkinson's disease. *Annals of Neurology, 52*(3), 276–284. http://dx.doi.org/10.1002/ana.10277.

Herning, R. I., Better, W., Nelson, R., Gorelick, D., & Cadet, J. L. (1999). The regulation of cerebral blood flow during intravenous cocaine administration in cocaine abusers. *Annals of the New York Academy of Sciences, 890*, 489–494.

Hobbs, W. E., Moore, E. E., Penkala, R. A., Bolgiano, D. D., & Lopez, J. A. (2013). Cocaine and specific cocaine metabolites induce von Willebrand factor release from endothelial cells in a tissue-specific manner. *Arteriosclerosis, Thrombosis, and Vascular Biology, 33*(6), 1230–1237. http://dx.doi.org/10.1161/ATVBAHA.113.301436.

Inaba, T., Stewart, D. J., & Kalow, W. (1978). Metabolism of cocaine in man. *Clinical Pharmacology and Therapeutics, 23*(5), 547–552.

Iwanami, A., Sugiyama, A., Kuroki, N., Toda, S., Kato, N., Nakatani, Y., et al. (1994). Patients with methamphetamine psychosis admitted to a psychiatric hospital in Japan. A preliminary report. *Acta Psychiatrica Scandinavica, 89*(6), 428–432.

Jaffe, J. (1985). Drug addiction and drug abuse. In G. L. Goodman, A. Gilman, T. W. Rall, & F. Murad (Eds.), *Pharmacological basis of therapeutics* (7th ed., pp. 532–581). New York: MacMillan Publishing Company.

Johanson, C. E., Frey, K. A., Lundahl, L. H., Keenan, P., Lockhart, N., Roll, J., et al. (2006). Cognitive function and nigrostriatal markers in abstinent methamphetamine abusers. *Psychopharmacology, 185*(3), 327–338. http://dx.doi.org/10.1007/s00213-006-0330-6.

Johnson, B., Lamki, L., Fang, B., Barron, B., Wagner, L., Wells, L., et al. (1998). Demonstration of dose-dependent global and regional cocaine-induced reductions in brain blood flow using a novel approach to quantitative single photon emission computerized tomography. *Neuropsychopharmacology, 18*(5), 377–384. http://dx.doi.org/10.1016/S0893-133X(97)00168-1.

Kendrick, W. C., Hull, A. R., & Knochel, J. P. (1977). Rhabdomyolysis and shock after intravenous amphetamine administration. *Annals of Internal Medicine, 86*(4), 381–387. http://dx.doi.org/10.1089/ten.2005.11.1085.

Klawans, H. L., & Weiner, W. J. (1974). The effect of d-amphetamine on choreiform movement disorders. *Neurology, 24*(4), 312–318.

Kleven, M. S., & Seiden, L. S. (1992). Methamphetamine-induced neurotoxicity: Structure activity relationships. *Annals of the New York Academy of Sciences, 654*, 292–301.

Knochel, J. P. (1981). Serum calcium derangements in rhabdomyolysis. *The New England Journal of Medicine, 305*(3), 161–163. http://dx.doi.org/10.1056/NEJM198107163050307.

Knuepfer, M. M., Rowe, K. D., Schwartz, J. A., & Lomax, L. L. (2005). Role of angiotensin II and corticotropin-releasing hormone in hemodynamic responses to cocaine and stress. *Regulatory Peptides, 127*(1–3), 1–10. http://dx.doi.org/10.1016/j.regpep.2004.12.010.

Konno, C., Taguchi, T., Tamada, M., & Hikino, H. (1979). Ephedroxane, antiinflammatory principle of Ephedra herbs. *Phytochemistry, 18*, 697–698.

Kumor, K., Sherer, M., & Jaffe, J. (1986). Haloperidol-induced dystonia in cocaine addicts. *Lancet, 2*(8519), 1341–1342.

Lake, C. R., & Quirk, R. S. (1984). CNS stimulants and the look-alike drugs. *The Psychiatric Clinics of North America*, 7(4), 689–701.

Lieberman, J. A., Kinon, B. J., & Loebel, A. D. (1990). Dopaminergic mechanisms in idiopathic and drug-induced psychoses. *Schizophrenia Bulletin, 16*(1), 97–110.

Lowenstein, D. H., Massa, S. M., Rowbotham, M. C., Collins, S. D., McKinney, H. E., & Simon, R. P. (1987). Acute neurologic and psychiatric complications associated with cocaine abuse. *The American Journal of Medicine, 83*(5), 841–846.

Lucena, J., Blanco, M., Jurado, C., Rico, A., Salguero, M., Vazquez, R., et al. (2010). Cocaine-related sudden death: A prospective investigation in south-west Spain. *European Heart Journal, 31*(3), 318–329. http://dx.doi.org/10.1093/eurheartj/ehp557.

Lundh, H., & Tunving, K. (1981). An extrapyramidal choreiform syndrome caused by amphetamine addiction. *Journal of Neurology, Neurosurgery, and Psychiatry, 44*(8), 728–730.

Madden, J. A., & Powers, R. H. (1990). Effect of cocaine and cocaine metabolites on cerebral arteries in vitro. *Life Sciences, 47*(13), 1109–1114.

Mahoney, J. J., 3rd., Kalechstein, A. D., De La Garza, R., 2nd., & Newton, T. F. (2008). Presence and persistence of psychotic symptoms in cocaine- versus methamphetamine-dependent participants. *The American Journal on Addictions, 17*(2), 83–98. http://dx.doi.org/10.1080/10550490701861201.

Mathew, R. J., Wilson, W. H., Lowe, J. V., & Humphries, D. (1996). Acute changes in cranial blood flow after cocaine hydrochloride. *Biological Psychiatry, 40*(7), 609–616.

Matsumoto, R. R., Seminerio, M. J., Turner, R. C., Robson, M. J., Nguyen, L., Miller, D. B., et al. (2014). Methamphetamine-induced toxicity: An updated review on issues related to hyperthermia. *Pharmacology & Therapeutics, 144*(1), 28–40. http://dx.doi.org/10.1016/j.pharmthera.2014.05.001.

Matsumura, K., Tsuchihashi, T., & Abe, I. (2001). Central human cocaine- and amphetamine-regulated transcript peptide 55–102 increases arterial pressure in conscious rabbits. *Hypertension, 38*(5), 1096–1100.

McCann, U. D., Kuwabara, H., Kumar, A., Palermo, M., Abbey, R., Brasic, J., et al. (2008). Persistent cognitive and dopamine transporter deficits in abstinent methamphetamine users. *Synapse, 62*(2), 91–100. http://dx.doi.org/10.1002/syn.20471.

Merab, J. (1988). Acute dystonic reaction to cocaine. *The American Journal of Medicine, 84*(3 Pt. 1), 564.

Merkel, P. A., Koroshetz, W. J., Irizarry, M. C., & Cudkowicz, M. E. (1995). Cocaine-associated cerebral vasculitis. *Seminars in Arthritis and Rheumatism, 25*(3), 172–183.

Mittleman, R. E., & Wetli, C. V. (1984). Death caused by recreational cocaine use. An update. *JAMA, 252*(14), 1889–1893.

Mo, W., Arruda, J. A., Dunea, G., & Singh, A. K. (1999). Cocaine-induced hypertension: Role of the peripheral sympathetic system. *Pharmacological Research, 40*(2), 139–145. http://dx.doi.org/10.1006/phrs.1999.0503.

Morgan, J. C., Winter, W. C., & Wooten, G. F. (2004). Amphetamine-induced chorea in attention deficit-hyperactivity disorder. *Movement Disorders, 19*(7), 840–842. http://dx.doi.org/10.1002/mds.20081.

Moszczynska, A., Fitzmaurice, P., Ang, L., Kalasinsky, K. S., Schmunk, G. A., Peretti, F. J., et al. (2004). Why is parkinsonism not a feature of human methamphetamine users? *Brain, 127*(Pt. 2), 363–370. http://dx.doi.org/10.1093/brain/awh046.

Nakamura, K., Nakagawa, H., Sakurai, M., Murakami, Y., Irie, F., Fujiyoshi, A., et al. (2012). Influence of smoking combined with another risk factor on the risk of mortality from coronary heart disease and stroke: Pooled analysis of 10 Japanese cohort studies. *Cerebrovascular Diseases, 33*(5), 480–491. http://dx.doi.org/10.1159/000336764.

National Institute of Neurological Disorders and Stroke, NIH. (2012). Final Report of the Stroke Progress Review Group – January 2012. *National Institute of Neurological Disorders and Stroke (NINDS-NIH).* Retrieved from http://www.ninds.nih.gov/about_ninds/groups/stroke_prg/2012-stroke-prg-full-report.htm.

NIDA. (2011). *Drug facts: Drug-related hospital emergency room visits.* Rockville, MD: Drug Abuse Warning Network (DAWN).

NIDA. (2014). *Nationwide trends in drug abuse.* from, http://www.drugabuse.gov/publications/drugfacts/nationwide-trends.

Nolte, K. B. (1991). Rhabdomyolysis associated with cocaine abuse. *Human Pathology, 22*(11), 1141–1145.

O'Connor, A. D., Rusyniak, D. E., & Bruno, A. (2005). Cerebrovascular and cardiovascular complications of alcohol and sympathomimetic drug abuse. *The Medical Clinics of North America*, *89*(6), 1343–1358. http://dx.doi.org/10.1016/j.mcna.2005.06.010.

O'Donnell, M. J., Xavier, D., Liu, L., Zhang, H., Chin, S. L., Rao-Melacini, P., et al. (2010). Risk factors for ischaemic and intracerebral haemorrhagic stroke in 22 countries (the INTERSTROKE study): a case-control study. *Lancet*, *376*(9735), 112–123. http://dx.doi.org/10.1016/S0140-6736(10)60834-3.

Office of National Drug Control Policy. (2011). *America's drug use profile*. http://www.ncjrs.gov/ondcppubs/publications/policy/ndcs01/chap2.html.

O'Leary, M. E., & Hancox, J. C. (2010). Role of voltage-gated sodium, potassium and calcium channels in the development of cocaine-associated cardiac arrhythmias. *British Journal of Clinical Pharmacology*, *69*(5), 427–442. http://dx.doi.org/10.1111/j.1365-2125.2010.03629.x.

O'Sullivan, S. S., Evans, A. H., & Lees, A. J. (2009). Dopamine dysregulation syndrome: An overview of its epidemiology, mechanisms and management. *CNS Drugs*, *23*(2), 157–170. http://dx.doi.org/10.2165/00023210-200923020-00005.

Pascual-Leone, A., Dhuna, A., Altafullah, I., & Anderson, D. C. (1990). Cocaine-induced seizures. *Neurology*, *40*(3 Pt. 1), 404–407.

Patra, J., Taylor, B., Irving, H., Roerecke, M., Baliunas, D., Mohapatra, S., et al. (2010). Alcohol consumption and the risk of morbidity and mortality for different stroke types—A systematic review and meta-analysis. *BMC Public Health*, *10*, 258. http://dx.doi.org/10.1186/1471-2458-10-258.

Peng, W., & Duan, S. F. (1989). The acute effects of ligustrazini on hemodynamics and right cardiac function in pulmonary arterial hypertension secondary to chronic obstructive pulmonary disease. *Journal of Tongji Medical University*, *9*(2), 100–102.

Pierce, R. C., & Kalivas, P. W. (1997). A circuitry model of the expression of behavioral sensitization to amphetamine-like psychostimulants. *Brain Research. Brain Research Reviews*, *25*(2), 192–216.

Pulay, E. (1922). Cocaine poisoning. *JAMA*, *78*, 1855.

Randrup, A., & Munkvad, I. (1967). Stereotyped activities produced by amphetamine in several animal species and man. *Psychopharmacologia*, *11*(4), 300–310.

Rhee, K. J., Albertson, T. E., & Douglas, J. C. (1988). Choreoathetoid disorder associated with amphetamine-like drugs. *The American Journal of Emergency Medicine*, *6*(2), 131–133.

Rinder, H. M., Ault, K. A., Jatlow, P. I., Kosten, T. R., & Smith, B. R. (1994). Platelet alpha-granule release in cocaine users. *Circulation*, *90*(3), 1162–1167.

Rippeth, J. D., Heaton, R. K., Carey, C. L., Marcotte, T. D., Moore, D. J., Gonzalez, R., et al. (2004). Methamphetamine dependence increases risk of neuropsychological impairment in HIV infected persons. *Journal of the International Neuropsychological Society*, *10*(1), 1–14. http://dx.doi.org/10.1017/S1355617704101021.

Ritchie, J. M., & Greene, N. M. (1985). Local anesthetics. In A. G. Gilman, L. S. Goodman, & T. W. Rall (Eds.), *The pharmacological basis of therapeutics* (p. 302). New York: MacMillan.

Ritz, M. C., Lamb, R. J., Goldberg, S. R., & Kuhar, M. J. (1987). Cocaine receptors on dopamine transporters are related to self-administration of cocaine. *Science*, *237*(4819), 1219–1223.

Ross, B. M., Moszczynska, A., Peretti, F. J., Adams, V., Schmunk, G. A., Kalasinsky, K. S., et al. (2002). Decreased activity of brain phospholipid metabolic enzymes in human users of cocaine and methamphetamine. *Drug and Alcohol Dependence*, *67*(1), 73–79.

Roth, D., Alarcon, F. J., Fernandez, J. A., Preston, R. A., & Bourgoignie, J. J. (1988). Acute rhabdomyolysis associated with cocaine intoxication. *The New England Journal of Medicine*, *319*(11), 673–677. http://dx.doi.org/10.1056/NEJM198809153191103.

Rothwell, P. M., Howard, S. C., Dolan, E., O'Brien, E., Dobson, J. E., Dahlof, B., et al. (2010). Prognostic significance of visit-to-visit variability, maximum systolic blood pressure, and episodic hypertension. *Lancet, 375*(9718), 895–905. http://dx.doi.org/10.1016/S0140-6736(10)60308-X.

Rumbaugh, C. L., Bergeron, R. T., Scanlan, R. L., Teal, J. S., Segall, H. D., Fang, H. C., et al. (1971). Cerebral vascular changes secondary to amphetamine abuse in the experimental animal. *Radiology, 101*(2), 345–351. http://dx.doi.org/10.1148/101.2.345.

Russell, R. D., & Stripling, J. S. (1987). Monoaminergic and local anesthetic components of cocaine's effects on kindled seizure expression. *Pharmacology, Biochemistry, and Behavior, 22*, 427–434.

Rusyniak, D. E. (2011). Neurologic manifestations of chronic methamphetamine abuse. *Neurologic Clinics, 29*(3), 641–655. http://dx.doi.org/10.1016/j.ncl.2011.05.004.

Rusyniak, D. E. (2013). Neurologic manifestations of chronic methamphetamine abuse. *The Psychiatric Clinics of North America, 36*(2), 261–275. http://dx.doi.org/10.1016/j.psc.2013.02.005.

Rylander, G. (1972). Psychoses and the punding and choreiform syndromes in addiction to central stimulant drugs. *Psychiatria, Neurologia, Neurochirurgia, 75*(3), 203–212.

Sanchez-Ramos, J. R. (1993). Psychostimulants. *Neurologic Clinics, 11*(3), 535–553.

Sato, M. (1992). A lasting vulnerability to psychosis in patients with previous methamphetamine psychosis. *Annals of the New York Academy of Sciences, 654*, 160–170.

Schep, L. J., Slaughter, R. J., & Beasley, D. M. (2010). The clinical toxicology of metamfetamine. *Clinical Toxicology (Philadelphia, Pa.), 48*(7), 675–694. http://dx.doi.org/10.3109/15563650.2010.516752.

Scott, J. C., Woods, S. P., Matt, G. E., Meyer, R. A., Heaton, R. K., Atkinson, J. H., et al. (2007). Neurocognitive effects of methamphetamine: A critical review and meta-analysis. *Neuropsychology Review, 17*(3), 275–297. http://dx.doi.org/10.1007/s11065-007-9031-0.

Shuster, L., Garhart, C. A., Powers, J., Grunfeld, Y., & Kanel, G. (1988). Hepatotoxicity of cocaine. *NIDA Research Monograph, 88*, 250–275.

Sordo, L., Indave, B. I., Barrio, G., Degenhardt, L., de la Fuente, L., & Bravo, M. J. (2014). Cocaine use and risk of stroke: A systematic review. *Drug and Alcohol Dependence, 142*, 1–13. http://dx.doi.org/10.1016/j.drugalcdep.2014.06.041.

Sperling, L. S., & Horowitz, J. L. (1994). Methamphetamine-induced choreoathetosis and rhabdomyolysis. *Annals of Internal Medicine, 121*(12), 986.

Srisurapanont, M., Ali, R., Marsden, J., Sunga, A., Wada, K., & Monteiro, M. (2003). Psychotic symptoms in methamphetamine psychotic in-patients. *The International Journal of Neuropsychopharmacology, 6*(4), 347–352. http://dx.doi.org/10.1017/S1461145703003675.

Stork, C. M., & Cantor, R. (1997). Pemoline induced acute choreoathetosis: Case report and review of the literature. *Journal of Toxicology. Clinical Toxicology, 35*(1), 105–108.

Stripling, J. S. (1983). Cocaine and "pharmacological kindling" in the rat. *Experimental Neurology, 82*(2), 499–503.

Su, J., Li, J., Li, W., Altura, B. T., & Altura, B. M. (2003). Cocaine induces apoptosis in cerebral vascular muscle cells: Potential roles in strokes and brain damage. *European Journal of Pharmacology, 482*(1–3), 61–66.

Suwaki, H., Fukui, S., & Konuma, K. (1997). Methamphetamine abuse in Japan: Its 45 year history and the current situation. In H. Klee (Ed.), *Amphetamine misuse: International perspectives on current trends*. Reading, UK: Harwood Academic Publisher.

Suzuki, O., Hattori, H., Asano, M., Oya, M., & Katsumata, Y. (1980). Inhibition of monoamine oxidase by d-methamphetamine. *Biochemical Pharmacology, 29*(14), 2071–2073.

Truong, J. G., Wilkins, D. G., Baudys, J., Crouch, D. J., Johnson-Davis, K. L., Gibb, J. W., et al. (2005). Age-dependent methamphetamine-induced alterations in vesicular monoamine transporter-2 function: Implications for neurotoxicity. *The Journal of Pharmacology and Experimental Therapeutics, 314*(3), 1087–1092. http://dx.doi.org/10.1124/jpet.105.085951.

Tulving, E. (2002). Episodic memory: From mind to brain. *Annual Review of Psychology, 53*, 1–25. http://dx.doi.org/10.1146/annurev.psych.53.100901.135114.

UNDOC. (2008). *Annual report 2008.* http://www.unodc.org/documents/about-unodc/AR08_WEB.pdf.

Volkow, N. D., Chang, L., Wang, G. J., Fowler, J. S., Ding, Y. S., Sedler, M., et al. (2001). Low level of brain dopamine D2 receptors in methamphetamine abusers: Association with metabolism in the orbitofrontal cortex. *The American Journal of Psychiatry, 158*(12), 2015–2021.

Volkow, N. D., Chang, L., Wang, G. J., Fowler, J. S., Franceschi, D., Sedler, M., et al. (2001). Loss of dopamine transporters in methamphetamine abusers recovers with protracted abstinence. *The Journal of Neuroscience, 21*(23), 9414–9418.

Volkow, N. D., Chang, L., Wang, G. J., Fowler, J. S., Leonido-Yee, M., Franceschi, D., et al. (2001). Association of dopamine transporter reduction with psychomotor impairment in methamphetamine abusers. *The American Journal of Psychiatry, 158*(3), 377–382.

Weinberger, A. H., & Sofuoglu, M. (2009). The impact of cigarette smoking on stimulant addiction. *The American Journal of Drug and Alcohol Abuse, 35*(1), 12–17. http://dx.doi.org/10.1080/00952990802326280.

Weiner, W. J., & Sanchez-Ramos, J. (1992). Movement disorders and dopaminomimetic stimulant drugs. In A. E. Lang, & W. J. Weiner (Eds.), *Drug induced movement disorders* (pp. 315–337). Mount Kisco, NY: Futura Publishing Co.

Westover, A. N., McBride, S., & Haley, R. W. (2007). Stroke in young adults who abuse amphetamines or cocaine: A population-based study of hospitalized patients. *Archives of General Psychiatry, 64*(4), 495–502. http://dx.doi.org/10.1001/archpsyc.64.4.495.

Wilson, J. M., Kalasinsky, K. S., Levey, A. I., Bergeron, C., Reiber, G., Anthony, R. M., et al. (1996). Striatal dopamine nerve terminal markers in human, chronic methamphetamine users. *Nature Medicine, 2*(6), 699–703.

Yamamoto, B. K., Moszczynska, A., & Gudelsky, G. A. (2010). Amphetamine toxicities: Classical and emerging mechanisms. *Annals of the New York Academy of Sciences, 1187*, 101–121. http://dx.doi.org/10.1111/j.1749-6632.2009.05141.x.

Yonetani, M., Huang, C. C., Lajevardi, N., Pastuszko, A., Delivoria-Papadopoulous, M., & Anday, E. (1994). Effect of acute cocaine injection on the extracellular level of dopamine, blood flow, and oxygen pressure in brain of newborn piglets. *Biochemical Medicine and Metabolic Biology, 51*(1), 91–97.

Young, R., & Glennon, R. A. (1986). Discriminative stimulus properties of amphetamine and structurally related phenalkylamines. *Medicinal Research Reviews, 6*(1), 99–130.

Yui, K., Ikemoto, S., Ishiguro, T., & Goto, K. (2000). Studies of amphetamine or methamphetamine psychosis in Japan: Relation of methamphetamine psychosis to schizophrenia. *Annals of the New York Academy of Sciences, 914*, 1–12.

CHAPTER EIGHT

Neurobehavioral Sequelae of Psychostimulant Abuse

Atbin Djamshidian[1]
Department of Neurology, Innsbruck Medical University, Innsbruck, Austria
Reta Lila Weston Institute of Neurological Studies, University of London, London, United Kingdom
[1]Corresponding author: e-mail address: a.djamshidian-tehrani@ucl.ac.uk

Contents

Abstract

Psychostimulants are a heterogeneous group of drugs known not only for its arousal and motor activity enhancing effects but also for its high risk of abuse. In susceptible individuals, chronic use can cause addiction leading to devastating physical, psychological, and social health consequences. This chapter will focus on the neurobehavioral consequences of psychostimulant abuse. Different models and theories of addiction and possible underlying mechanisms as well as changed in decision making on neuropsychological tasks have been discussed. Prevention and early behavioral intervention are of paramount importance given the lack of approved drug therapies for these patients.

1. INTRODUCTION

Psychostimulants and their behavioral side effects are known for centuries. According to a legend, written by Antonius Faustus Naironus in his book "De saluberrima potione cahve," in Abyssinia (Ethiopia) the shepherd

International Review of Neurobiology, Volume 120
ISSN 0074-7742
http://dx.doi.org/10.1016/bs.irn.2015.01.002

Kaldi observed that his goats were more energetic, restless, dancing around, and sleepless when eating berries from a certain green bush that later turned out to contain caffeine. The shepherd then also tasted the berries and joined in the dance (Chou, 1992). Although this story is probably a myth, coffee is indeed the world's most used psychostimulant and is consumed daily by 90% of North Americans (Hausser, Schlemmer, Kaiser, Kalis, & Mojzisch, 2014).

As with any psychostimulants, in higher doses, caffeine can induce tolerance, dependence, and withdrawal symptoms. Sensitive subjects can experience a variety of different side effects, such as anxiety, restlessness, dysphoria, insomnia, and psychomotor agitation, collectively termed as caffeinism.

However, in the majority of individuals even chronic use is usually harmless. In fact, it has been proposed that caffeine is neuroprotective (de Lau & Breteler, 2006; Ribeiro & Sebastiao, 2010) and its beneficial effects on attention have been described in several studies, for a review, see Einother and Giesbrecht (2013).

2. PSYCHOSTIMULANT ADDICTION

Drug addiction is defined as a chronic relapsing disorder that goes through three stages: (a) the compulsive drug seeking, (b) the loss of control in amount of intake, and (c) the occurrence of negative side effects during withdrawal symptoms (Koob & Volkow, 2010). Although drug addiction can present in several different ways, these general concepts largely apply to all psychostimulant abusers.

The initial administration of the drug is rewarding, largely mediated via dopamine release. Psychostimulants increase these dopamine levels in the limbic system (mesolimbic dopamine levels) in a dose-dependent manner. Higher doses of the drug initially induce euphoria and satisfaction. However, as the dopamine levels reduce and hence the enjoyable feeling diminishes, individuals crave to administer another dose to replicate the same feeling of euphoria (Taylor, Lewis, & Olive, 2013). Thus, abusers tend to administer psychostimulants repeatedly which leads to addiction (e.g., loss of drug control). Individuals are prone to withdraw socially and work performance and personal relationships deteriorate. They start lying and concealing their behavior and are at risk of getting arrested for drug-related criminal activities.

Particularly, adolescents are vulnerable and sensitive to addiction and outside influences (Gulley & Juraska, 2013). Furthermore, they are known to be higher novelty and sensation seeking (Spear, 2000) and risk prone. This heightened vulnerability has been attributed to slow maturation of the cognitive control mechanisms, which are necessary for inhibition (Steinberg, 2004). Exposure to psychostimulants during puberty also negatively affects prefrontal cortex (PFC) maturation (Nyberg, 2014), which in turn further increases the vulnerability to disadvantageous decisions.

2.1 Amphetamines

Amphetamines are a group of stimulants containing methamphetamine, D-amphetamine, and 3,4-methylenedioxymethamphetamine (ecstasy). In contrast to cocaine, amphetamines are synthetically derived and have a long duration of action (Nordahl, Salo, & Leamon, 2003). At lower doses and in drug-naïve individuals, amphetamines increase alertness, attentiveness, and energy. At higher doses, they cause well-being, euphoria, high self-esteem, hypomania, and increase sexual activity (Nordahl et al., 2003). Acute doses of methamphetamine in drug-naïve individuals may also improve long-term memory processes via enhanced memory consolidation. A study from the 1950s demonstrated that amphetamines reduced reaction times and improved overall performance in sleep-deprived subjects (Kornetsky, Mirsky, Kessler, & Dorff, 1959).

Repetitive use, however, causes reduced libido and low appetite with weight loss. Patients get restless, suffer from insomnia, and may develop suspiciousness that can lead to acute paranoia (Nordahl et al., 2003). They also show more risk-taking behavior, have more sexual partners, and have higher rates of sexual transmitted diseases (Molitor, Truax, Ruiz, & Sun, 1998). Patients often become distractible and have difficulties sustaining attention. Visual, auditory, and tactile hallucinations as well as illusions are common and are sometimes associated with skin picking (Nordahl et al., 2003; Schiorring, 1981). In some, these acute paranoid reactions can become chronic, despite abstinence from illicit substances (Nordahl et al., 2003).

2.2 Cocaine

Cocaine derives from the leaves of the coca plant and blocks the reuptake of monoamine neurotransmitters such as serotonin, norepinephrine, and dopamine. About 10–15% of individuals become addicted after initial use (Gawin, 1991). It is either injected, snorted, or smoked (crack) (Wood, Sage, Shuman, & Anagnostaras, 2014). Initially, similarly to amphetamine users, subjects report profound well-being together with increased alertness. Self-confidence and positive emotions are increased, while anxiety and social inhibitions are reduced (Gawin, 1991). With regular use, however, these behavioral changes subside and patients usually mix other drugs (alcohol, heroin, and marijuana) to decrease unpleasant components of the cocaine experience, such as anxiety (Gawin, 1991). Once addiction occurs subjects readminister drugs in a compulsive uncontrolled way. Euphoria and phases of dysphoria during drug craving occur.

2.3 Methcathinone

Methcathinone also sometimes called ephedrone is a synthetic derivate that stems from the leaves of the khat bush which contains cathinone. Similar to amphetamines and cocaine it also inhibits the uptake of catecholamines in the brain and causes euphoria, agitation, anxiety, and hallucinations (Sikk, Haldre, Aquilonius, & Taba, 2011; Zhingel, Dovensky, Crossman, & Allen, 1991). Typically, it is used in a binge pattern, injecting several times a day, followed by 1–2 days of abstinence. The ingestion of potassium permanganate during the process of oxidation of pseudoephedrine (Emerson & Cisek, 1993) causes pallidal signal abnormalities leading to devastating neurological side effects including generalized dystonia, postural instability, dopaminergic unresponsive bradykinesia, and a typical "cock gait" (Sanotsky et al., 2007). These side effects are most likely a consequence of chronic manganese toxicity (Colosimo & Guidi, 2009; de Bie, Gladstone, Strafella, Ko, & Lang, 2007; Sikk et al., 2011).

2.4 Legal Highs

"Legal highs," psychoactive chemicals, which are sold from "head shops," street suppliers, are getting increasingly popular and are designed to mimic traditional drugs of abuse but do not underlie legal restriction (Gibbons, 2012). A variety of different stimulants are used such as mephedrone, khat, calamas root, betel, and ephedrine. Other names include "meow-meow," "MCAT," "bubbles," and "drone." All these substances are chemically similar to khat and induce acute euphoria. It is often found as a compound in ecstasy tablets and is responsible for strong feelings of craving (Brunt, Poortman, Niesink, & van den Brink, 2011). Over time subjects often suffer from depression, poor working memory, and impulsivity. Furthermore, chronic users scored higher on schizotypy rating scales, which is a personality trait related to schizophrenia (Freeman et al., 2012). Similarly, khat leaves when chewed release cathinone and induce euphoria. Long-term use causes a variety of different complications including depression, aggressive behavior, anorexia, paranoia, delusions, and hallucinations (Balint, Falkay, & Balint, 2009).

3. PSYCHIATRIC COMPLICATIONS SEEN IN PSYCHOSTIMULANT ABUSERS

Psychiatric symptoms, such as depression, anxiety, and psychosis as well as sleep deprivation, are common in psychostimulant abusers (Dawe, Davis, Lapworth, & McKetin, 2009; Zweben et al., 2004). After chronic use physical and sexual aggression toward partner and spouses occur frequently, even in the absence of recent exposure (Dawe et al., 2009; Moore et al., 2008). Psychosis may occur at higher doses and resembles psychosis seen in schizophrenia. Paranoia and auditory hallucinations as well as tactile hallucinations (insects crawling on or underneath the skin) and visual hallucinations have been described (MacKenzie & Heischober, 1997).

In contrast to other substances of abuse, such as alcohol or opioids, where patients experience physical withdrawal symptoms, psychostimulant abusers mainly experience psychological withdrawal symptoms such as hypersomnolence, sadness, fatigue, anhedonia, and dysphoria (D'Souza & Markou, 2010). These affective and psychological symptoms are likely due to neuroplastic changes within the PFC which is necessary for self-control and the ability to inhibit impulsive action. Compelling evidence for serotonin dysfunction is in seen cocaine addicts, who exhibit psychiatric symptoms such as major depression, suicidal ideation, and suicide attempts during withdrawal (Rothman, Blough, & Baumann, 2006).

4. THEORIES OF ADDICTION

There are several different theories to explain the underlying mechanisms of addiction. The *incentive sensitization* theory suggests that drug users become more sensitive to drugs and drug-related cues, which correlate with higher mesolimbic dopamine release. This change of stimuli perception causes enhanced "wanting" rather than "liking" the drugs. This discrepancy of "wanting" versus "liking" is typical for drug craving (Robinson & Berridge, 1993). Others have suggested that during chronic drug abuse reduced functioning of reward brain areas and an upregulation of the "antireward" stress circuitries may occur (*antireward theory*) (Koob & Le Moal, 2008). Another theory involves *habit formation*. In a classical learning paradigm an action is directed to achieve a goal or outcome. This is called goal-directed behavior

(Dickinson & Balleine, 1994). However, in stimulus-response behavior, the outcome becomes less relevant and the stimulus drives the behavior, which leads to habitual learning. The habit formation theory suggests that chronic drug abuse changes from voluntary control to habitual and compulsive use and that this behavioral shift correlates with a transition from initially ventral to dorsal striatal activation with reduction in PFC inhibition (Everitt & Robbins, 2005). The *negative reinforcement theory* proposes that addicts seek drugs in order to avoid unpleasant withdrawal effects and dysphoria, due to repeated cycles of highs and withdrawal symptoms (Newton, De La Garza, Kalechstein, Tziortzis, & Jacobsen, 2009).

Finally, impulsivity is likely to contribute to chronic drug abuse. Whether it is a cause or consequence of drug addiction is, however, unclear. Impulsivity can be described as a failure to resist and an impulse (Newton et al., 2009) but is a broad term and can be further divided into several categories (a–e) (Dalley, Everitt, & Robbins, 2011; Evenden, 1999):

(a) Reflection impulsivity, the inability to gather more information and "jump to conclusions."
(b) Impulsive action, the failure to inhibit a motor response.
(c) Temporal discounting, the preference of small immediate over large delayed rewards.
(d) Risk-prone behavior, the tendency to overestimate that small unlikely probabilities happen.
(e) Aggression can also be part of impulsive behavior.

Although all these theories are involving different mechanisms, it is now clear that chronic drug abuse causes long-term complex neuroplastic and behavioral changes. Each of these models has its strengths and weaknesses and each alone cannot fully explain the psychological mechanisms why some individuals are prone to get addicted to illicit substances. Other risk factors, such as environmental and social factors, genetic predisposition, and the influence of social media, have to be taken into account (Kreek, Nielsen, Butelman, & LaForge, 2005). Furthermore, not only acute but also chronic stress plays a crucial role and is known to increase the risk of developing an addiction and is also responsible for relapses (Schwabe, Dickinson, & Wolf, 2011).

The transition from sporadic drug use to addiction is a progressive evolution and contains mainly three distinct phases. Phase 1 is the sporadic drug use, phase 2 is an intensive escalated and sustained use, and phase 3 is the loss of control of drug intake. It has been proposed that each phase is independent but consecutive, e.g., one phase follows the other. A *drug escalation-prone* personality is more likely to shift into phase 2 and a *loss of control-prone* person is necessary to shift into phase 3 which is the full addiction phase (Deroche-Gamonet & Piazza, 2014). Furthermore, to enter phase 1 individual, susceptibility and an element on novelty seeking/sensation seeking is necessary (Zuckerman, 1986).

5. NEUROCIRCUITRY OF ADDICTION

Psychostimulants cause a wide variety of different structural changes. The ventral tegmental area, the nucleus accumbens (Nac), the PFC, the dorsal striatum (DS), the amygdala, and the hippocampus (Hipp) all play a major role in addictive behaviors (Fig. 1). The PFC is important for several cognitive functions such as the inhibition of inappropriate behavior (top-down control), cognitive flexibility, modulating drug-seeking behavior, and emotional control (Taylor et al., 2013). Among several other glutamatergic projections, the PFC also projects to the ventral tegmental area and the Nac, both rich on dopamine (Sesack & Pickel, 1992; Taylor et al., 2013), and to the limbic system including the amygdala and the Hipp (Kalivas & Volkow, 2005; Vertes, Hoover, Szigeti-Buck, & Leranth, 2007). Consistent with this, PFC atrophy with lower gray matter tissue as well as reduction in orbitofrontal dysfunction in positron emission tomography scans have been found in cocaine addicts (Bolla et al., 2003; Fein, Di Sclafani, & Meyerhoff, 2002; Matochik, London, Eldreth, Cadet, & Bolla, 2003) and amphetamine users (Berman, O'Neill, Fears, Bartzokis, & London, 2008; Thompson et al., 2004).

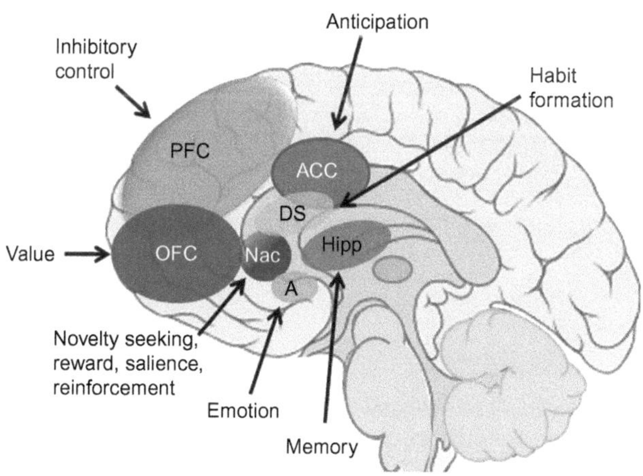

Figure 1 Brain circuits involved in addictions. Psychostimulants induce neuroplastic changes in a variety of different brain areas. DS, dorsal striatum; Nac, nucleus accumbens; A, amygdala; Hipp, hippocampus. *Figure adapted from Lee, Carter, Owen, and Hall (2012).*

Apart from PFC atrophy, the temporal lobes as well as the parietal, occipital, and Hipp have been shown to be atrophic in chronic psychostimulant users (Berman et al., 2008). Furthermore, microstructural white matter changes on diffusion tensor imaging are common and may involve gliosis (Berman et al., 2008; Romero, Asensio, Palau, Sanchez, & Romero, 2010). In contrast, higher striatal volumes have been described in amphetamine users, which may reflect compensation for neurotoxicity (Berman et al., 2008).

The DS is important for habit formation and leads to a stimulus-response learning (Everitt & Robbins, 2005). Although the initial rewarding effects of psychostimulants are mediated via a dopamine release in the Nac shell, after prolonged use dopamine release shifts to the DS leading to habitual compulsive drug use (Everitt & Robbins, 2005; Taylor et al., 2013). In addition to memory processes, the Hipp is also involved in motivational processes and in rodents the CA3 regions has been found to be in involved in cocaine seeking (Xie, Ramirez, Lasseter, & Fuchs, 2010).

The orbitofrontal cortex (OFC) modulates value of choices and is important for motivation (Aron, Robbins, & Poldrack, 2004). In healthy controls, it has been postulated that these brain areas are critical to prevent addictions. In contrast, in patients with poor self-control dysfunction of the PFC together with impaired OFC function and an upregulation of mesolimbic dopamine release cause aberrant motivation (Fig. 2; Lee et al.,

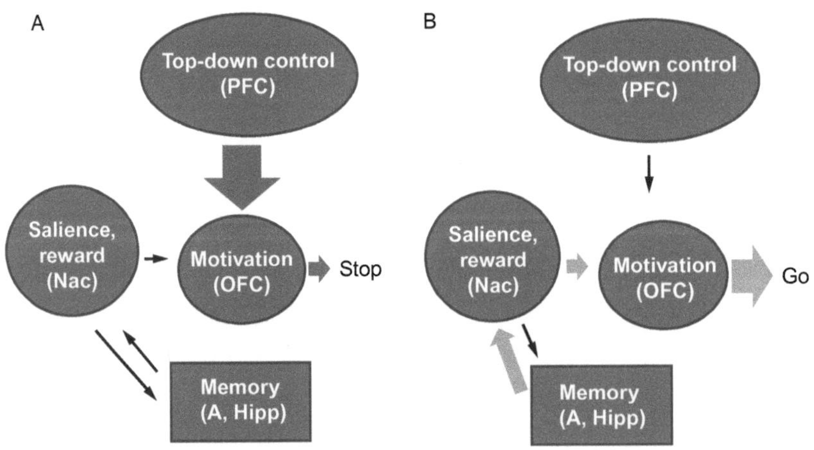

Figure 2 Simplified schematic overview of mechanisms underlying addictive behavior. (A) In healthy volunteers, inhibitory control from the PFC and assessing of the value of choices is sufficient to refrain from addiction. These regulatory mechanisms are impaired in patients with addictions (B). Increased mesolimbic dopamine levels are thought to be responsible for an overvalue of an immediate action, causing aberrant motivation. PFC, prefrontal cortex; OFC, orbitofrontal cortex; A, amygdala; Hipp, hippocampus; Nac, nucleus accumbens. *Figure adapted from Lee, Carter, Owen, and Hall (2012).*

2012). Furthermore, mesolimbic dopamine, originating from the ventral tegmental area and projecting to the PFC via the ventral striatum, can reduce the reward threshold (Koob & Volkow, 2010), causing the feeling of pleasure, which is necessary to reinforce an addictive behavior. However, as the addiction continues withdrawal symptoms and anxiety, depression, and other psychiatric complications frequently occur (Koob & Volkow, 2010).

6. NEUROPSYCHOLOGICAL CHANGES

The majority of psychostimulant abusers show abnormalities on neuropsychological tests.

For example, learning plays a pivotal role in adapting to the environment. Thus, it is not surprising that several studies found impairments in learning behavior in patients with psychostimulant abuse. Early studies from the 1960s showed slower learning in amphetamine users compared to a placebo group (Burns, House, Fensch, & Miller, 1967). More recent studies assessed probabilistic reversal learning in cocaine and amphetamine users. In probabilistic learning tasks, participants usually need to learn which of two stimuli is rewarded and are told to pick the rewarded stimuli as many times as possible.

However, in about 20% of the trials, the computer provides a false feedback (e.g., selecting a correct stimulus is followed by an incorrect feedback). Furthermore, after a certain amount of trials reward contingencies change (e.g., the previously rewarded stimuli become unrewarded and vice versa) (Swainson et al., 2000). Cocaine abusers, but not amphetamine abusers had significant impairment in changing their behavior when reward contingencies were reversed. This result demonstrates response perseveration in the cocaine group, although the mechanisms are still unclear (Ersche, Roiser, Robbins, & Sahakian, 2008). Several other studies assessing cognitive flexibility, where suppression of task irrelevant distractors is necessary, have demonstrated poorer performance in psychostimulant abusers compared to controls. For example, amphetamine users were impaired on the Stroop test, were participants need to respond to the ink color, rather than reading the word, and on a Go/Nogo test, where motor suppression is required (Nordahl et al., 2003). Performance on the Stroop test requires selective attention and cognitive control that allows selecting the weaker task relevant response rather than responding to the stronger, but task irrelevant stimuli. Poorer scores on the Stroop test may also identify cocaine-dependent users who are at risk for treatment dropouts in recovery programs (Streeter et al., 2008).

Furthermore, chronic psychostimulant abusers had slower reaction times on the pegboard task and made more errors on the trail making tests (Rosselli, Ardila, Lubomski, Murray, & King, 2001; Volkow et al., 2001).

Clinically, perseveration and stereotypies are often seen in cocaine and amphetamine users (Fasano et al., 2008; Rylander, 1972). These include bizarre movements, such as excessive grooming, fidgeting with clothes, hoarding, and walkabouts. Others repeat single words or phrases (Schiorring, 1981). This behavior is called "punding" and was first described in 40 out of 152 methylphenidate users (Rylander, 1972). The term "punding" derives from the Swedish slang and means "blockhead" to illustrate the purposeless of this behavior, where voluntary control of the behavior is lost (Rylander, 1972). Punding, also called "knick-knacking" in the United States, is a nongoal orientated complex stereotype behavior driven by an intense fascination (Ellinwood, Sudilovsky, & Nelson, 1973) and can also be seen in patients with Parkinson's disease (PD) under levodopa therapy. In PD patients, punding often occurs in combination with overuse of levodopa (dopamine dysregulation syndrome) (O'Sullivan, Evans, & Lees, 2009). Although dopamine plays a role in punding behavior, the exact mechanisms are unclear (Fasano & Petrovic, 2010). Levodopa mainly stimulates the dopamine D1 and D2 receptors (Evans et al., 2004; Fasano & Petrovic, 2010) leading to increased mesolimbic dopamine levels. This increased "bottom-up" dopamine levels (either via levodopa in PD or via psychostimulants in abusers) together with reduced "top-down" PFC control is likely responsible for punding. Although behaviorally there are many similarities between PD punders and psychostimulant punders, there are also key differences. In PD therapy is necessary to remedy depleted striatal dopamine levels, while in illicit drug abusers no deficits in dopamine levels exist. This may explain why punding in drug addicts is frequently seen after the first drug intake (Fasano & Petrovic, 2010), while in PD punding usually take several months or years to develop.

Time perception is another key area that has been shown to be distorted in patients with psychostimulant abuse. Time perception varies depending on attention, mood, memories of past events, and compromises several scales ranging from milliseconds to years (Teixeira et al., 2013). Although several different areas are necessary for time perception, the striatum and the PFC are particularly important. This fronto-striatal network may be the neural basis of the "internal clock" which is necessary for time estimation and time reproduction (Hinton & Meck, 2004). The circadian rhythm, which regulates sleep and wakefulness (Teixeira et al., 2013), is often dysregulated in cocaine (Valladares & Irwin, 2007) and amphetamine abusers (Rechtschaffen & Maron, 1964). Furthermore, cocaine and methamphetamine abusers overestimated the duration of a stimulus, had impairment in time discrimination, and accelerated on time reproduction tests (Wittmann, Leland, Churan, & Paulus, 2007). Moreover, temporal discounting, the preference of a small immediate, over a delayed larger reward is a hallmark of addiction. Several studies have shown that cocaine abusers as well as methamphetamine abusers discount future larger rewards more than controls (Coffey, Gudleski, Saladin, & Brady, 2003; Hoffman et al., 2006, 2008; Monterosso et al., 2007). Thus, these studies suggest that participants have difficulties in waiting, often also described as "waiting impulsivity" (Dalley et al., 2011). Furthermore, information sampling seems to be a core behavioral deficit in drug addiction. Amphetamine, cocaine abusers as well as methcathinone patients and opioid-dependent patients demonstrated "reflection impulsivity" and gathered significantly less evidence and made more irrational decisions than healthy controls (Clark, Robbins, Ersche, & Sahakian, 2006; Djamshidian et al., 2013). This inability to gather information did not improve after drug abstinence. In fact, abstinent abusers also "jumped to conclusions," suggesting that poor information sampling is a persistent cognitive marker for substance abuse (Clark et al., 2006).

Novelty and "thrill" seeking plays an important role in drug addiction and is also associated with alcohol, unsafe sex, and smoking (Bardo, Donohew, & Harrington, 1996; Wagner, 2001). Sensation seeking is defined as "the need for varied, novel, and complex sensations and experiences and the willingness to take physical and social risks for the sake of such experience" (Zuckerman, 1979). It is likely that novelty and sensation seeking as well as impulsivity predict the risk for addiction. Furthermore, reward processing is impaired in sensation seekers which may underlie the increased tendency of thrill seeking (Jupp & Dalley, 2014). It is likely that novelty seeking in combination with impulsivity is necessary for addictive behavior. One study demonstrated that novelty seekers alone were able to control drug use, while those with novelty seeking and impulsive personality traits could not (Ersche et al., 2013).

Several studies have also demonstrated poor working memory and attention in patients with stimulant abuse (Djamshidian et al., 2013; Freeman et al., 2012; George, Mandyam, Wee, & Koob, 2008; Rosselli et al., 2001). These deficits may be due to changes in hippocampal neurogenesis

Table 1 Overview of Neuropsychological Tests Done in Patients with Psychostimulant Abuse

Abnormalities on Neuropsychological Tests	References
Jumping to conclusions	Clark et al. (2006) and Djamshidian et al. (2013)
Poorer working memory and attention	Djamshidian et al. (2013), George et al. (2008), and Rosselli et al. (2001)
Increased novelty seeking	Bardo et al. (1996) and Wagner (2001)
Impaired time perception	Teixeira et al. (2013)
Increased temporal discounting	Coffey et al. (2003), Hoffman et al. (2006, 2008), and Monterosso et al. (2007)
Poorer learning	Burns et al. (1967)
Impaired reversal learning[a]	Ersche et al. (2008)
Impaired Stroop test/motor inhibition	Nordahl et al. (2003)

[a]Abnormality found in cocaine but not amphetamine users.

(Nyberg, 2014). Whether poor working memory is the cause or a consequence of addiction remains elusive (Table 1).

7. CONCLUSIONS

Drug addiction leads to complex alterations in a variety of different brain networks, leading to profound behavioral and personality changes. Preliminary results from computer-based training programs, albeit in patients with schizophrenia, and general anxiety disorders have shown improvement in PFC function lasting for several months (Amir & Taylor, 2012; Subramaniam et al., 2012). Whether these behavioral interventions are also useful in patients with psychostimulant addiction is, however, unknown. Cognitive behavior therapy and contingency management to shift the focus away from addictive behaviors have proven to be effective in methamphetamine users (Lee & Rawson, 2008) and other substance abusers and remain the mainstay of treatment (Phillips, Epstein, & Preston, 2014).

Given the lack of approved treatments, early behavioral interventions are necessary to avoid long-term neuroplastic changes in brain addiction networks to prevent subjects from devastating psychosocial consequences.

REFERENCES

Amir, N., & Taylor, C. T. (2012). Combining computerized home-based treatments for generalized anxiety disorder: An attention modification program and cognitive behavioral therapy. *Behavior Therapy*, *43*, 546–559.

Aron, A. R., Robbins, T. W., & Poldrack, R. A. (2004). Inhibition and the right inferior frontal cortex. *Trends in Cognitive Science*, *8*(4), 170–177. http://dx.doi.org/10.1016/j.tics.2004.02.010.

Balint, E. E., Falkay, G., & Balint, G. A. (2009). Khat—A controversial plant. *Wiener Klinische Wochenschrift*, *121*(19–20), 604–614. http://dx.doi.org/10.1007/s00508-009-1259-7.

Bardo, M. T., Donohew, R. L., & Harrington, N. G. (1996). Psychobiology of novelty seeking and drug seeking behavior. *Behavioural Brain Research*, *77*, 23–43.

Berman, S., O'Neill, J., Fears, S., Bartzokis, G., & London, E. D. (2008). Abuse of amphetamines and structural abnormalities in the brain. *Annals of the New York Academy of Sciences*, *1141*, 195–220.

Bolla, K. I., Eldreth, D. A., London, E. D., Kiehl, K. A., Mouratidis, M., Contoreggi, C., et al. (2003). Orbitofrontal cortex dysfunction in abstinent cocaine abusers performing a decision-making task. *NeuroImage*, *19*, 1085–1094.

Brunt, T. M., Poortman, A., Niesink, R. J., & van den Brink, W. (2011). Instability of the ecstasy market and a new kid on the block: Mephedrone. *Journal of Psychopharmacology*, *25*, 1543–1547.

Burns, J. T., House, R. F., Fensch, F. C., & Miller, J. G. (1967). Effects of magnesium pemoline and dextroamphetamine on human learning. *Science*, *155*, 849–851.

Chou, T. (1992). Wake up and smell the coffee. Caffeine, coffee, and the medical consequences. *Western Journal of Medicine*, *157*, 544–553.

Clark, L., Robbins, T. W., Ersche, K. D., & Sahakian, B. J. (2006). Reflection impulsivity in current and former substance users. *Biological Psychiatry*, *60*, 515–522.

Coffey, S. F., Gudleski, G. D., Saladin, M. E., & Brady, K. T. (2003). Impulsivity and rapid discounting of delayed hypothetical rewards in cocaine-dependent individuals. *Experimental and Clinical Psychopharmacology*, *11*, 18–25.

Colosimo, C., & Guidi, M. (2009). Parkinsonism due to ephedrone neurotoxicity: A case report. *European Journal of Neurology*, *16*, 114–115.

Dalley, J. W., Everitt, B. J., & Robbins, T. W. (2011). Impulsivity, compulsivity, and top-down cognitive control. *Neuron*, *69*, 680–694.

Dawe, S., Davis, P., Lapworth, K., & McKetin, R. (2009). Mechanisms underlying aggressive and hostile behavior in amphetamine users. *Current Opinion in Psychiatry*, *22*, 269–273.

de Bie, R. M., Gladstone, R. M., Strafella, A. P., Ko, J. H., & Lang, A. E. (2007). Manganese-induced Parkinsonism associated with methcathinone (Ephedrone) abuse. *Archives of Neurology*, *64*, 886–889.

de Lau, L. M., & Breteler, M. M. (2006). Epidemiology of Parkinson's disease. *Lancet Neurology*, *5*, 525–535.

Deroche-Gamonet, V., & Piazza, P. V. (2014). Psychobiology of cocaine addiction: Contribution of a multi-symptomatic animal model of loss of control. *Neuropharmacology*, *76*, 437–449.

Dickinson, A., & Balleine, B. (1994). Motivational control of goal-directed action. *Animal Learning & Behavior*, *22*, 1–18.

Djamshidian, A., Sanotsky, Y., Matviyenko, Y., O'Sullivan, S. S., Sharman, S., Selikhova, M., et al. (2013). Increased reflection impulsivity in patients with ephedrone-induced Parkinsonism. *Addiction*, *108*, 771–779.

D'Souza, M. S., & Markou, A. (2010). Neural substrates of psychostimulant withdrawal-induced anhedonia. *Current Topics in Behavioral Neurosciences*, *3*, 119–178.

Einother, S. J., & Giesbrecht, T. (2013). Caffeine as an attention enhancer: Reviewing existing assumptions. *Psychopharmacology*, *225*, 251–274.

Ellinwood, E. H., Jr., Sudilovsky, A., & Nelson, L. M. (1973). Evolving behavior in the clinical and experimental amphetamine (model) psychosis. *The American Journal of Psychiatry, 130*, 1088–1093.

Emerson, T. S., & Cisek, J. E. (1993). Methcathinone: A Russian designer amphetamine infiltrates the rural midwest. *Annals of Emergency Medicine, 22*, 1897–1903.

Ersche, K. D., Jones, P. S., Williams, G. B., Smith, D. G., Bullmore, E. T., & Robbins, T. W. (2013). Distinctive personality traits and neural correlates associated with stimulant drug use versus familial risk of stimulant dependence. *Biological Psychiatry, 74*, 137–144.

Ersche, K. D., Roiser, J. P., Robbins, T. W., & Sahakian, B. J. (2008). Chronic cocaine but not chronic amphetamine use is associated with perseverative responding in humans. *Psychopharmacology, 197*, 421–431.

Evans, A. H., Katzenschlager, R., Paviour, D., O'Sullivan, J. D., Appel, S., Lawrence, A. D., et al. (2004). Punding in Parkinson's disease: Its relation to the dopamine dysregulation syndrome. *Movement Disorders, 19*, 397–405.

Evenden, J. L. (1999). Varieties of impulsivity. *Psychopharmacology, 146*, 348–361.

Everitt, B. J., & Robbins, T. W. (2005). Neural systems of reinforcement for drug addiction: From actions to habits to compulsion. *Nature Neuroscience, 8*, 1481–1489.

Fasano, A., Barra, A., Nicosia, P., Rinaldi, F., Bria, P., Bentivoglio, A. R., et al. (2008). Cocaine addiction: From habits to stereotypical-repetitive behaviors and punding. *Drug and Alcohol Dependence, 96*, 178–182.

Fasano, A., & Petrovic, I. (2010). Insights into pathophysiology of punding reveal possible treatment strategies. *Molecular Psychiatry, 15*, 560–573.

Fein, G., Di Sclafani, V., & Meyerhoff, D. J. (2002). Prefrontal cortical volume reduction associated with frontal cortex function deficit in 6-week abstinent crack-cocaine dependent men. *Drug and Alcohol Dependence, 68*, 87–93.

Freeman, T. P., Morgan, C. J., Vaughn-Jones, J., Hussain, N., Karimi, K., & Curran, H. V. (2012). Cognitive and subjective effects of mephedrone and factors influencing use of a 'new legal high'. *Addiction, 107*, 792–800.

Gawin, F. H. (1991). Cocaine addiction: Psychology and neurophysiology. *Science, 251*, 1580–1586.

George, O., Mandyam, C. D., Wee, S., & Koob, G. F. (2008). Extended access to cocaine self-administration produces long-lasting prefrontal cortex-dependent working memory impairments. *Neuropsychopharmacology, 33*, 2474–2482.

Gibbons, S. (2012). 'Legal highs'—Novel and emerging psychoactive drugs: A chemical overview for the toxicologist. *Clinical Toxicology (Philadelphia, Pa.), 50*, 15–24.

Gulley, J. M., & Juraska, J. M. (2013). The effects of abused drugs on adolescent development of corticolimbic circuitry and behavior. *Neuroscience, 249*, 3–20.

Hausser, J. A., Schlemmer, A., Kaiser, S., Kalis, A., & Mojzisch, A. (2014). The effects of caffeine on option generation and subsequent choice. *Psychopharmacology, 18*, 3719–3727.

Hinton, S. C., & Meck, W. H. (2004). Frontal-striatal circuitry activated by human peak-interval timing in the supra-seconds range. *Brain Research. Cognitive Brain Research, 21*, 171–182.

Hoffman, W. F., Moore, M., Templin, R., McFarland, B., Hitzemann, R. J., & Mitchell, S. H. (2006). Neuropsychological function and delay discounting in methamphetamine-dependent individuals. *Psychopharmacology, 188*, 162–170.

Hoffman, W. F., Schwartz, D. L., Huckans, M. S., McFarland, B. H., Meiri, G., Stevens, A. A., et al. (2008). Cortical activation during delay discounting in abstinent methamphetamine dependent individuals. *Psychopharmacology, 2012*, 183–193.

Jupp, B., & Dalley, J. W. (2014). Behavioral endophenotypes of drug addiction: Etiological insights from neuroimaging studies. *Neuropharmacology, 76*, 487–497.

Kalivas, P. W., & Volkow, N. D. (2005). The neural basis of addiction: A pathology of motivation and choice. *The American Journal of Psychiatry*, *162*, 1403–1413.

Koob, G. F., & Le Moal, M. (2008). Addiction and the brain antireward system. *Annual Review of Psychology*, *59*, 29–53.

Koob, G. F., & Volkow, N. D. (2010). Neurocircuitry of addiction. *Neuropsychopharmacology*, *35*, 217–238.

Kornetsky, C., Mirsky, A., Kessler, E., & Dorff, J. (1959). The effects of d-amphetamine on behavioral deficits produced by sleep loss in humans. *Journal de Pharmacologie*, *127*, 46–50.

Kreek, M. J., Nielsen, D. A., Butelman, E. R., & LaForge, K. S. (2005). Genetic influences on impulsivity, risk taking, stress responsivity and vulnerability to drug abuse and addiction. *Nature Neuroscience*, *8*, 1450–1457.

Lee, N. M., Carter, A., Owen, N., & Hall, W. D. (2012). The neurobiology of overeating. Treating overweight individuals should make use of neuroscience research, but not at the expense of population approaches to diet and lifestyle. *EMBO Reports*, *13*, 785–790.

Lee, N. K., & Rawson, R. A. (2008). A systematic review of cognitive and behavioural therapies for methamphetamine dependence. *Drug and Alcohol Review*, *27*, 309–317.

MacKenzie, R. G., & Heischober, B. (1997). Methamphetamine. *Pediatrics in Review*, *18*, 305–309.

Matochik, J. A., London, E. D., Eldreth, D. A., Cadet, J. L., & Bolla, K. I. (2003). Frontal cortical tissue composition in abstinent cocaine abusers: A magnetic resonance imaging study. *NeuroImage*, *19*, 1095–1102.

Molitor, F., Truax, S. R., Ruiz, J. D., & Sun, R. K. (1998). Association of methamphetamine use during sex with risky sexual behaviors and HIV infection among non-injection drug users. *Western Journal of Medicine*, *168*, 93–97.

Monterosso, J. R., Ainslie, G., Xu, J., Cordova, X., Domier, C. P., & London, E. D. (2007). Frontoparietal cortical activity of methamphetamine-dependent and comparison subjects performing a delay discounting task. *Human Brain Mapping*, *28*, 383–393.

Moore, T. M., Stuart, G. L., Meehan, J. C., Rhatigan, D. L., Hellmuth, J. C., & Keen, S. M. (2008). Drug abuse and aggression between intimate partners: A meta-analytic review. *Clinical Psychology Review*, *28*, 247–274.

Newton, T. F., De La Garza, R., 2nd, Kalechstein, A. D., Tziortzis, D., & Jacobsen, C. A. (2009). Theories of addiction: Methamphetamine users' explanations for continuing drug use and relapse. *The American Journal on Addictions*, *18*, 294–300.

Nordahl, T. E., Salo, R., & Leamon, M. (2003). Neuropsychological effects of chronic methamphetamine use on neurotransmitters and cognition: A review. *Journal of Neuropsychiatry and Clinical Neurosciences*, *15*, 317–325.

Nyberg, F. (2014). Structural plasticity of the brain to psychostimulant use. *Neuropharmacology*, *14*, 254–258.

O'Sullivan, S. S., Evans, A. H., & Lees, A. J. (2009). Dopamine dysregulation syndrome: An overview of its epidemiology, mechanisms and management. *CNS Drugs*, *23*, 157–170.

Phillips, K. A., Epstein, D. H., & Preston, K. L. (2014). Psychostimulant addiction treatment. *Neuropharmacology*, *14*, 128–132.

Rechtschaffen, A., & Maron, L. (1964). The effect of amphetamine on the sleep cycle. *Electroencephalography and Clinical Neurophysiology*, *16*, 438–445.

Ribeiro, J. A., & Sebastiao, A. M. (2010). Caffeine and adenosine. *Journal of Alzheimer's Disease*, *20*(Suppl. 1), S3–S15.

Robinson, T. E., & Berridge, K. C. (1993). The neural basis of drug craving: An incentive-sensitization theory of addiction. *Brain Research. Brain Research Reviews*, *18*, 247–291.

Romero, M. J., Asensio, S., Palau, C., Sanchez, A., & Romero, F. (2010). Cocaine addiction: Diffusion tensor imaging study of the inferior frontal and anterior cingulate white matter. *Psychiatry Research*, *181*, 57–63.

Rosselli, M., Ardila, A., Lubomski, M., Murray, S., & King, K. (2001). Personality profile and neuropsychological test performance in chronic cocaine-abusers. *International Journal of Neuroscience, 110*, 55–72.
Rothman, R. B., Blough, B. E., & Baumann, M. H. (2006). Dual dopamine-5-HT releasers: Potential treatment agents for cocaine addiction. *Trends in Pharmacological Sciences, 27*, 612–618.
Rylander, G. (1972). Psychoses and the punding and choreiform syndromes in addiction to central stimulant drugs. *Psychiatria, Neurologia, Neurochirurgia, 75*, 203–212.
Sanotsky, Y., Lesyk, R., Fedoryshyn, L., Komnatska, I., Matviyenko, Y., & Fahn, S. (2007). Manganic encephalopathy due to "ephedrone" abuse. *Movement Disorders, 22*, 1337–1343.
Schiorring, E. (1981). Psychopathology induced by "speed drugs". *Pharmacology, Biochemistry, and Behavior, 14*(Suppl. 1), 109–122.
Schwabe, L., Dickinson, A., & Wolf, O. T. (2011). Stress, habits, and drug addiction: A psychoneuroendocrinological perspective. *Experimental and Clinical Psychopharmacology, 19*, 53–63.
Sesack, S. R., & Pickel, V. M. (1992). Prefrontal cortical efferents in the rat synapse on unlabeled neuronal targets of catecholamine terminals in the nucleus accumbens septi and on dopamine neurons in the ventral tegmental area. *Journal of Comparative Neurology, 320*, 145–160.
Sikk, K., Haldre, S., Aquilonius, S. M., & Taba, P. (2011). Manganese-induced Parkinsonism due to ephedrone abuse. *Parkinson's Disease, 2011*, 865319.
Spear, L. P. (2000). The adolescent brain and age-related behavioral manifestations. *Neuroscience and Biobehavioral Reviews, 24*, 417–463.
Steinberg, L. (2004). Risk taking in adolescence: What changes, and why? *Annals of the New York Academy of Sciences, 1021*, 51–58. http://dx.doi.org/10.1196/annals.1308.005.
Streeter, C. C., Terhune, D. B., Whitfield, T. H., Gruber, S., Sarid-Segal, O., Silveri, M. M., et al. (2008). Performance on the Stroop predicts treatment compliance in cocaine-dependent individuals. *Neuropsychopharmacology, 33*, 827–836.
Subramaniam, K., Luks, T. L., Fisher, M., Simpson, G. V., Nagarajan, S., & Vinogradov, S. (2012). Computerized cognitive training restores neural activity within the reality monitoring network in schizophrenia. *Neuron, 73*, 842–853.
Swainson, R., Rogers, R. D., Sahakian, B. J., Summers, B. A., Polkey, C. E., & Robbins, T. W. (2000). Probabilistic learning and reversal deficits in patients with Parkinson's disease or frontal or temporal lobe lesions: Possible adverse effects of dopaminergic medication. *Neuropsychologia, 38*, 596–612.
Taylor, S. B., Lewis, C. R., & Olive, M. F. (2013). The neurocircuitry of illicit psychostimulant addiction: Acute and chronic effects in humans. *Substance Abuse and Rehabilitation, 4*, 29–43. http://dx.doi.org/10.2147/SAR.S39684.
Teixeira, S., Machado, S., Paes, F., Velasques, B., Silva, J. G., Sanfim, A. L., et al. (2013). Time perception distortion in neuropsychiatric and neurological disorders. *CNS & Neurological Disorders Drug Targets, 12*, 567–582.
Thompson, P. M., Hayashi, K. M., Simon, S. L., Geaga, J. A., Hong, M. S., Sui, Y., et al. (2004). Structural abnormalities in the brains of human subjects who use methamphetamine. *Journal of Neuroscience, 24*, 6028–6036.
Valladares, E. M., & Irwin, M. R. (2007). Polysomnographic sleep dysregulation in cocaine dependence. *ScientificWorldJournal, 7*, 213–216.
Vertes, R. P., Hoover, W. B., Szigeti-Buck, K., & Leranth, C. (2007). Nucleus reuniens of the midline thalamus: Link between the medial prefrontal cortex and the hippocampus. *Brain Research Bulletin, 71*, 601–609.
Volkow, N. D., Chang, L., Wang, G. J., Fowler, J. S., Leonido-Yee, M., Franceschi, D., et al. (2001). Association of dopamine transporter reduction with psychomotor impairment in methamphetamine abusers. *The American Journal of Psychiatry, 158*, 377–382.

Wagner, M. K. (2001). Behavioral characteristics related to substance abuse and risk-taking, sensation-seeking, anxiety sensitivity, and self-reinforcement. *Addictive Behaviors, 26*, 115–120.

Wittmann, M., Leland, D. S., Churan, J., & Paulus, M. P. (2007). Impaired time perception and motor timing in stimulant-dependent subjects. *Drug and Alcohol Dependence, 90*, 183–192.

Wood, S., Sage, J. R., Shuman, T., & Anagnostaras, S. G. (2014). Psychostimulants and cognition: A continuum of behavioral and cognitive activation. *Pharmacological Reviews, 66*, 193–221.

Xie, X., Ramirez, D. R., Lasseter, H. C., & Fuchs, R. A. (2010). Effects of mGluR1 antagonism in the dorsal hippocampus on drug context-induced reinstatement of cocaine-seeking behavior in rats. *Psychopharmacology, 208*, 1–11.

Zhingel, K. Y., Dovensky, W., Crossman, A., & Allen, A. (1991). Ephedrone: 2-methylamino-1-phenylpropan-1-one (Jeff). *Journal of Forensic Sciences, 36*, 915–920.

Zuckerman, M. (1979). *Sensation seeking: Beyond the optimal level of arousal*. Hillsdale, NJ: Lawrence Erlbaum Associates.

Zuckerman, M. (1986). Sensation seeking and the endogenous deficit theory of drug abuse. *NIDA Research Monograph, 74*, 59–70.

Zweben, J. E., Cohen, J. B., Christian, D., Galloway, G. P., Salinardi, M., Parent, D., et al. (2004). Psychiatric symptoms in methamphetamine users. *The American Journal on Addictions, 13*, 181–190.

CHAPTER NINE

Neuropsychiatric Adverse Effects of Amphetamine and Methamphetamine

Jaanus Harro[1]
Division of Neuropsychopharmacology, Department of Psychology, University of Tartu, Tartu, Estonia
[1]Corresponding author: e-mail address: jaanus.harro@ut.ee

Contents

Abstract

Administration of amphetamine and methamphetamine can elicit psychiatric adverse effects at acute administration, binge use, withdrawal, and chronic use. Most troublesome of these are psychotic states and aggressive behavior, but a large variety of undesirable changes in cognition and affect can be induced. Adverse effects occur more frequently with higher dosages and long-term use. They can subside over time but some persist long-term. Multiple alterations in the gray and white matter of the brain assessed as changes in tissue volume or metabolism, or at molecular level, have been associated with amphetamine and methamphetamine use and the psychiatric adverse effects, but further studies are required to clarify their causal role, specificity, and relationship with preceding states and traits and comorbidities. The latter include other substance use disorders, mood and anxiety disorders, attention deficit hyperactivity disorder, and antisocial personality disorder. Amphetamine- and methamphetamine-related psychosis is similar to schizophrenia in terms of symptomatology and pathogenesis, and these two disorders share predisposing genetic factors.

International Review of Neurobiology, Volume 120
ISSN 0074-7742
http://dx.doi.org/10.1016/bs.irn.2015.02.004

1. INTRODUCTORY REMARKS

While the numbers of users of stimulants such as amphetamine and methamphetamine can be assessed with some precision and validity, obvious difficulties are encountered if trying to quantitatively assess the levels of occurrence of adverse effects of these substances in any population, as their use is illegal and this places serious obstacles on the way of performing studies with balanced design and adequate consideration of potential confounding factors. Nevertheless, neuropsychiatric adverse effects are known to have a strong impact on quality of life of drug users, and with the existing high number of them the burden on medical resources is felt. Similarly, and even more so, systematic research on the central nervous system (CNS) effects of such illicit drugs, and on the impact of their chronic use (see Table 1 for overview), is a daunting task: subjects with a drug problem have multiple mental and physical health issues but they may be less cooperative, and their background and lifestyle present various confounders. Cross-sectional studies of long-term effects of (meth)amphetamine may be severely confounded, as pathways to illicit drug use include genetic and environmental factors that may have independent effects on the CNS structure and function, produce lifestyle changes that are reflected in symptomatology, and lead to the substantial comorbidity of amphetamine and methamphetamine use disorders with other psychiatric disorders and somatic conditions. Psychiatry is still relying on interview-based expert decision and no diagnostic test of physiological activity has been introduced; hence, all research on the neural function underlying adverse effects is specific to scientific aims, therefore, limited in scope and volume, and until recently very modest in terms of technology that could be applied to a living patient. As to postmortem research that accesses the brain tissue, drug-related deaths are typically referred to medico-legal autopsies that may limit the possibility to collect tissue samples, and often the pathologist is dealing with polydrug use that is increasingly common (Cadet, Bisagno, & Milroy, 2014). Much of the available literature that presents information with sufficient scope or modern technology is fairly recent and therefore devoted specifically to methamphetamine use that has become a dominant drug problem in many regions, and in many studies amphetamine and methamphetamine are used synonymously.

Bearing these limitations in mind, one can appreciate the sheer amount of information that has been collected on the psychiatric conditions connected to amphetamine and methamphetamine use and their neural

Table 1 Main Neuropsychiatric Adverse Effects, Comorbidities, and Neurobiological Changes Associated with Amphetamine and Methamphetamine Use

Symptoms/Syndromes			**Neurobiological Findings**		**Comorbidities**
Acute/Binge	**Withdrawal**	**Chronic Use**	**Molecular**	**Regional**	
Cognitive bias (e.g., memory retrieval errors)	Depression	Amphetamine/methamphetamine use disorder	Reduced levels of tyrosine hydroxylase, dopamine transporter, serotonin transporter, and dopamine D_2 receptor	Increases and decreases in energy metabolism	Other substance use disorders
Psychotic symptoms	Fatigue	Psychosis	Sensitized dopamine release	Changes in gray matter density	Mood disorders
Anxiety	Sleep disturbance	(Schizophrenia?)		Reduced neuronal integrity	Anxiety disorders
Insomnia	Agitation	Anxiety, insomnia		Changes in white-matter density	Attention deficit hyperactivity disorder
Aggressiveness	Irritability	Cognitive decline		Microglial activation	Antisocial personality disorder
	Poor concentration	Suicidality		Altered EEG patterns	Parkinson's disease (?)

substrate. Psychopharmacology has always devoted much energy to making use of the study of drug action for learning about the function of the brain and the mental faculties. While in case of illicit drugs, the possibilities for controlled experiments are limited, much can be inferred from the examination of drug users who have, notwithstanding their original intentions while self-administering the substance, become participants in analysis of the harm to mental health that these substances can bring. Similarly, studies on drug users can help to reveal predictive and associated factors and underlying pathogenetic mechanisms.

2. SHORT-TERM EFFECTS

Amphetamine-like drugs facilitate attention and performance of various tasks if taken as single doses and especially in conditions that are taxing to the subject. It also appears in recent studies that such single doses can increase memory retrieval errors by biasing recall toward positively rated stimuli that may be relevant to their potential of abuse (Ballard, Gallo, & de Wit, 2014). The acute euphorigenic- and alertness-enhancing effects of amphetamine and methamphetamine usually transform to psychiatric conditions during their binge use, in which the drug is repeatedly administrated over a period of hours or days. This pattern of administration occurs commonly in chronic drug users (Scott et al., 2007). The nature of the mechanism of action of amphetamine and methamphetamine facilitates tachyphylactic reduction of effect and this in turn supports progressive increasing of doses: an amphetamine addict may take up to 1 g of the drug daily (Crossland, 1970). During such a binge, within 2 days, anxiety, irritability, insomnia, paranoid ideation, hallucinations, and delirium may develop (Smith & Fischer, 1970). Psychotic conditions frequently include auditory hallucinations and bizarre delusions (Harris & Batki, 2000). Very often, the delusions are of persecutory nature (Srisurapanont et al., 2003). Stereotypic behavior may develop, and may include some complexity like assembling and dissembling devices, without ability to stop even if the activity is perceived as meaningless (King & Ellinwood, 1992). Some patients with paranoid states will need to remain in hospital for months, and despite of abstinence from the stimulant and treatment with antipsychotic drugs, symptoms tend to persist in a few subjects (Iwanami et al., 1994).

Withdrawal period can be subjectively highly distressing but not a life-threatening condition (McGregor et al., 2005; Scott et al., 2007; Watson, Hartmann, & Schildkraut, 1972). Depression, fatigue, insomnia or hypersomnia, and increased appetite or agitation are common symptoms. A prospective study of abstinence concluded that while moderate levels of depression are reported by methamphetamine users during the first several days of abstinence, these symptoms (most prominently anhedonia, irritability, and poor concentration) subsided thereafter, and while the abstinence syndrome was individually variable with regard to intensity and duration, it was generally mild and resolved quickly in most of the subjects (Newton, Kalechstein, Duran, Vansluis, & Ling, 2004).

One particular concern over the use of amphetamine and methamphetamine is aggressive behavior. Methamphetamine use has been associated with impulsive, aggressive, antisocial, and in cases, with homicidal behavior in many studies (Anglin, Burke, Perrochet, Stamper, & Dawud-Noursi, 2000; Freese, Miotto, & Reback, 2002; Scott et al., 2007; Sekine et al., 2006). This behavior often brings the addicts into conflict with law, and drug users have high odds of receiving assault and weapons charges (Zweben et al., 2004). Hostility is partly coincident with psychotic symptoms elicited by methamphetamine: it has been found co-occurring and is more common with severe and longer lasting episodes of methamphetamine-associated psychosis (McKetin, McLaren, Lubman, & Hides, 2008). Amphetamine- and methamphetamine-linked aggressive behavior is facilitated by combination with alcohol use that increases the unprovoked violent behavior (Asnis & Smith, 1978).

3. DRUG USE DISORDER AND PREDISPOSITION

Of the neuropsychiatric conditions associated with chronic use of amphetamine and methamphetamine, the most obviously causally related is the respective drug use disorder. This develops as the subject becomes dependent on the drug, and the symptomatology revolves around craving the drug, and its usage (Perez-Mana, Castells, Torrens, Capella, & Farre, 2013). The patient will become engaged in dysfunctional behavior but lose control over the quantities of drug used and use frequency and continues drug use despite of persistent problems with health and social functioning. The addicted person is to a high degree preoccupied with the drug and gives up formerly pleasurable and even important activities. Attempts can be made to curb this preoccupation and to reduce use, but in vain. While the causal factor here clearly is the substance, disposition to the pathogenetic process triggered by the stimulant involves preexistent brain vulnerability that is at least in part genetic.

The genes and pathways that predispose to stimulant use and consequent neuropsychiatric symptoms still need to be identified, even though a number of genes have been nominally associated with methamphetamine use disorders (Bousman, Glatt, Everall, & Tsuang, 2009). Nevertheless, some of the genes already identified as having variants associated with neuropsychiatric adverse effects of amphetamine and methamphetamine are informative with regard to the underlying brain mechanisms of both addiction and other psychiatric disorders. For example, variants of the dopamine D_2 receptor encoding gene have been found to predispose to earlier onset of methamphetamine psychosis and to spontaneous relapses of psychosis after remission (Ujike et al., 2009). Because dopamine release and subsequent D_2 receptor activation are implicated in the action of amphetamine and derivatives, and in pathogenesis of addiction and schizophrenia, this molecular genetic mechanism may serve as one of the common links between drug use and psychotic symptoms. A variant of the gene encoding the type 1 receptor of neuropeptide Y (*NPYR1*) has been associated with methamphetamine use and psychosis (Okahisa et al., 2009), and this may be pathogenetically relevant as the blockade of NPY Y_1 receptors strongly reduces the effects of dopamine receptor agonists and dopamine-releasing drugs (Kask & Harro, 2000). Several genes contributing to the function of glutamatergic synapses have been associated with methamphetamine use disorder and other neuropsychiatric conditions related to stimulant effects. One such a gene that has a variant associated with increased risk for methamphetamine-related psychosis is *G72*, that encodes a protein possibly activating the D-amino acid oxidase and hence moderating the D-serine-dependent NMDA receptor activation (Kotaka et al., 2009) that in turn is implicated in glutamate-mediated pathway to schizophrenia, and affected by methamphetamine treatment (Lee, Kim, Lee, & Jang, 2011). Other glutamate-related genes that have variants associated with methamphetamine include the glycine transporter 1 gene (*GLYT1*) that was linked with the prevalence of the methamphetamine use disorder (Morita et al., 2008); the dysbindin gene, a gene that has been associated not only with schizophrenia and psychosis in bipolar disorder but also with methamphetamine psychosis (Kishimoto et al., 2008); and a gene for a subunit of the NMDA receptor itself, *GRIN1*, that had a variant more frequently found in patients with methamphetamine psychosis (Chanasong, Thanoi, Watiktinkorn, Reynolds, & Nudmamud-Thanoi, 2013).

4. PSYCHOSIS

Other long-term adverse effects of amphetamine and methamphetamine range from such transient conditions as anxiety and insomnia to paranoid ideation and convulsions (Krasnova & Cadet, 2009; Murray, 1998), but the particular concern with amphetamine and methamphetamine use is their association with psychosis. Chronic use enhances the risk for psychosis, and this risk is dependent on dose and, inversely, the age of onset of drug use (Farrell et al., 2002).

Abused psychoactive substances of all classes have been implicated in psychosis, but amphetamine and methamphetamine use is clinically highly significant in this regard, and 26–46% of patients with methamphetamine dependence have been estimated to develop methamphetamine-associated psychosis (Grant et al., 2012). While psychosis that occurs during a binge episode or withdrawal is usually transient, susceptibility to psychotic disorders is increasing with chronic methamphetamine use (Ujike & Sato, 2004). In a community sample of methamphetamine users in the Sydney area, 13% of subjects appeared to have psychosis at a structured interview and 23% had experienced clinically significant symptoms of psychosis (McKetin, McLaren, Lubman, & Hides, 2006). Signs of psychosis were three times more prevalent in methamphetamine-dependent subjects compared to non-dependent users. Psychosis is more frequent in addicts who inject the drug, either amphetamine (Hall, Hando, Darke, & Ross, 1996) or methamphetamine (McKetin et al., 2006).

Methamphetamine-associated psychosis is frequently characterized by persecutory delusions and auditory hallucinations, but also delusions of reference, visual hallucinations, and thought broadcasting (Akiyama, 2006; Grant et al., 2012). The psychotic state can be resolved with dopamine receptor antagonists (Grant et al., 2012). Some patients with methamphetamine psychosis do not remit psychotic symptoms for weeks or months, exhibiting the so-called "prolonged type of methamphetamine-induced psychosis" (Ujike & Sato, 2004). In Japan, where amphetamine and subsequently methamphetamine use have historically been a great concern, and attracted much research and clinical interest, the opinion prevails that methamphetamine psychosis is not reflecting a precipitation of psychosis in subjects with preexisting schizoid trait but rather a genuine drug-induced schizophrenia-type psychosis (Ikeda et al., 2013). In Thailand, follow-up of patients with methamphetamine psychosis revealed that one-quarter of them had been given the diagnosis of schizophrenia within the next 5 years after their first hospitalization (Kittirattanapaiboon et al., 2010). Psychotic reaction in users of amphetamine and its analogs is also more common in subjects with schizotypal or schizoid traits (Chen et al., 2003) and in subjects with family history of psychotic disorders (Chen et al., 2005). One recent study followed 15 methamphetamine users and their 15 siblings who all had family background of schizophrenia for 5 years, and found that while just one of the control siblings developed schizophrenia, seven methamphetamine users were diagnosed of schizophrenia (Li et al., 2014). This result would suggest a causal role of methamphetamine in schizophrenia but does not necessarily generalize to people without family history of this disorder.

The average difference between age of onset of amphetamine use and the onset of psychotic disorders has been estimated at slightly more than 5 years (Power et al., 2014). Once developed, methamphetamine-related psychosis is predictive of poor outcomes: more than half of those who could be reached at follow-up about 6 years after the index episode had experienced a relapse of psychosis or had current alcohol use disorder (Kittirattanapaiboon et al., 2010).

5. COGNITION, AFFECT, AND SUICIDALITY

Cognitive function is, expectedly, disturbed in subjects abusing methamphetamine (Dean, Groman, Morales, & London, 2013). This has been well documented in domains of episodic memory; executive functions; and information processing speed, motor skills, language, and visuoconstructional abilities (Scott et al., 2007). These impairments would be consistent with alterations in frontostriatal and limbic circuits (see below). A complex question to be addressed is to what extent the cognitive and emotional dysfunction in stimulant abusers is related to dependence and other neuropsychiatric issues. Neither is it clear to which extent the latter are caused by the repeated exposure to the drug versus reflecting comorbidity. The preponderance of evidence however supports the notion that methamphetamine use is causal to cognitive decline in at least some users of the drug (Dean et al., 2013). One twin study (Toomey et al., 2003) has addressed the issue of whether amphetamine or methamphetamine use has a causal effect or is it the lower cognitive abilities that predispose to drug use. Because of the limitations to design the results were not conclusive, but still suggest that stimulant use may reduce some cognitive measures.

Cognitive impairments appear as persistent because former methamphetamine users who become abstinent show memory deficits months after discontinuation of drug use (Rendell, Mazur, & Henry, 2009). It is not only in psychological assessments that cognitive deficits become evident; everyday life also becomes disorganized, owing to limited coping skills and reduction of social support (Cretzmeyer, Sarrazin, Huber, Block, & Hall, 2003; Henry, Minassian, & Perry, 2010; Obermeit et al., 2013). By means of questionnaires covering such aspects of everyday functioning like financial management, shopping, housekeeping, telephone use, etc., the daily difficulties that the methamphetamine users experience have been demonstrated to be related to their cognitive decline, even when controlling for the confounding effect of depressive symptoms (Sadek, Vigil, Grant, & Heaton, 2007). This may become particularly relevant with aging, as a comparative study of formerly methamphetamine-dependent patients revealed the detrimental effect of methamphetamine use to become apparent at more advanced ages (Iudicello et al., 2014).

Methamphetamine users can present depression and suicidal ideation during active drug use and withdrawal period, but also increased risk during abstinence (Kalechstein et al., 2000; Scott et al., 2007). Again, injecting drug users are more vulnerable (Domier, Simon, Rawson, Huber, & Ling, 2000). Nevertheless, in some studies, negative affect is more strongly related to recent abstinence and higher quantity consumed than other variables (Montoya et al., 2013), and the link with major depression is relative weak. Mood transients and impulsive behavior seem to be a component in the variety of psychiatric syndromes methamphetamine use can lead to, with the most severe outcome laying in the increase in suicidality (Glasner-Edwards et al., 2008). A recent prospective study in Canada associated chronic injecting of amphetamine with suicide attempts with (adjusted) odds ratio of about 2 (Artenie et al., 2015). Also in the follow-up study of methamphetamine psychosis in Thailand quoted above (Kittirattanapaiboon et al., 2010), suicidality was very high.

6. NEUROPSYCHIATRIC CORRELATES OF ADVERSE EFFECTS

Subjects who are methamphetamine dependent are estimated to self-administer between 500 and 1400 mg of the drug daily in one to five doses, and more than 20 times per month (Dean et al., 2013; Simon et al., 2002). This becomes a remarkable load on the brain that takes the drug up fast. The easy entrance of amphetamine and its analogs, including methamphetamine, into the CNS and their high affinity for the cell membrane transporters of noradrenaline, dopamine, and serotonin leads upon administration of these stimulants to fast uptake by neurons that express the transporter proteins. It hence follows that brain regions enriched with monoamine transporters are most exposed to intracellular action of amphetamine and methamphetamine. Because much of the subsequent cellular toxicity is due to the release and auto-oxidation of dopamine (Krasnova & Cadet, 2009), dopamine-rich brain regions become particularly vulnerable and observable adverse effects are likely to reflect this.

Consistently, postmortem studies have also revealed significant biochemical and/or structural abnormalities in some addicted individuals (Cadet et al., 2014). On the other hand, the sympathomimetic effects of amphetamine derivatives are known to raise blood pressure, and the risk of ischemic strokes, and intracerebral and subarachnoid hemorrhages are high with methamphetamine use, the brain regions where the strokes occur coinciding with the pattern of hypertensive hemorrhages (Cadet et al., 2014; Olsen, 1977).

In postmortem studies, striatal levels of tyrosine hydroxylase, the rate-limiting enzyme in catecholamine synthesis, as well as levels of dopamine and the dopamine transporter have been found lower in chronic methamphetamine users (Wilson et al., 1996). Dopamine transporters have been labeled *in vivo* and these positron emission tomography (PET) studies agree with postmortem findings (Johanson et al., 2006; McCann et al., 1998; Volkow, Chang, Wang, Fowler, Leonido-Yee, et al., 2001). Reduction of dopamine binding capacity in caudate and putamen was about 20–30% in these studies, and this is quantitatively clearly lower than what occurs in patients with Parkinson's disease (McCann et al., 1998). Nevertheless, dopamine transporter reduction was found to be associated with motor slowing and memory impairment (Volkow, Chang, Wang, Fowler, Leonido-Yee, et al., 2001). Of note, a functional variant of the dopamine transporter gene has been associated with increased risk of development of psychosis after methamphetamine use (Ujike et al., 2003).

After abstinence for 1–1½ years, the dopamine transporter reduction in methamphetamine users, as measured by PET with [^{11}C]D-threo-methylphenidate, had shown some recovery as compared to short abstinence period (Volkow et al., 2001a). This study was longitudinal and the recovery of dopamine transporter availability was very strongly correlated with the duration of abstinence. Improvement in motor and cognitive functions was at trend levels, but the number of subjects was just five so any statistical assessment of both indicators of transporter binding and function measures should not be considered definitive. The fact that dopamine transporter levels increase suggests that either the reduction was not organic or that the damaged terminals can be replaced in humans, possibly after arborization. A small single-photon emission computed tomography (SPECT) study assessed dopamine transporter availability and performance in Wisconsin Card Sorting Test (WCST) at baseline when subjects screened positive for methamphetamine and after 2 weeks of abstinence (Chou et al., 2007) and also found an increase of both measures and a positive relationship between the gains (with dopamine transporter assessed in the striatum). The presence of the drug at initial measurements of course complicates the interpretation, and the smallness ($n=5$, plus seven control subjects) of the sample did not facilitate using of all desirable statistical control. Another small SPECT study recently compared dopamine transporter specific uptake ratios 24–48 h after the last administration of methamphetamine and then again 2 and 4 weeks later in the same subjects during continuous abstinence (Yuan et al., 2014). Some increase in the dopamine transporter function was observable in methamphetamine users but the measures were still lower as compared to the control group. Dopamine transporter function in striatum correlated with methamphetamine craving immediately after withdrawal, but this correlation was not strong and did not persist, hence not supporting a major role of dopamine transporters in craving. The difference between the two studies was in the age of the subjects and their drug use pattern: as the patients in Chou et al.'s (2007) study were younger and used methamphetamine less regularly, it can be hypothetized that reversibility of dopamine transporter function is less prominent if the drug users become older or they shift drug habit to regular use, or both.

Pertinent to the dynamics of dopamine transporter availability as a function of methamphetamine use is the issue of whether or not the on average lower cognitive function in methamphetamine users would improve with abstinence. Several studies have addressed this question but without a control group any increase may also be attributed to the common improvement over repeated testing. Comparisons of drug users with longer versus shorter abstinence periods have consistently found better performance in subjects with prolonged (grossly, more than 6 months) abstinence in measures such as the Stroop Task (Salo et al., 2009) and WCST (Kim et al., 2006). However, a longitudinal study with a healthy control group that administered a neuropsychological test battery twice with about 1 year in-between found that neither nonabstinent nor abstinent methamphetamine user group had a larger gain than controls (Iudicello et al., 2010). The authors, nevertheless, pointed out that those drug users who had performed the worst appeared to improve more.

In the postmortem study by Wilson and colleagues (1996), striatal levels of vesicular monoamine transporter type 2 (VMAT2) were not different in methamphetamine users as compared to controls, even though this could have been expected, at least in this brain region, if dopaminergic nerve terminals had been damaged. However, VMAT2 levels were reduced in chronic methamphetamine users who had been abstinent for, on average, 3 years, suggestive of occurrence of persistent nerve terminal damage, previously shown in animals, to occur also in human (Johanson et al., 2006). The very limited decline in neurocognitive functioning in these subjects however suggests that the cognitive symptoms improve over time and that these neurotoxic effects may have relationship with cognitive symptoms.

Serotonin transporter density was found reduced in methamphetamine users by PET in many brain regions including cerebral cortex, thalamus, caudate, putamen, and cerebellum (Sekine et al., 2006), and level of aggressiveness, as measured by the Buss and Perry Aggression Questionnaire, as well as the duration of methamphetamine use was found to correlate negatively with serotonin transporter availability in the orbitofrontal, anterior cingulate, and temporal cortex. This however was a study on 12 patients and no replication study appears to have been made. The psychiatric background was rather mixed, the sample including patients with persistent psychotic state, depression, or anxiety, and four patients had severe aggression but the correlation between aggressiveness and serotonin transporter binding did not appear to rest on these cases but rather characterize the whole sample. The reduction of serotonin transporter density did not appear to correlate with the length of abstinence, supporting persistent decline. As the subjects were confirmedly abstinent from the drug, this association of aggressiveness with methamphetamine use could not be attributed to the direct drug effect but rather to the persistent reduction in the capacity of serotonergic neurotransmission that has since long been known to contribute to increases in impulsivity and aggressive behavior (Linnoila et al., 1983), as are lesions of these brain regions and regional alterations of other serotonergic measures (Parsey, Oquendo, Simpson, Ogden, van Heertum, Arango, et al., 2002).

As little as three instances of amphetamine administration have in human experimental conditions led to increased dopamine release in striatum 1 year later (Boileau et al., 2006). While such a sensitization phenomenon is thought to contribute to the development of dependence, the increased capacity of dopamine release resembles the high dopamine response to amphetamine observed in schizophrenia patients (Laruelle et al., 1996). As discussed above, repeated administration of (meth)amphetamine in a brief period can elicit paranoid psychosis hard to distinguish from acute schizophrenic episode; in long-term methamphetamine users with psychosis, the clinical picture mimics the positive symptomatology of schizophrenia (Chen et al., 2003). Another key protein in the dopaminergic system, the dopamine D_2 receptor, has been found downregulated in methamphetamine users in PET studies, but this is a phenomenon in common with other addictions, as low dopamine D_2 receptor availability has also been found in alcoholics and heroin users (Lee et al., 2009; Volkow, Chang, Wang, Fowler, Ding, et al., 2001).

Glucose metabolism as measured by [^{18}F]fluorodeoxyglucose PET was found to be higher in methamphetamine users across the brain, and to the largest extent in parietal cortex (Volkow et al., 2001b). This latter finding has been confirmed by other PET studies (Berman, Voytek, et al., 2008). This would indicate a spread of neural alterations to other brain regions besides the primarily dopaminergic. When normalized for this overall higher metabolic activity, the patients had lower glucose uptake in thalamus and in striatum. Another study reported both reductions and increases of relative regional glucose metabolism in methamphetamine users: while an increase was found in orbitofrontal, and middle and posterior cingulate areas, amygdala, ventral striatum, and cerebellum, a reduction was present in anterior cingulate and insula (London et al., 2004). Particularly, the alterations in anterior cingulate and amygdala have been associated with the increase in depressive symptomatology in methamphetamine users (Scott et al., 2007). A longitudinal PET study in five methamphetamine-dependent patients reported a relative regional increase of metabolism in thalamus with continuation of abstinence from the start at less than 6 to more than 12 months (Wang et al., 2004). Some of the improvements in neuropsychological performance were correlated with the thalamic increase in glucose uptake.

Another *in vivo* technique that is based on CNS metabolism, proton magnetic resonance spectroscopy, provides indirect information on neuronal integrity by quantitating *N*-acetylaspartate. Methamphetamine users have been found with lower *N*-acetylaspartate levels in anterior cingulate, basal ganglia, and white matter (Ernst, Chang, Leonido-Yee, & Speck,

2000), and the reduction was found to correlate with greater drug use (Sung et al., 2007), but not all studies agree (Taylor et al., 2007).

Literature on brain structural abnormality in methamphetamine use is rich but contains many inconsistencies, probably owing to the multitude of technologies used and cross-sectional designs with their confounding factors (Berman, O'Neill, Fears, Bartzokis, & London, 2008; Salo & Fassbender, 2012). First imaging studies with magnetic resonance tomography suggested abnormalities at regional level in methamphetamine users, possibly selectively associated with medial part of the temporal lobe (Thompson et al., 2004). Severe gray matter deficits were described in the cingulate, limbic and paralimbic cortex, and hippocampus, while white matter was hypertrophic. In abstinent methamphetamine users, gray matter density was lower bilaterally in insula and in left middle frontal gyrus (Schwartz et al., 2010). Cortical gray matter loss in frontal lobe, temporal lobe, and insula was age dependent and significantly faster in methamphetamine users, and hence drug use could be associated with accelerated reduction of mental capacities (Nakama et al., 2011), e.g., with the marked detrimental effect of methamphetamine use on episodic memory (Scott et al., 2007). Alterations in insula, in particular, have been associated with changed motivational status of the addicted subjects (Schwartz et al., 2010), and indeed activation of insula (but also posterior cingulate and temporal cortex) have been reported to predict relapse in methamphetamine-dependent patients (Paulus, Tapert, & Schuckit, 2005).

In contrast, volume of caudate, putamen, globus pallidus, and nucleus accumbens has been found larger in methamphetamine users (Berman, O'Neill, et al., 2008; Chang et al., 2005; Jernigan et al., 2005). Chang and colleagues (2005) also reported larger mid-posterior corpus callosum in female methamphetamine users.

Exactly, how these volume changes may have bearance on neuropsychiatric conditions brought about by amphetamine or methamphetamine remains to be identified. During abstinence from a few days to 1 month postdrug, gray matter was increasing in methamphetamine-dependent patients in several brain regions, including the temporal gyrus, right angular gyrus, right insula, left precuneus, left inferior frontal gyrus, and left occipital pole (Morales, Lee, Hellemann, O'Neill, & London, 2012), but the functional relevance of these changes was not assessed.

White-matter abnormalities have been found manifold. MRI studies have found prominent temporal and occipital white-matter hypertrophy (Thompson et al., 2004). Diffusion tensor imaging studies have reported changes in prefrontal white matter, corpus callosum, corona radiata, and perforant fibers (Tobias et al., 2010). In prefrontal cortex, deoxyglucose uptake was reduced in left inferior frontal white matter (Kim et al., 2009), and this hypometabolism was related to the total cumulative dose of methamphetamine as well as to inferior performance in the WCST. Total and perseverative errors in the WCST have been found to correlate also with the gray matter volume in the right middle frontal gyrus (Kim et al., 2006).

Chronic methamphetamine use activates microglia in various brain regions, such as midbrain, striatum, thalamus, orbitofrontal, and insular cortex, but this microgliosis appears to subside during abstinence (Sekine et al., 2008). Microglial activation has been attributed a role in the pathogenesis of Parkinson's disease (Doorn, Lucassen, Boddeke, Berendse, & van Dam, 2012) and hence proposed to serve as the link for the increased risk of Parkinsonism in methamphetamine users (Granado, Ares-Santos, & Moratalla, 2013) but is also found in schizophrenia (Wierzba-Bobrowicz, Lewandowska, Lechowicz, Stepien, & Pasennik, 2005) and depression (Rajkowska & Miguel-Hidalgo, 2007). Nevertheless, there appear to be differences in regional patterns of microglial activation among these disorders, so even if microglial reaction is important either in the development of symptoms or in the adaptation to noxious effectors as a general syndrome for many neuropsychiatric conditions, there are distinct patterns consistent with the affected regions for each disorder. In animal experiments, methamphetamine-elicited microglial activation is preceding damage to striatal dopaminergic nerve terminals (LaVoie, Card, & Hastings, 2004) and hence microglial activation could trigger the neurodegenerative cascade through proinflammatory mechanisms. Protracted abstinence from methamphetamine use can lead to normalization of the microglia, as after an approximately 2 years of abstinence was sufficient to observe control levels of microglia activation (Sekine et al., 2008).

Brain imaging studies also suggest reductions specifically in subjects who have developed methamphetamine-associated psychosis. Significant gray matter volume reduction was found in left perisylvian structures (posterior inferior frontal gyrus and anterior superior temporal gyrus) and in frontopolar cortex (Aoki et al., 2013). White-matter volume was also lower in patients in the orbitofrontal area. Other brain regions reported to be affected include hippocampus and amygdala (Orikabe et al., 2011). In this study, the overall volumes and gray and white matter were found lower in subjects with methamphetamine psychosis, but in the temporal lobe regions, the reduction was significant even after correction for this. The reduction in amygdala was the most prominent finding and the authors suggested this alteration to be a relative specific symptom of methamphetamine psychosis, as it is not commonly found in schizophrenia.

EEG measures are also altered in methamphetamine users. A couple of small quantitative EEG studies during a brief abstinence period revealed increased theta power that correlated with reaction times in more difficult tasks and reduced accuracy of working memory, and measures in delayed recall tasks (Kalechstein et al., 2009; Newton, Kalechstein, Hardy, et al., 2004).

7. COMORBIDITY

As referred to above, the interdependence of distinct but comorbid psychiatric disorders has not been clarified to any great extent. Without prospective studies this issue will never be finally settled, but a few retrospective analyses have addressed methamphetamine-associated psychosis with the purpose to understand why some but not all methamphetamine abusers will develop psychotic symptoms. The psychotic methamphetamine users have been characterized as having been younger at initiation of drug use, having been using larger dosages, and at assessment produced higher scores of the premorbid schizoid and schizotypal traits inventory, and presented more psychiatric comorbidity (Chen et al., 2003). Principal component analysis of symptoms observed in methamphetamine psychosis yielded clusters of symptoms of anxiety and depression, and two psychotic symptoms clusters, negative and positive/disorganized syndromes (Srisurapanont et al., 2003). Presence of negative symptoms (poverty of speech, psychomotor retardation, and flattened or incongruous affect) is less frequent but still occurs in a substantial proportion, at least in one-fifth of the patients. Similarities between methamphetamine-related psychosis and schizophrenia that exist at clinical and neurobiological level recently received genetic support: a genome-wide association study comparing in a hypothesis-free manner the molecular genetics of methamphetamine dependence, methamphetamine psychosis and schizophrenia, and performing polygenic component analysis did find that the two psychotic conditions share much of the "risk alleles" (Ikeda et al., 2013).

Antisocial personality disorder that is more prevalent in methamphetamine users (Chen et al., 2003; Glasner-Edwards et al., 2010) is likely to represent a condition that may have rather preceded and contributed to initiation of drug use and subsequent development of the drug use disorder.

Indeed, the higher frequency of antisocial behavior preceding the methamphetamine-related as compared to schizophrenic psychosis (Grant et al., 2012) has been pointed out as an argument for keeping the pathogenesis of these two disorders separate (see Aoki et al., 2013).

Higher prevalence of bipolar disorder in drug users (Shoptaw, Peck, Reback, & Rotheram-Fuller, 2003) may also reflect at least the genetic predisposition either specific to mania or general to mental health vulnerability that possibly contributed to stimulant use. It can however also owe to difficulties with differential diagnosis between drug-related syndrome and the genuine bipolar disorder. In chronic methamphetamine users, mood disorders and anxiety disorders are fairly frequent (Conway, Compton, Stinson, & Grant, 2006), and a smaller proportion of these have been attributed directly to the use of the drug (Salo et al., 2011). Changes in self-reported depressive symptoms were in strong correlation with relative deoxyglucose uptake in ventral striatum, in a study with two measurements 4 weeks of supervised abstinence apart (Berman, Voytek, et al., 2008). Striatal dopamine D_2 receptor availability in striatum, at baseline or after amphetamine administration, was however not associated with depression (Parsey et al., 2001), but this remains to be investigated in drug users. Depressive symptoms in early abstinence were also associated with white-matter integrity in midcaudal superior corona radiata (Tobias et al., 2010).

Methamphetamine use is common in attention deficit hyperactivity disorder (ADHD) patients (Jaffe et al., 2005; Matsumoto, Kamijo, Yamaguchi, Iseki, & Hirayasu, 2005) and is associated with more severe cognitive symptomatology and less successful everyday functioning than with drug abuse or ADHD alone (Obermeit et al., 2013). ADHD develops earlier than methamphetamine use begins, and hence the co-occurrence has been interpreted as a kind of self-medication, even though it cannot be taken as certain that with the drug taking pattern as observed in illicit stimulant use, the cognitive abilities improve to any extent that would be relevant to better everyday functioning. ADHD is strongly genetic but there can be many mediating mechanisms that connect genes with different psychopathologies. One gene implicated in ADHD is encoding for cadherin 13, and it has also been found associated with both subjective responses to amphetamine and methamphetamine dependence (Hart et al., 2012). ADHD symptomatology is however dimensional in general population, and even if expressed at subsyndromal levels it is deteriorating to educational attainment (Kiive & Harro, 2013) that in turn can reduce social adjustment capabilities and predispose to drug abuse.

A common component in various psychiatric disorders, especially ADHD but also depression, and indeed possibly a predisposing factor, is impulsivity. Impulsive behavior in amphetamine and methamphetamine users may exacerbate their psychosocial behavior (Scott et al., 2007). Higher impulsivity may have already contributed to early experiences with illicit substances and can have been further aggravated by the drug itself. Methamphetamine-related impulsivity is common and has been attributed to striatal dopamine receptor availability (Lee et al., 2009). Methamphetamine users were reported to have fewer years of education than predicted by their cognitive abilities (Dean, Hellemann, Sugar, & London, 2012), and the discrepancy between actual and predicted educational attainment was in negative correlation with the age of first use of the drug. High trait impulsivity and lower skill training can facilitate development of risky decision-making that in methamphetamine-dependent individuals has been associated with higher resting-state functional connectivity of the midbrain with the putamen, amygdala, and hippocampus that in turn is coupled with reduced prefrontal connectivity in task conditions (Kohno, Morales, Grahremani, Hellemann, & London, 2014). In methamphetamine users, higher impulsivity is related to higher intensity drug craving (Tziortzis, Mahoney, Kalechstein, Newton, & De la Garza, 2011).

Even though relatively little is known about CNS alterations brought about by using combinations of addictive drugs, methamphetamine-dependent patients are known to often be polydrug users. About one-fifth to one-third of chronic methamphetamine users have been found to be dependent on alcohol (Simons, Oliver, Gaher, Ebel, & Brummels, 2005).

What is known about neurotoxicity of amphetamine and methamphetamine has served as a realistic background for proposing use of these drugs as a risk factor for developing the clinical picture of Parkinson's disease. Indeed, in subjects using amphetamine or methamphetamine, the risk for Parkinson's disease has been found increased (Callaghan, Cunningham, Sykes, & Kish, 2012). Both illnesses are also characterized by higher prevalence of depression and deterioration of cognitive function. Nevertheless, the prevalence of clinical signs of Parkinson's disease is still not remarkably high in methamphetamine users (Scott et al., 2007), suggesting that the underlying neuropathology is sufficiently distinct. Dopamine levels may not be severely enough reduced in the majority of chronic methamphetamine users, and caudate is affected more than putamen (Moszczynska et al., 2004), which is the opposite pattern to Parkinson's disease. No evidence has been presented that amphetamine and methamphetamine could damage the dopaminergic cell bodies in the substantia nigra and by this means directly cause Parkinsonism. It is conceivable, however, that drug use could contribute to the development of Parkinson's disease when the brain ages, and the trends in drug use and sociodemographic changes may bring about an increase of Parkinson's disease in future. Indeed, recent studies have observed impressive odds ratios for increased risk of Parkinson's disease in amphetamine and methamphetamine users (Curtin et al., 2015).

A special case of psychiatric adverse effects of amphetamine and methamphetamine that deserves attention is the possible deterioration of early development after prenatal exposure. A recent comparison of 412 mother–infant pairs reported that while at age of 7.5 years, children exposed *in utero* to methamphetamine did not exhibit any increase in ADHD or conduct disorder symptomatology, they had much more frequently cognitive problems as measured by the Conners Parent Rating Scale (Diaz et al., 2014).

Conclusively, amphetamine and methamphetamine use is, similarly to abuse of several other intoxicants, leading to long-lasting alterations in cortico-limbic-striatal circuitries that are directly mediating the addictive potential of these substances, but changes in brain are found also in many other cortical and subcortical regions. These alterations may be elicited by drug-induced vascular changes, oxidative stress, and other biochemical cascades (Cadet et al., 2014). Pathological structural changes develop as the addict is intermittently exposing the brain to the often increasing doses of these substances over a period of time, and these are responsible for the plethora of symptoms observed in patients with stimulant use disorders, ranging from changes in behavior to the multitude of somatic deficits. Addiction to amphetamine and methamphetamine is hence a brain disease that comprises symptoms of many other neurological and psychiatric conditions.

REFERENCES

Akiyama, K. (2006). Longitudinal clinical course following pharmacological treatment of methamphetamine psychosis which persists after long-term abstinence. *Annals of the New York Academy of Sciences*, *801*, 136–147.

Anglin, M. D., Burke, C., Perrochet, B., Stamper, E., & Dawud-Noursi, S. (2000). History of the methamphetamine problem. *Journal of Psychoactive Drugs*, *32*, 137–141.

Aoki, Y., Orikabe, L., Tajayanagi, Y., Yahata, N., Mozue, Y., Sudo, Y., et al. (2013). Volume reductions in frontopolar and left perisylvian cortices in methamphetamine induced psychosis. *Schizophrenia Research*, *147*, 355–361.

Artenie, A. A., Bruneau, J., Zang, G., Lesperance, F., Renaud, J., Tremblay, J., et al. (2015). Associations of substance use patterns with attempted suicide among persons who inject drugs: Can distinct use patterns play a role? *Drug and Alcohol Dependence*, *147*, 208–214. http://dx.doi.org/10.1014/j.drugalcdep.2014.11.011.

Asnis, S. F., & Smith, R. C. (1978). Amphetamine abuse and violence. *Journal of Psychedelic Drugs*, *10*, 371–377.

Ballard, M. E., Gallo, D. A., & de Wit, H. (2014). Amphetamine increases errors during episodic memory retrieval. *Journal of Clinical Psychopharmacology*, *34*, 85–92.

Berman, S., O'Neill, J., Fears, S., Bartzokis, G., & London, E. D. (2008). Abuse of amphetamines and structural abnormalities in the brain. *Annals of the New York Academy of Sciences*, *1141*, 195–220.

Berman, S. M., Voytek, B., Mandelkern, M. A., Hassid, B. D., Isaacson, A., Monterosso, J., et al. (2008). Changes in cerebral glucose metabolism during early abstinence from chronic methamphetamine abuse. *Molecular Psychiatry*, *13*, 897–908.

Boileau, I., Dagher, A., Leyton, M., Gunn, R. N., Baker, G. B., Diksic, M., et al. (2006). Modeling sensitization to stimulants in humans. An [^{11}C]-raclopride/positron emission tomography study in healthy men. *Archives of General Psychiatry*, *63*, 1386–1395.

Bousman, C. A., Glatt, S. J., Everall, I. P., & Tsuang, M. T. (2009). Genetic association studies of methamphetamine use disorders: A systematic review and synthesis. *American Journal of Medical Genetics. Part B, Neuropsychiatric Genetics*, *150B*, 1025–1049.

Cadet, J. L., Bisagno, V., & Milroy, C. M. (2014). Neuropathology of substance use disorders. *Acta Neuropathologica*, *127*, 91–107.

Callaghan, R. C., Cunningham, J. K., Sykes, J., & Kish, S. J. (2012). Increased risk of Parkinson's disease in individuals hospitalized with conditions related to the use of methamphetamine or other amphetamine-type drugs. *Drug and Alcohol Dependence*, *120*, 35–40.

Chanasong, R., Thanoi, S., Watiktinkorn, P., Reynolds, G. P., & Nudmamud-Thanoi, S. (2013). Genetic variation of GRIN1 confers vulnerability to methamphetamine-dependent psychosis in a Thai population. *Neuroscience Letters*, *551*, 58–61.

Chang, L., Cloak, C., Patterson, K., Grob, C., Miller, E. N., & Ernst, T. (2005). Enlarged striatum in abstinent methamphetamine abusers: A possible compensatory response. *Biological Psychiatry*, *57*, 967–974.

Chen, C. K., Lin, S. K., Sham, P. C., Ball, D., Loh, E., Hsiao, C. C., et al. (2003). Pre-morbid characteristics and co-morbidity of methamphetamine users with and without psychosis. *Psychological Medicine*, *33*, 1407–1414.

Chen, C. K., Lin, S. K., Sham, P. C., Ball, D., Loh, E., & Murray, R. M. (2005). Morbid risk for psychiatric disorder among the relatives of methamphetamine users with and without psychosis. *American Journal of Medical Genetics Part B, Neuropsychiatric Genetics*, *136*, 87–91.

Chou, Y. H., Huang, W. S., Su, T. P., Lu, R. B., Wan, F. J., & Fu, Y. K. (2007). Dopamine transporters and cognitive function in methamphetamine abuser after a short abstinence: A SPECT study. *European Neuropsychopharmacology*, *17*, 46–52.

Conway, K. P., Compton, W., Stinson, F. S., & Grant, B. F. (2006). Lifetime comorbidity of DSM-IV mood and anxiety disorders and specific drug use disorders: Results from the National Epidemiologic Survey on Alcohol and Related Conditions. *Journal of Clinical Psychiatry*, *67*, 247–257.

Cretzmeyer, M., Sarrazin, M. V., Huber, D. L., Block, R. I., & Hall, J. A. (2003). Treatment of methamphetamine abuse: Research findings and clinical directions. *Journal of Substance Abuse Treatment*, *24*, 267–277.

Crossland, J. (1970). *Lewis's pharmacology* (4th ed.). Edinburgh and London: E. & S. Livingstone (chapter 4).

Curtin, K., Fleckenstein, A. E., Robison, R. J., Crookston, M. J., Smith, K. R., & Hanson, G. R. (2015). Methamphetamine/amphetamine abuse and risk of Parkinson's disease in Utah: A population-based assessment. *Drug and Alcohol Dependence*, *146*, 30–38. http://dx.doi.org/10.1016/j.drugalcdep.2014.10.027.

Dean, A. C., Groman, S. M., Morales, A. M., & London, E. D. (2013). An evaluation of the evidence that methamphetamine abuse causes cognitive decline in humans. *Neuropsychopharmacology, 38*, 256–274.

Dean, A. C., Hellemann, G., Sugar, C. A., & London, E. D. (2012). Educational attainment is not a good proxy for cognitive function in methamphetamine dependence. *Drug and Alcohol Dependence, 123*, 249–254.

Diaz, S. D., Smith, L. M., LaGasse, L. L., Derauf, C., Newman, E., Shah, R., et al. (2014). Effects of prenatal methamphetamine exposure on behavioural and cognitive findings at 7.5 years of age. *Journal of Pediatrics, 164*, 1333–1338.

Domier, C. P., Simon, S. L., Rawson, R. A., Huber, A., & Ling, W. (2000). A comparison of injecting and noninjecting methamphetamine users. *Journal of Psychoactive Drugs, 32*, 229–232.

Doorn, K. J., Lucassen, P. J., Boddeke, H. W., Berendse, H. W., & van Dam, A. M. (2012). Emerging roles of microglial activation and non-motor symptoms in Parkinson's disease. *Progress in Neurobiology, 98*, 222–238.

Ernst, T., Chang, L., Leonido-Yee, M., & Speck, O. (2000). Evidence for long-term neurotoxicity associated with methamphetamine abuse: A ^{1}H MRS study. *Neurology, 54*, 1344–1349.

Farrell, M., Boys, P., Bebbington, T., Brugha, J., Coid, R., Jenkins, G., et al. (2002). Psychosis and drug dependence: Results from a national survey of prisoners. *American Journal of Psychiatry, 181*, 393–398.

Freese, T. E., Miotto, K., & Reback, C. J. (2002). The effects and consequences of selected club drugs. *Journal of Substance Abuse Treatment, 23*, 151–156.

Glasner-Edwards, S., Mooney, L. J., Marinelli-Casey, P., Hillhouse, M., Ang, A., & Rawson, R. (2008). Risk factors for suicide attempts in methamphetamine-dependent patients. *The American Journal on Addictions, 17*, 24–27.

Glasner-Edwards, S., Mooney, L. J., Marinelli-Casey, P., Hillhouse, M., Ang, A., Rawson, R., et al. (2010). Psychopathology in methamphetamine-dependent adults 3 years after treatment. *Drug and Alcohol Review, 29*, 12–20.

Granado, N., Ares-Santos, S., & Moratalla, R. (2013). Methamphetamine and Parkinson's disease. *Parkinson's Disease, 2013*, 308052. http://dx.doi.org/10.1155/2013/308052 (ID308052).

Grant, K. M., LeVan, T. D., Wells, S. M., Li, M., Stoltenberg, S. F., Gendelman, H. E., et al. (2012). Methamphetamine-associated psychosis. *Journal of Neuroimmune Pharmacology, 7*, 113–139.

Hall, C. D., Hando, J., Darke, S., & Ross, J. (1996). Psychological morbidity and route of administration among amphetamine users in Sydney, Australia. *Addiction, 9*, 81–87.

Harris, D., & Batki, S. L. (2000). Stimulant psychosis: Symptom profile and acute clinical course. *The American Journal on Addictions, 9*, 28–37.

Hart, A. B., Engelhardt, B. E., Wardle, M. C., Sokoloff, G., Stephens, M., de Wit, H., et al. (2012). Genome-wide association study of D-amphetamine response in healthy volunteers identifies putative associations, including cadherin 13 (*CDH13*). *PLoS One, 7*, e42646.

Henry, B. L., Minassian, A., & Perry, W. (2010). Effect of methamphetamine dependence on everyday functional abilities. *Addictive Behaviors, 35*, 593–598.

Ikeda, M., Okahisa, Y., Aleksic, B., Won, M., Kondo, N., Naruse, N., et al. (2013). Evidence for shared genetic risk between methamphetamine-induced psychosis and schizophrenia. *Neuropsychopharmacology, 38*, 1864–1870.

Iudicello, J. E., Morgan, E. E., Gongvatana, A., Letendre, S. L., Grant, I., Woods, S. P., et al. (2014). Detrimental impact of remote methamphetamine dependence on neurocognitive and everyday functioning in older but not younger HIV+ adults: Evidence for a legacy effect? *Journal of Neurovirology, 20*, 85–98.

Iudicello, J. E., Woods, S. P., Vigil, O., Scott, J. C., Cherner, M., Heaton, R. K., et al. (2010). Longer term improvement in neurocognitive functioning and affective distress among methamphetamine users who achieve stable abstinence. *Journal of Clinical and Experimental Neuropsychology*, *32*, 704–718.

Iwanami, A., Sugiyama, A., Kuroki, N., Toda, S., Kato, N., Nakatani, Y., et al. (1994). Patients with methamphetamine psychosis admitted to a psychiatric hospital in Japan. A preliminary study. *Acta Psychiatrica Scandinavica*, *89*, 428–432.

Jaffe, C., Bush, K. R., Straits-Tröster, K., Meredith, C., Romwall, L., Rosenbaum, G., et al. (2005). A comparison of methamphetamine-dependent inpatients childhood attention deficit hyperactivity disorder symptomatology. *Journal of Addictive Diseases*, *24*, 133–152.

Jernigan, T. L., Gamst, A. C., Archibald, S. L., Fennema-Notestine, C., Mindt, M. R., Marcotte, T. D., et al. (2005). Effects of methamphetamine dependence and HIV infection on cerebral morphology. *American Journal of Psychiatry*, *162*, 1461–1472.

Johanson, C. E., Frey, K. A., Lundahl, L. H., Keenan, P., Lockhart, N., Roll, J., et al. (2006). Cognitive function and nigrostriatal markers in abstinent methamphetamine abusers. *Psychopharmacology*, *185*, 327–338.

Kalechstein, A. D., De La Garza, R., Newton, T. F., Green, M. F., Cook, I. A., & Leuchter, A. F. (2009). Quantitative EEG abnormalities are associated with memory impairment in recently abstinent methamphetamine-dependent individuals. *Journal of Neuropsychiatry and Clinical Neurosciences*, *21*, 254–258.

Kalechstein, A. D., Newton, T. F., Longshore, D., Anglin, M. D., van Gorp, W. G., & Gawin, F. H. (2000). Psychiatric comorbidity of methamphetamine dependence in a forensic sample. *Journal of Neuropsychiatry and Clinical Neurosciences*, *12*, 215–220.

Kask, A., & Harro, J. (2000). Inhibition of amphetamine- and apomorphine-induced behavioural effects by neuropeptide Y Y_1 receptor antagonist BIBO3304. *Neuropharmacology*, *39*, 1292–1302.

Kiive, E., & Harro, J. (2013). The effect of serotonin transporter gene promoter polymorphism on adolescent and adult ADHD symptoms and educational attainment: A longitudinal study. *European Psychiatry*, *28*, 372–378.

Kim, Y.-T., Lee, S.-W., Kwon, D.-H., Seo, J.-H., Ahn, B.-C., & Lee, J. (2009). Dose-dependent frontal hypometabolism on FDG-PET in methamphetamine abusers. *Journal of Psychiatric Research*, *43*, 1166–1170.

Kim, S. J., Lyoo, I. K., Hwang, J., Chung, A., Hoon, S. Y., Kim, J., et al. (2006). Prefrontal grey-matter changes in short-term and long-term abstinent methamphetamine abusers. *International Journal of Neuropsychopharmacology*, *9*, 221–228.

King, G. R., & Ellinwood, E. H., Jr. (1992). Amphetamines and other stimulants. In J. H. Lowinson, P. Ruiz, R. B. Millman, & J. G. Langrod (Eds.), *Substance abuse: A comprehensive textbook* (pp. 247–270). Baltimore, MD: Williams & Wilkins.

Kishimoto, M., Ujike, H., Motohashi, Y., Tanaka, Y., Okahisa, Y., Kotaka, T., et al. (2008). The dysbindin gene (*DTNBP1*) is associated with methamphetamine psychosis. *Biological Psychiatry*, *63*, 191–196.

Kittirattanapaiboon, P., Mahatnirunkul, S., Booncharoen, H., Thummawomg, P., Dumrongchai, U., & Chutha, W. (2010). Long-term outcomes in methamphetamine psychosis after first hospitalization. *Drug and Alcohol Review*, *29*, 456–461.

Kohno, M., Morales, A. M., Grahremani, D. G., Hellemann, G., & London, E. D. (2014). Risky decision-making, prefrontal cortex, and mesocorticolimbic functional connectivity in methamphetamine dependence. *JAMA Psychiatry*, *71*, 812–820.

Kotaka, T., Ujike, H., Okahisa, Y., Takaki, M., Nakata, K., Kodama, M., et al. (2009). *G72* gene is associated with susceptibility to methamphetamine psychosis. *Progress in Neuro-Psychopharmacology and Biological Psychiatry*, *33*, 1046–1049.

Krasnova, I. N., & Cadet, J. L. (2009). Methamphetamine toxicity and messengers of death. *Brain Research Reviews*, *60*, 379–407.

Laruelle, M., Abi-Dargham, A., van Dyck, C. H., Gil, R., D'Souza, C. D., Erdos, J., et al. (1996). Single emission computerized tomography imaging of amphetamine-induced dopamine release in drug-free schizophrenic patients. *Proceedings of the National Academy of Sciences of the United States of America*, *93*, 9235–9240.

LaVoie, M. J., Card, J. P., & Hastings, T. G. (2004). Microglial activation precedes dopamine terminal pathology in methamphetamine-induce neurotoxicity. *Experimental Neurology*, *187*, 47–57.

Lee, K. W., Kim, H. C., Lee, S. Y., & Jang, C. G. (2011). Methamphetamine-sensitized mice are accompanied by memory impairment and reduction of N-methyl-D-aspartate receptor ligand binding in the prefrontal cortex and hippocampus. *Neuroscience*, *178*, 101–107.

Lee, B., London, E. D., Poldrack, R. A., Farahi, J., Nacca, A., Monterosso, J. R., et al. (2009). Striatal dopamine D2/D3 receptor availability is reduced in methamphetamine dependence and is linked to impulsivity. *Journal of Neuroscience*, *29*, 14734–14740.

Li, H., Lu, Q., Xiao, E., Li, Q., He, Z., & Mei, X. (2014). Methamphetamine enhances the development of schizophrenia in first-degree relatives of patients with schizophrenia. *Canadian Journal of Psychiatry*, *59*, 107–113.

Linnoila, M., Virkkunen, M., Scheinin, M., Nuuttila, A., Rimon, R., & Goodwin, F. K. (1983). Low cerebrospinal fluid 5-hydroxyindoleacetic acid concentration differentiates impulsive from nonimpulsive violent behavior. *Life Sciences*, *33*, 2609–2614.

London, E. D., Simon, S. L., Berman, S. M., Mandelkern, M. A., Lichtman, A. M., Bramen, J., et al. (2004). Mood disturbances and regional cerebral metabolic abnormalities in recently abstinent methamphetamine abusers. *Archives of General Psychiatry*, *61*, 73–84.

Matsumoto, T., Kamijo, A., Yamaguchi, A., Iseki, E., & Hirayasu, Y. (2005). Childhood histories of attention-deficit hyperactivity disorders in Japanese methamphetamine and inhalant abusers: Preliminary report. *Journal of Neuropsychiatry and Clinical Neurosciences*, *59*, 102–105.

McCann, U. D., Wong, D. F., Yokoi, F., Villemagne, V., Dannals, R. F., & Ricaurte, G. A. (1998). Reduced striatal dopamine transporter density in abstinent methamphetamine and methcathinone users: Evidence from positron emission tomography studies with [^{11}C]WIN35,428. *Journal of Neuroscience*, *18*, 8417–8422.

McGregor, C., Srisurapanont, M., Jittiwutikarn, J., Laobhripatr, S., Wongtan, T., & White, J. M. (2005). The nature, time course and severity of methamphetamine withdrawal. *Addiction*, *100*, 1320–1329.

McKetin, R., McLaren, J., Lubman, D. I., & Hides, L. (2006). The prevalence of psychotic symptoms among methamphetamine users. *Addiction*, *101*, 1473–1478.

McKetin, R., McLaren, J., Lubman, D. I., & Hides, L. (2008). Hostility among methamphetamine users experiencing psychotic symptoms. *The American Journal on Addictions*, *17*, 235–240.

Montoya, J. L., Umlauf, A., Abramson, I., Badiee, J., Woods, S. P., Atkinson, J. H., et al. (2013). Dynamic indices of methamphetamine dependence and HIV infection predict fluctuations in affective distress: A five-year longitudinal analysis. *Journal of Affective Disorders*, *151*, 728–737.

Morales, A. M., Lee, B., Hellemann, G., O'Neill, J., & London, E. D. (2012). Gray-matter volume in methamphetamine dependence: Cigarette smoking and changes with abstinence from methamphetamine. *Drug and Alcohol Dependence*, *125*, 230–238.

Morita, Y., Ujike, H., Tanaka, Y., Kishimoto, M., Okahisa, Y., Kotaka, T., et al. (2008). The glycine transporter 1 gene (GLYT1) is associated with methamphetamine-use disorder. *American Journal of Medical Genetics. Part B, Neuropsychiatric Genetics*, *147B*, 54–58.

Moszczynska, A., Fitzmaurice, P., Ang, L., Kalasinsky, K. S., Schmunk, G. A., Peretti, F. J., et al. (2004). Why is Parkinsonism not a feature of human methamphetamine users? *Brain*, *127*, 363–370.

Murray, J. B. (1998). Psychophysiological aspects of amphetamine-methamphetamine abuse. *Journal of Psychology: Interdisciplinary and Applied, 132*, 227–237.

Nakama, H., Chang, L., Fein, G., Shimotsu, R., Jiang, C. S., & Ernst, T. (2011). Methamphetamine users show greater than normal age-related cortical gray matter loss. *Addiction, 106*, 1474–1483.

Newton, T. F., Kalechstein, A. D., Duran, S., Vansluis, N., & Ling, W. (2004). Methamphetamine abstinence syndrome: Preliminary findings. *The American Journal on Addictions, 13*, 248–255.

Newton, T. F., Kalechstein, A. D., Hardy, D. J., Cook, I. A., Nestor, L., Ling, W., et al. (2004). Association between quantitative EEG and neurocognition in methamphetamine-dependent volunteers. *Clinical Neurophysiology, 115*, 194–198.

Obermeit, L. C., Cattie, J. E., Bolden, K. A., Marquine, M. J., Morgan, E. E., Franklin, D. E., Jr., et al. (2013). Attention-deficit/hyperactivity disorder among chronic methamphetamine users: Frequency, persistence, and adverse effects on everyday functioning. *Addictive Behaviors, 38*, 2874–2878.

Okahisa, Y., Ujike, H., Kotaka, T., Morita, Y., Kodama, M., Inada, T., et al. (2009). Association between neuropeptide Y gene and its receptor Y_1 gene and methamphetamine dependence. *Psychiatry and Clinical Neurosciences, 2009*(63), 417–422.

Olsen, E. R. (1977). Intracranial hemorrhage and amphetamine usage. Review of the effects of amphetamines on the central nervous system. *Angiology, 28*, 464–471.

Orikabe, L., Yamasue, H., Inoue, H., Takayanagi, Y., Mozue, Y., Sudo, Y., et al. (2011). Reduced amygdala and hippocampal volumes in patients with methamphetamine psychosis. *Schizophrenia Research, 132*, 183–189.

Parsey, R. V., Oquendo, M. A., Zea-Ponce, Y., Rodenhiser, J., Kegeles, L. S., Pratap, M., et al. (2001). Dopamine D_2 receptor availability and amphetamine-induced dopamine release in unipolar depression. *Biological Psychiatry, 50*, 313–322.

Parsey, R. V., Oquendo, M. A., Simpson, N. R., Ogden, R. T., Van Heertum, R., Arango, V., & Mann, J. J. (2002). Effects of age, sex and aggressive traits in man on serotonin 5-HT1A binding potential measured by PET using [11C]WAY100-635. *Brain Research, 954*, 173–182.

Paulus, M. P., Tapert, S. F., & Schuckit, M. A. (2005). Neural activation patterns of methamphetamine-dependent subjects during decision making predict relapse. *Archives of General Psychiatry, 62*, 761–768.

Perez-Mana, C., Castells, X., Torrens, M., Capella, D., & Farre, M. (2013). Efficacy of psychostimulant drugs for amphetamine abuse or dependence. *The Cochrane Database of Systematic Reviews, 9*, CD009695. http://dx.doi.org/10.1002/14651858.CD009695.pub2.

Power, B. D., Stefanis, N. C., Dragovic, M., Jablensky, A., Castle, D., & Morgan, V. (2014). Age at initiation of amphetamine use and the age at onset of psychosis: The Australian Survey of High Impact Psychosis. *Schizophrenia Research, 152*, 300–302.

Rajkowska, G., & Miguel-Hidalgo, J. J. (2007). Gliogenesis and glial pathology in depression. *CNS & Neurological Disorders Drug Targets, 6*, 219–233.

Rendell, P. G., Mazur, M., & Henry, J. D. (2009). Prospective memory impairment in former users of methamphetamine. *Psychopharmacology, 203*, 609–616.

Sadek, J. R., Vigil, O., Grant, I., & Heaton, R. K. (2007). The impact of neuropsychological functioning and depressed mood on functional complaints in HIV-1 infection and methamphetamine dependence. *Journal of Clinical and Experimental Neuropsychology, 29*, 266–276.

Salo, R., & Fassbender, C. (2012). Structural, functional and spectroscopic MRI studies of methamphetamine addiction. *Current Topics in Behavioral Neurosciences, 11*, 321–363.

Salo, R., Flower, K., Kielsten, A., Leamon, M. H., Nordahl, T. E., & Galloway, G. P. (2011). Psychiatric comorbidity in methamphetamine dependence. *Psychiatry Research, 186*, 356–361.

Salo, R., Nordahl, T. E., Galloway, G. P., Moore, C. D., Waters, C., & Leamon, M. H. (2009). Drug abstinence and cognitive control in methamphetamine-dependent individuals. *Journal of Substance Abuse Treatment, 37*, 292–297.

Schwartz, D. L., Mitchell, A. D., Lahna, D. L., Luber, H. S., Huckans, M. S., Mitchell, S. H., et al. (2010). Global and local morphometric differences in recently abstinent methamphetamine-dependent individuals. *NeuroImage, 50*, 1392–1401.

Scott, J. C., Woods, S. P., Matt, G. E., Meyer, R. A., Heaton, R. K., Atkinson, J. H., et al. (2007). Neurocognitive effects of methamphetamine: A critical review and meta-analysis. *Neuropsychology Review, 17*, 275–297.

Sekine, Y., Ouchi, Y., Sugihara, G., Takei, N., Yoshikawa, E., Nakamura, K., et al. (2008). Methamphetamine causes microglial activation in the brains of human abusers. *Journal of Neuroscience, 28*, 5756–5761.

Sekine, Y., Ouchi, Y., Takei, N., Yoshikawa, E., Nakamura, K., Futatsubashi, M., et al. (2006). Brain serotonin transporter density and aggression in abstinent methamphetamine abusers. *Archives of General Psychiatry, 63*, 90–100.

Shoptaw, S., Peck, J., Reback, C. J., & Rotheram-Fuller, E. (2003). Psychiatric and substance dependence comorbidities, sexually transmitted diseases, and risk behaviors among methamphetamine-dependent gay and bisexual men seeking outpatient drug abuse treatment. *Journal of Psychoactive Drugs, 35*, 161–168.

Simon, S. L., Richardson, K., Dacey, J., Glynn, S., Domier, C. P., Rawson, R. A., et al. (2002). A comparison of patterns of methamphetamine and cocaine use. *The American Journal on Addictions, 9*, 222–231.

Simons, J. S., Oliver, M. N., Gaher, R. M., Ebel, G., & Brummels, P. (2005). Methamphetamine and alcohol abuse and dependence symptoms: Associations with affect lability and impulsivity in a rural treatment population. *Addictive Behaviors, 30*, 1370–1381.

Smith, D. E., & Fischer, C. M. (1970). An analysis of 310 cases of acute high-dose methamphetamine toxicity in Haight-Ashbury. *Clinical Toxicology, 3*, 117–124.

Srisurapanont, M., Ali, R., Marsden, J., Sunga, A., Wada, K., & Monteiro, M. (2003). Psychotic symptoms in methamphetamine psychotic in-patients. *International Journal of Neuropsychopharmacology, 6*, 347–352.

Sung, Y. H., Cho, S. C., Hwang, J., Kim, S. J., Kim, H., Bae, S., et al. (2007). Relationship between N-acetyl-aspartate in gray and white matter of abstinent methamphetamine abusers and their history of drug abuse: A proton magnetic resonance spectroscopy study. *Drug and Alcohol Dependence, 88*, 28–35.

Taylor, M., Schweinsburg, B., Alhassoon, O., Gongvatana, A., Brown, G., Young-Casey, C., et al. (2007). Effects of human immunodeficiency virus and methamphetamine on cerebral metabolites measured with magnetic resonance spectroscopy. *Journal of Neurovirology, 13*, 150–159.

Thompson, P. M., Hayashi, K. M., Simon, S. L., Geaga, J. A., Hong, M. S., Sui, Y., et al. (2004). Structural abnormalities in the brains of human subjects who use methamphetamine. *Journal of Neuroscience, 24*, 6028–6036.

Tobias, M. C., O'Neill, J., Hudkins, M., Bartzokis, G., Dean, A. C., & London, E. D. (2010). White-matter abnormalities in brain during early abstinence from methamphetamine abuse. *Psychopharmacology, 209*, 13–24.

Toomey, R., Lyons, M. J., Eisen, S. A., Xian, H., Chantarujikapong, S., Seidman, L. J., et al. (2003). A twin study of the neuropsychological consequences of stimulant abuse. *Archives of General Psychiatry, 60*, 303–310.

Tziortzis, D., Mahoney, J. R., Kalechstein, A. D., Newton, T. F., & De la Garza, R. N. (2011). The relationship between impulsivity and craving in cocaine- and methamphetamine-dependent volunteers. *Pharmacology, Biochemistry, and Behavior, 98*, 196–202.

Ujike, H., Harano, M., Inada, T., Yamada, M., Komiyama, T., Sekine, Y., et al. (2003). Nine- or fewer repeat alleles in VNTR polymorphism of the dopamine transporter gene is a strong risk factor for prolonged methamphetamine psychosis. *Pharmacogenomics Journal, 3*, 242–247.

Ujike, H., Katsu, T., Okahisa, Y., Takaki, M., Kodama, M., Inada, T., et al. (2009). Genetic variants of D2 but not D3 or D4 dopamine receptor gene are associated with rapid onset and poor prognosis of methamphetamine psychosis. *Progress in Neuro-Psychopharmacology and Biological Psychiatry, 33*, 625–629.

Ujike, H., & Sato, M. (2004). Clinical features of sensitization to methamphetamine observed in patients with methamphetamine dependence and psychosis. *Annals of the New York Academy of Sciences, 1025*, 279–287.

Volkow, N. D., Chang, L., Wang, G. J., Fowler, J. S., Ding, Y. S., Sedler, M., et al. (2001). Low level of brain dopamine D2 receptors in methamphetamine abusers: Association with metabolism in orbitofrontal cortex. *American Journal of Psychiatry, 158*, 2015–2021.

Volkow, N. D., Chang, L., Wang, G. J., Fowler, J. S., Franceschi, M., Sedler, M., et al. (2001a). Loss of dopamine transporters in methamphetamine abusers recovers with protracted abstinence. *Journal of Neuroscience, 21*, 9414–9418.

Volkow, N. D., Chang, L., Wang, G. J., Fowler, J. S., Franceschi, M., Sedler, M., et al. (2001b). Higher cortical and lower subcortical metabolism in detoxified methamphetamine abusers. *American Journal of Psychiatry, 158*, 383–389.

Volkow, N. D., Chang, L., Wang, G. J., Fowler, J. S., Leonido-Yee, M., Franceschi, M., et al. (2001). Association of dopamine transporter reduction with psychomotor impairment in methamphetamine abusers. *American Journal of Psychiatry, 158*, 377–382.

Wang, G. J., Volkow, N. D., Chang, L., Miller, E., Sedler, M., Hitzemann, R., et al. (2004). Partial recovery of brain metabolism in methamphetamine abusers after protracted abstinence. *American Journal of Psychiatry, 161*, 242–248.

Watson, R., Hartmann, E., & Schildkraut, J. J. (1972). Amphetamine withdrawal: Affective state, sleep patterns, and MHPG excretion. *American Journal of Psychiatry, 129*, 263–269.

Wierzba-Bobrowicz, T., Lewandowska, E., Lechowicz, W., Stepien, T., & Pasennik, E. (2005). Quantitative analysis of activated microglia, ramified and damage of processes in the frontal and temporal lobes of chronic schizophrenics. *Folia Neuropathologica, 43*, 81–89.

Wilson, J. M., Kalasinsky, K. S., Levey, A. I., Bergeron, C., Reiber, G., Anthony, R. M., et al. (1996). Striatal dopamine nerve terminal markers in human, chronic methamphetamine users. *Nature Medicine, 2*, 699–703.

Yuan, J., Lv, R., Brasic, J. R., Han, M., Liu, X., Wang, Y., et al. (2014). Dopamine transporter dysfunction in Han Chinese people with chronic methamphetamine dependence after a short-term abstinence. *Psychiatry Research: Neuroimaging, 221*, 92–96.

Zweben, J. E., Cohen, J. B., Christian, D., Galloway, G. P., Salinardi, M., Parent, D., et al. (2004). Psychiatric symptoms in methamphetamine users. *The American Journal on Addictions, 13*, 181–190.

CHAPTER TEN

"Addicted to Euphoria": The History, Clinical Presentation, and Management of Party Drug Misuse

Jenny Bearn[*,†,1], **Matthew O'Brien**[*]
[*]Addictions Clinical Academic Group, South London and Maudsley NHS Foundation Trust, Maudsley Hospital, London, United Kingdom
[†]Institute of Psychiatry, Psychology and Neuroscience, King's College, London, United Kingdom
[1]Corresponding author: e-mail address: jenny.bearn@slam.nhs.uk

Contents

Abstract

Eating, drinking, sexual activity, and parenting invoke pleasure, an emotion that promotes repetition of these behaviors, are essential for survival. Euphoria, a feeling or state of intense excitement and happiness, is an amplification of pleasure, aspired to one's essential biological needs that are satisfied.

People use party drugs as a shortcut to euphoria. Ecstasy (3,4-methylenedioxymethamphetamine), γ-hydroxybutyric acid, and ketamine fall under the umbrella of the term "party drugs," each with differing neuropharmacological and physiological actions. This chapter seeks to survey the history and epidemiology of party drug use; we will then discuss the pharmacological characteristics of each drug to provide a platform for understanding the difficulties that party drug users encounter through intoxication, harmful use, dependence, and withdrawal and how these should be clinically managed.

International Review of Neurobiology, Volume 120
ISSN 0074-7742
http://dx.doi.org/10.1016/bs.irn.2015.02.005

1. HISTORICAL ASPECTS OF PARTY DRUG USE

1.1 3,4-Methylenedioxymethamphetamine

3,4-Methylenedioxymethamphetamine (MDMA) or ecstasy was the first party drug, the term being adopted in the late 1980s (Saunders, 1993). As with many of the defining pharmacological discoveries of the twentieth century, it began with a mistake. Kollish described the synthesis of MDMA in 1912 while working for the German pharmaceutical company Merck in Darmstadt. Later, three Merck chemists became interested in MDMA: Max Oberlin in 1927, Albert van Schoor in 1952, and Wolfgang Fruhstorfer in 1959, each explored its pharmacological characteristics, though no studies were carried out on humans. Their most salient finding was that they were toxic to fruit flies (Freudenmann, Oxler, & Bernschneider-Reif, 2006).

MDMA reemerged in the United States in 1953 in the context of Cold War paranoia. Projects supported by the Army Chemical Center at the University of Michigan between 1953 and 1954 investigated physiological characteristics of MDMA in mice, rats, snakes, monkeys, and dogs, although there is no evidence that it was tested in man. The results of these tests were declassified in 1969 and published 4 years later (Hardman, Haavik, & Seevers, 1973). These studies were directed by Sidney Gottlieb director of the MK-ULTRA Project, the CIA's fabled "mind control program," which tested various psychedelic compounds for potential military use.

The first recorded human ingestion of MDMA was in the mid-1970s, by the Californian psychedelic chemist Alexander Shulgin, often referred to as the stepfather of ecstasy. He synthesized MDMA and recorded titration experiments in his Lab Notebooks (Erowid, 2009), involving his wife, friends, and colleagues, with commentaries on their subjective experiences. Subsequently, MDMA was applied both as an adjunct to the exploration of new drugs and as a subjective "control" for the assessment of new psychedelic drugs. He later published the seminal paper *Characterization of Three New Psychotomimetics*, in which he remarked "*Qualitatively, the drug (MDMA) appears to evoke an easily controlled altered state of consciousness with emotional and sensual overtones. It can be compared in its effects to marijuana, to psilocybin devoid of the hallucinatory component, or to low levels of MDMA*" (Shulgin & Nichols, 1978).

MDMA acquired an underground following among hippies, psychedelic chemists, and unconventional psychiatrists and psychotherapists in the late 1970s and early 1980s. The earliest published advocate of the use of MDMA in psychotherapy was George Greer (Greer, 1985), who investigated the potential use of MDMA as a psychotherapeutic adjunct and is still actively involved in the therapeutic psychedelic movement at the Heffter Research Institute in Zürich. He anonymously published "*The legal, safe, and effective use of MDMA*" and later a "*Recommended protocol for MDMA sessions*" (Greer & Tolbert, 1986). Viewed as an empathogen (and labeled "empathy") by radical psychiatrists, it was thought to lower patient's defenses, thus aiding the psychotherapeutic process (Greer, 1985).

As a brand name, "ecstasy" the name coined by members of an underground East Coast distribution network in 1981 had greater consumer appeal than "empathy." Used primarily on the East and West Coasts of United States, MDMA use rapidly escalated in the 1980s among "New Age" Americans. Media attention followed and one of the first nonscientific articles was published anonymously in the counterculture magazine *Wet* in 1981. In 1984, the San Francisco Chronicle dubbed MDMA "the yuppie psychedelic." Public controversy in the United States followed with popular magazines including Newsweek and TIME magazine publishing articles, which reported recreational use among the "American middle classes" (Shulgin, 1989). The Drug Enforcement Administration used emergency measures to add MDMA to Schedule 1 of the controlled substance list in 1985, in a response to concern about its growing use. MDMA was deemed as having a "high risk of addictive abuse potential" and a New York Times article reported that it had been shown to cause brain damage. The UK followed suit, though the Misuse of Drugs Act 1971 had already been altered in 1977 to include all ring-substituted amphetamines such as MDMA and 3,4-methylenedioxyamphetamine (MDA); a further amendment was made in 1985 to refer specifically to ecstasy, which was subsequently designated as class C drug.

At this time, the United States was bearing witness to the birth of a new cultural phenomenon that would define the history and popularity of ecstasy. In Chicago, DJs such as Frankie Knuckles, at the Warehouse nightclub, created the early fusion of disco and electronic music that would become house and dance music. By 1987, house music had spread to Ibiza with a group of UK DJs exporting the Balearic mix of house sound to the United Kingdom. Clubs including the Hacienda in Manchester started hosting house music parties, ecstasy followed the music, and the United Kingdom rave scene was born (Saunders, 1993).

Having ushered in the Thatcher era in 1979, the intervening years (1978–1988) brought the Brixton riots, rising youth unemployment, reduced manufacturing output, and the miner's strikes. The changes in fortunes for some were stoked by widening societal inequalities creating fertile ground for the emergence of a new British youth counterculture movement. Outdoor unlicensed acid house parties took place in and around the M25, and ecstasy rather than alcohol became the drug of choice as the United Kingdom experienced a melting pot of politics, music, and drugs that spawned the "Second Summer of Love" in 1988, mirroring the narrative of social change brought about by the youth counterculture movement of 1960s America that had opposed the Vietnam War and the nuclear arms race and spawned the first "Summer of Love" in 1967.

The use of ecstasy mushroomed in the United Kingdom; the oral route of administration labeling (the smiley face) and the underground marketing methods reduced the fear of harm by users. The press reaction was initially neutral, and images of the smiley face that parodied ravers as harmless hedonists were common during the early reporting of the acid house movement. Reports of harm, gangland involvement in distribution of ecstasy, and moral concern later prompted police action. The police developed a task force to close down illegal parties, often engaging in a cat and mouse game with those organizing illegal parties. Later, the Criminal Justice and Public Order Act 1994 provided the police with new powers to close down illegal parties, acknowledging the role house music played in its use. The act made public gatherings where music or "sounds wholly or predominantly characterized by the emission of a succession of repetitive beats" illegal. Acid house moved into clubs and licensed bars, but the use of ecstasy continued and disseminated further into the UK mainstream. Public concern reached its peak following the death of Leah Betts, a teenager and the daughter of a policeman, in 1995 (Davison & Parrott, 1997). In response to her death, "the Public Entertainments Licences (Drug Misuse) Act 1997" provided the police with new powers that included the ability to close venues thought to contain persons consuming illegal drugs. The global dance scene is now worth 6.2 billion pounds worldwide and is expected to be worth 18 billion pounds within the next 10 years.

1.2 γ-Hydroxybutyric Acid

Henri Laborit synthesized γ-hydroxybutyric acid (GHB) in 1960 as a potential anesthetic agent (Laborit, Buchard, Laborit, Kind, & Weber, 1960). His team subsequently synthesized GHB from butyrolactone and carried out extensive *in vivo* testing, finding that at dose of 250 mg/kg, it caused sleepiness in several animal species and had little effect on respiration and oxygen consumption (Basil, Blair, & Holmes, 1964). His work was expanded on by Dr. Margaret Blumenfeld who noted that induction was slow (up to 45 min), sleep was indistinguishable from natural sleep (both in appearance and on the electroencephalogram), respiratory depression occurred (Cheyne–Stokes respiration in some subjects), and bradycardia and mild elevation of the arterial blood pressure were also noted. They also observed that GHB appeared to potentiate or be potentiated by hypnotic drugs, tranquilizers, and narcotics as evidenced by markedly reduced amounts of these agents necessary for anesthesia, the so-called sparing effect (Blumenfeld, Suntay, & Harmel, 1962).

Subsequent research focused on the sleep-modifying effects leading to therapeutic interventions in the form of sodium oxybate for sleep disturbances, particularly in Gelineau's syndrome of narcolepsy and cataplexy (Alshaikh et al., 2012). It was also shown to be effective in the treatment of the alcohol withdrawal syndrome (Leone, Vigna-Taglianti, Avanzi, Brambilla, & Faggiano, 2010). In contrast to its use as an anesthetic, it is limited by its lack of analgesic and muscle relaxant properties (Schep, Knudsen, Slaughter, Vale, & Mégarbane, 2012). The effects on respiration and cardiac functions and the sparing effect began to be recognized by doctors in accident and emergency departments (Galicia, Nogue, & Miró, 2011) and users of GHB on the dance floor (Wood, Nicolaou, & Dargan, 2009).

GHB reemerged as a food and dietary supplement and was sold in health food stores in tablet, capsule, and liquid forms during the 1980s and early 1990s throughout the United States (Dyer, 1991), popular with bodybuilders (Steele & Watson, 1995), due to its growth hormone-releasing properties (Van Cauter et al., 1997). Concerns about its safety as a food supplement began to surface, with reports of altered levels of consciousness and seizures being reported (Dyer, 1991; Steele & Watson, 1995). Recreational users then chanced upon euphoria and increased libido as side effects, a discovery that intersected with the emergence of the club scene.

GHB's potential as a party drug has been recognized since the early 1990s (Dyer, 1991; Steele & Watson, 1995). Ingested orally, GHB and its analogs, γ-butyrolactone (GBL) and 1,4-butanediol, are available via the Internet and drug dealers and can be readily synthesized from a number of household products. GBL and 1,4-butanediol continue to be used as industrial solvents and are important components in the production of polyurethane and pesticides and are found in nail polish removal products (Gonzalez & Nutt, 2005).

Rapidly converted to GHB once ingested, the industrial use of GBL and 1,4-butanediol has had a marked impact on the legal classification, price, and availability of GHB. In many ways, GHB is the first drug of the Internet age, with the distribution and means of preparation disseminated via the web and social media (Anderson et al., 2006). It is known by various street names including GHB, "liquid ecstasy," "liquid E," "grievous bodily harm," "fantasy," "G," "Georgia home boy," "Mils," "liquid X," and "liquid G."

Increased media attention, public health concerns, and clinical scrutiny eventually led to a change in the legal classification of GHB, GBL, and 1,4-butanediol in Europe and the United States (Anderson, Kim-Katz, Dyer, & Blanc, 2010). The deaths of American teenagers, Hillory Farias and Samantha Reid, caught the public imagination in the United States and with fears growing about the role of GHB in assisted sexual assault (the rape drug) that led to its classification under Schedule 1 in the United States. The UK followed suit and GHB was classified as a class C drug, though the discrepancy in the legal classification of GHB and its analogs between 2003 and 2009 led to the substitution of GHB with its precursors GBL and to a lesser extent 1,4-butanediol (Anderson et al., 2010).

1.3 Ketamine

Ketamine was discovered in 1962 at the University of Michigan by the chemist Calvin Stevens in a quest to find an alternative to phencyclidine (aka "PCP" or "angel dust") (Teltzrow & Bosch, 2012). Labeled CI-581, ketamine was first trialed in prisoners in 1965. Domino's description of the experiment is illuminating: "*So unique were these effects that we had to invent a new set of words to describe its anaesthetic properties. The drug produced 'zombies' who were totally disconnected from their environment, with their eyes open, and yet in a complete anesthetic and analgesic state. The observation of being disconnected from the environment gave rise to the term 'dissociative anesthesia'*" (Domino, Chodoff, & Corssen, 1965). The term "dissociative anesthesia" had also been used to describe the effects of GHB, although its lack of analgesic properties limited it to be used as an induction agent. In contrast to GHB, ketamine demonstrated properties of rapid induction, rapid recovery, and effective analgesia while having a limited effect on respiratory and cardiovascular functioning (Teltzrow & Bosch, 2012).

Its first use as a recreational drug occurred as early as 1967, acquiring street names including "mean green" and "rock masculine" by a psychedelic chemist in Michigan (Jansen, 2001), though it has been suggested that a major catalyst for the recreational ketamine use was the Vietnam War (Sewell, 2007). Ketamine can be administered by almost any route and made an ideal battlefield anesthetic. It has continued to be used on the battlefield and in areas that have limited medical equipment (Bonanno, 2002; Mercer, 2008). From 1970s onward, ketamine was used clinically as an anesthetic, although in recent years, this has been declined mainly due to the dissociative effects (Pai & Heining, 2007).

By the early 1980s, ketamine moved from the hospital setting to the private consulting room for use by "New Age therapists" and later for recreational purposes. Karl Jansen recounts the history of ketamine in "Ketamine: Dreams and Realities" (Jansen, 2001) noting that its recreational use was relatively rare until the late 1990s when it started to be used on the United Kingdom dance and rave scene (Moore & Miles, 2004). This owes something to the variable purity of ecstasy tablets, so that experimentation with ketamine may have been as a result of taking ecstasy tablets containing little or no MDMA. Known as "K," "special K," "kit-kat," or "vitamin K," it is also sometimes referred to as "the horse tranquilizer" (Dillon & Degenhardt, 2001) due to its use by vets as an animal tranquilizer. Recreational use has grown rapidly in the last 20 years (Morgan & Curran, 2012), particularly in Asia.

More recently, ketamine has been used as a neuropharmacological simulator of psychosis in functional MRI studies (Hashimoto, 2014). It had been noted in the 1960s that PCP and ketamine produced schizophrenia-like symptoms in some healthy volunteers and cause the exacerbation of symptoms in schizophrenic patients (Lahti, Weiler, & Tamara, 2001; Pomarol-Clotet et al., 2006), supporting the glutamate dysfunction model of schizophrenia (Coyle, 2001). For example, atypical antipsychotic drugs block the neuropsychiatric symptoms of ketamine (Duncan & Miyamoto, 2000). These findings have led to ketamine being used in functional neuroimaging studies to assess the efficacy of existing and new antipsychotic drugs (Large, 2007).

2. EPIDEMIOLOGY OF PARTY DRUG USE

Ecstasy is by far the most popular "party drug" worldwide with between 19 and 29 million users and is the fourth most popular drug after cannabis, opioids, and amphetamines (and stimulants), with world prevalence estimates of between 0.4% and 0.6%. Prevalences in Europe, the United States, and Oceania (New Zealand and Australia) are higher than the world average at 0.5%, 0.9%, and 2.9%, respectively. In the United Kingdom, the use of ecstasy is declining, with evidence that new designer drugs are taking its place. In contrast, the use of ecstasy and club drugs is increasing in Asia and developing world, though there are difficulties in obtaining accurate prevalence data (World drug report, 1997).

GHB is a relatively new drug on the party scene, becoming more popular in the last decade (McCambridge, Winstock, Hunt, & Mitcheson, 2007). Prevalence estimates of GHB in industrialized countries are 0.1–2% (WHO, 2012), with an increased prevalence among subgroups including young adults who use it in combination with other party (or designer) drugs (McCambridge et al., 2007), bodybuilders (Gonzalez & Nutt, 2005), men who have sex with men (MSM) (Palamar & Halkitis, 2006; Wood & Beaumont, 2010), and clubbers (Anderson et al., 2010; Dillon & Degenhardt, 2001). A typical GHB user is a male, in his midtwenties to early thirties and active on the party scene, though among MSM, the age range is wider as they are more likely to use GHB as a prosocial drug (Palamar & Halkitis, 2006).

Ketamine use has also been growing in Southeast Asia. It is the second most commonly used illicit drug in Hong Kong (Kalsi, Wood, & Dargan, 2011), and its use on mainland China is growing. Its use in the United Kingdom and industrialized countries remains low with UK population-based studies reporting lifetime use of 4% for 16–24-year-olds and 2% for 16–59-year-olds; this contrasts with Australia and America who report significantly lower lifetime use of below 0.5% among all age groups (World drug report, 1997). Recreational use is most prevalent in ravers, MSM, young injecting drug users, and those who work in the medical or veterinary fields. Subjects interviewed in the party drug setting report lifetime use of 67.8% in the United Kingdom, 16.4% in France, and 10.8% in Italy (Kalsi et al., 2011).

3. RECREATIONAL USE VERSUS DEPENDENCE

"Recreational drug" use is a nonclinical term describing the use of a drug with the intention of enhancing life, inducing euphoria, or creating pleasure. It is a relatively new way of describing drug use and likely came into common usage as a way of describing patterns of drug use among young people and clubbers. The term contrasts with "drug dependence" that is characterized by a cluster of physiological, behavioral, and cognitive symptoms that drive repeated drug use in the face of harmful consequences and is a clinically defined entity that came into common usage 50 years ago.

In 1964, the WHO Expert Committee on Addiction-Producing Drugs introduced the term "dependence" to replace the terms addiction (a state of periodic or chronic intoxication produced by the repeated consumption of a drug) and habituation (a condition resulting from repeated consumption of the drug) (Berridge & Mars, 2004). WHO defined drug dependence as "a state arising from repeated administration of a drug on periodic or continuous basis" (WHO, 1964).

The diagnostic criteria for alcohol and drug dependence have evolved over time, though they remain largely derived from Edwards and Gross seminal paper on alcohol dependence (Edwards & Gross, 1976), which highlighted the key features as a narrowing in the repertoire of drug use, salience of drug-seeking behavior, increased tolerance, repeated withdrawal symptoms, repeated relief or avoidance of withdrawal symptoms by further use, subjective awareness of a compulsion to use (or cravings), and reinstatement of the use after abstinence. Both international classification of diseases (ICD) and diagnostic and statistical manual of mental disorders (DSM) criteria for drug and alcohol dependency and abuse continue to be based on these principles. Additionally, Edwards and Gross commented on the way that social processes impact on the rate of development of dependence, the secondary consequences, seeking treatment, and stigmatization (Edwards & Gross, 1976). These ideas are fundamental to understanding the nature of party drug use in its novel social settings. The history and social narrative of club culture, music, unique social settings of nightclubs, flashing lights, and restricted licensing hours (mostly open at weekends) all impact on the rates of drug dependency, consequences of drug use, pattern of use, and treatment options.

Not all drugs are equally likely to cause dependence and the influence of a party drugs' potential to cause dependence is both contextual and pharmacological (Nutt, King, Saulsbury, & Blakemore, 2007). The pleasurable effects of the drug and its propensity to produce dependent behavior are likely the most important factors, as this is the first step in the behavioral cycle of repeated administration. Drug-induced pleasure has two components—the initial, rapid effect (the rush), followed by a period of euphoria (Nutt et al., 2007). The initial rush of euphoria provides a psychological drive for repeated administration, mediated by activation of mesocorticolimbic dopaminergic reward networks underpinning abuse and dependence potential.

The faster an euphoriant drug reaches the brain, the greater the reinforcing effect or "rush" and the greater potential to cause dependence. This can be influenced by both neuropharmacological profile and route of administration. If a drug is smoked or injected, this provides rapid bioavailability by crossing the blood–brain barrier. In contrast, orally administered drugs are absorbed more slowly and present a less intense rush, though the euphoric effects may last longer. An intense rush combined with a marked experience of euphoria and short duration of action increases the likelihood of dependence (Nutt et al., 2007).

Physiological tolerance also plays a major role in the dependency potential of a drug (Edwards & Gross, 1976; Nutt et al., 2007), such that the continuing use is driven by the prevention of withdrawal symptoms coupled with compulsive drug-seeking behavior (craving). This leads to a cycle of escalating use. Drugs that are rapidly metabolized tend to produce greater tolerance and withdrawal symptoms (Nutt et al., 2007). Placing this in context, an orally administered drug (i.e., ecstasy) with a long half-life and generating limited physiological tolerance is significantly less likely to cause dependence when compared to an orally administered drug (i.e., GHB) with a short half-life and that generates marked physiological tolerance.

There has been a major conceptual shift in the latest version of the Diagnostic and Statistical Manual of Mental Disorders (DSM-5) (American Psychiatric Pub Inc., 2013). The concepts of abuse and dependence have been combined under the single diagnostic entity, substance use disorder, on a continuum from mild to severe depending on the number of symptoms experienced, which now includes craving as a diagnostic feature (Hasin et al., 2013).

4. PARTY DRUGS: SUBJECTIVE EFFECTS AND HAZARDS OF USE

4.1 MDMA (Ecstasy)

4.1.1 Administration, Metabolism, and Elimination

MDMA is usually orally ingested. Ecstasy in tablet form contains 30–150 mg of MDMA (Hall & Henry, 2006). In powder form, it is often dissolved in an alcoholic beverage or soft drink. The purity of ecstasy tablets is variable, although there is evidence that the purity of tablets is increasing (Giraudon & Bello, 2007; Tanner-Smith, 2006; Wolff, Hay, Sherlock, & Conner, 1995). MDMA can also be snorted, though this requires grinding to produce a fine powder and can result in intranasal trauma, and so is relatively rare. A minority of regular users report nasal and intravenous administration (up to 16% reporting having injected once or more); intravenous use is associated with a greater risk of overdose and physical harm (Degenhardt & Hall, 2010). When ingested orally, peak serum levels are reached 2 h postadministration (Degenhardt & Hall, 2010; Torre & Farré, 2004) and the elimination half-life of 100 mg is 8–9 h, though the effects of ecstasy may last between 2 and 12 h due to its complex metabolism (Torre & Farré, 2004).

Metabolism is hepatic and produces a number of active metabolites including MDA, making it difficult to predict the dose–response relationship in individuals. Cytochrome P450 family enzymes play a central role in the metabolism of MDMA, with the isoform 2D6-mediated O-demethylation and N-demethylation in humans (Torre & Farré, 2004). MDMA metabolism involves N-demethylation to 3,4-methylenedioxyamphetamine (MDA). This important pathway is influenced by CYPD polymorphism, for example, up to 10% of the Caucasian population has deficiency in the *CYP2D6* gene and has a reduced ability to metabolize MDMA (De La Torre et al., 2002), potentially prolonging drug effects and increasing the risk of toxicity. The major metabolites of MDMA are 3,4-dihydroxymethamphetamine, 4-hydroxy-3-methoxymethamphetamine, and 4-hydroxy-3-methoxyamphetamine that are excreted in the urine as conjugated glucuronide or sulfate metabolites (Abraham et al., 2009).

4.1.2 Neuropharmacology

MDMA is a ring-substituted amphetamine (Shulgin, 1986) and lies some where between traditional amphetamines (speed) and hallucinogens (mescaline) in its neuropharmacological effects; it offers mild stimulation and mild reality distortion to recreational users. In contrast to traditional amphetamines, it is a potent releaser of serotonin (5-HT) and inhibits 5-HT reuptake (Maxwell, 2005; Schifano, 2004; Torre & Farré, 2004), though unlike traditional hallucinogens, it does not directly activate postsynaptic 5-HT receptors. Its pharmacological activity results from its interaction with monoamine transporters, the serotonin transporter (SERT), norepinephrine transporter (NET), and dopamine transporter (DAT) (Verrico, Miller, & Madras, 2007).

MDMA reverses the actions of SERT, redirecting 5-HT stores into the synapse. A single dose of ecstasy can release up to 80% of the available serotonin into the synaptic cleft, acutely increasing serotonergic activity. MDMA also inhibits tryptophan hydroxylase, the rate-limiting enzymes in the synthesis of 5-HT (Green, Mechan, Elliott, O'Shea, & Colado, 2003). Animal models suggest that after acute administration, the inhibitory effects on tryptophan hydroxylase can last for up to 1 week (Green et al., 2003). It is likely that the combination of the depletion of neuronal serotonin (SERT activity) and the inhibition of tryptophan hydroxylase contributes to the ecstasy "comedown" symptoms of sleep disturbance, low mood, and irritability reported by users (Parrott, 2013). There is evidence for long term serotonergic neural toxity (Parrott, 2002; Benningfield & Cowan, 2013).

Like other amphetamines, it also potentiates dopamine and noradrenaline activity. MDMA increases dopamine and noradrenaline levels by reversing the action of DAT and NET, though MDMA-induced release of 5-HT is higher compared with the release of dopamine or norepinephrine and depletion of neuronal stores less pronounced Verrico et al., 2007. MDMA also mediates a mild inhibition of monoamine oxidase preventing the breakdown of 5-HT, noradrenaline, and dopamine. Prefrontal and dorsal hippocampus release of acetylcholine has been reported, and there is also an evidence for the activation of glutamate and interaction with gamma-aminobutyric acid (GABA) system (Torre & Farré, 2004).

4.1.3 Use, Harmful Use, and Dependence

The subjective experience of users has been important in the investigation of ecstasy's neuropharmacological and physiological actions. The acute psychological effects of ecstasy include a sense of well-being, euphoria, and increased sense of closeness with others (or empathy), leading to ecstasy being dubbed "the love drug." A range of negative psychological effects have also been reported and these include anxiety, depressed mood, irritability, and paranoia. A dose–response relationship related to the cardiovascular effects of ecstasy occurs at doses above 1 mg/kg, whereby significant increases in heart rate, blood pressure, and cardiac output occur. Nausea and vomiting, teeth grinding, headaches, body temperature changes, palpitations, muscle aches, fatigue, dizziness, dry mouth, increase energy, sweating, and paresthesia are the most common side effects (Baylen & Rosenberg, 2006) and are more pronounced in acute intoxication.

Ecstasy use in contrast to GHB or ketamine carries a low risk of dependence. There is limited evidence to suggest that physiological dependence occurs in animal studies, but in practice, people can stop using ecstasy without the need for specific medical intervention (Degenhardt, Bruno, & Topp, 2010). Typically, ecstasy is used one to two times per week in the context of partying, clubbing, or social gatherings. Ecstasy is often used with a number of other recreational drugs including alcohol, ketamine, GHB, cocaine, and methamphetamine. Escalation of recreational use to a level where it is deemed harmful is the most common scenario.

Bingeing behaviors include "stacking," the use of several tablets all at once, and "boosting," the use of successive tablets taken over an evening or over successive days. Comorbid psychiatric syndromes such as anxiety disorders may also play a role in facilitating the escalating use of ecstasy. People exhibiting these behaviors have reported mild/moderate subjective withdrawal symptoms during the comedown period including low mood and reduced appetite, which may be associated with taking days off work. Ecstasy dependence syndrome has been described applying the DSM-IV criteria that places an emphasis on compulsive use (use despite problems, giving up important activities because of ecstasy, unsuccessful attempts to stop, withdrawal, and excessive time spent obtaining or using it) and escalating use (tolerance and using it more often and longer than intended) (Degenhardt et al., 2010). However, presentation to treatment services with primary ecstasy dependence is rare. Ecstasy is normally the secondary or tertiary problematic drug reported by polydrug users. The course of ecstasy dependence has a tendency to differ from that of other drugs. Studies indicate that after 3 years, those initially meeting DSM-IV criteria for ecstasy dependence syndrome, 43% were still using the drug, though the majority no longer met the criteria for dependence (Degenhardt et al., 2010).

4.1.4 Intoxication and Overdose

Ecstasy use can result in acute physical health problems and psychiatric morbidity, though death is very rare (Hall & Henry, 2006). Psychiatric symptoms including an acute psychosis, flashback phenomena similar to those seen with lysergic acid diethylamide (LSD), anxiety/panic states, and depressive mood disorders may all occur (Green et al., 2003). Ecstasy can additionally precipitate psychotic and manic episodes in those with preexisting psychotic illness or precipitate a first psychosis (Rugani et al., 2012).

Clinically significant toxicity is rare and the presentation is usually in the context of polydrug use. As with other club drugs, ecstasy is often coingested with a range of other party drugs including alcohol, GHB, ketamine, methadone, cocaine, and methamphetamine. The major risks are around cardiovascular compromise. A combination of ecstasy use, hyperthermia, prolonged physical activity (in the form of vigorous dancing), and dehydration can lead to potentially fatal rhabdomyolysis and subsequent multiorgan failure and disseminated intravascular coagulation. Disturbances in sodium and water balance also occur and can be precipitated by acute water intoxication, which may present as an acute confusional state, impaired consciousness, and seizures. This is the main cause of ecstasy-associated mortality, is a medical emergency, and may require intensive care unit support.

4.2 GHB and GBL

4.2.1 Administration, Metabolism, and Elimination

GHB is oral ingested in the form of capsules, powder, tablets, or liquid. The powder is typically dissolved in water or alcoholic beverages to hide its salty taste. Its lipophilic properties potentiate a rapid absorption by the gastrointestinal tract with a bioavailability of about 25% (Schep et al., 2012). It reaches peak plasma concentrations in 20–60 min postingestion and has a relatively short half-life of between 20 and 60 min, with its lack of hangover effect cited as a reason for use among recreation users. Intravenous use has been reported, but this is rare (Gonzalez & Nutt, 2005; Wood, Brailsford, & Dargan, 2011).

All of the neurophysiological effects of GBL and 1,4-butanediol are attributable to GHB. GBL is metabolized to GHB via serum lactonase and 1,4-butanediol in the liver by alcohol dehydrogenase. GBL conversion to GHB is measurable within 5 min postingestion; in contrast, the conversion of 1,4-butanediol requires both alcohol dehydrogenase and aldehyde dehydrogenase enzymes party to zero-order kinetics, prolonging the conversion times when ingested with alcohol.

GHB is metabolized by GHB dehydrogenase and converted to succinic semialdehyde, which is then metabolized to succinic acid by succinic semialdehyde dehydrogenase. Succinic acid then enters the Krebs cycle and is further metabolized to CO_2 and water (Parviza, Vogelb, Gibsonb, & Pearl, 2014). The elimination is mostly via the lungs in the form of CO_2. Less than 2% of GHB is excreted in urine and is not detectable in urine after 12 h, presenting a challenge for drug monitoring, and GHB is reported to be a drug favored by airline pilots (Gonzalez & Nutt, 2005; Schep et al., 2012; Fig. 1).

4.2.2 Neuropharmacology

A short-chain fatty acid is similar in structure to GABA, for which it is both a precursor and a metabolite (Wong, Gibson, & Snead, 2004), though unlike GABA, it is able to cross the blood–brain barrier (Ryan & Stell, 1997; Van Cauter et al., 1997). GHB has both a stimulatory action and a sedative action, which can be partly explained by its high affinity to GHB receptors and low affinity to GABA-B receptors. It is an agonist at the excitatory

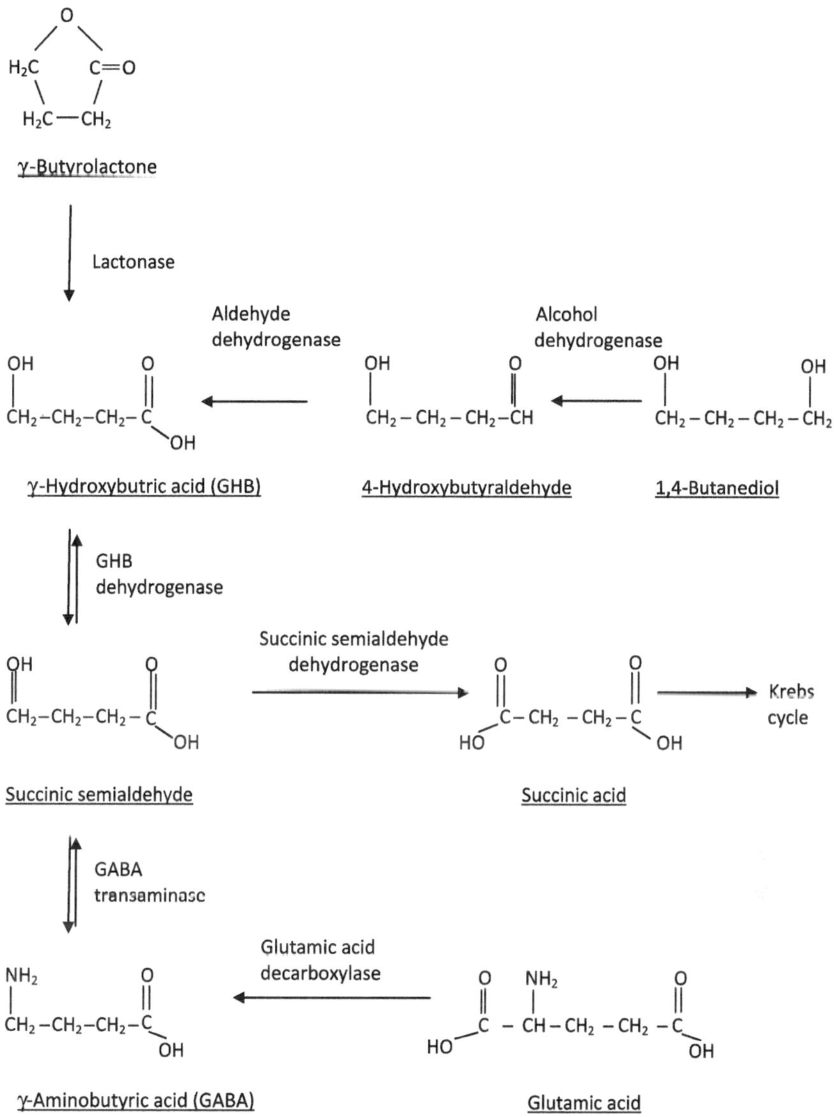

Figure 1 The metabolic pathway of GHB and precursors.

G protein-coupled GBH receptor that is widely distributed throughout the brain, with highest receptor density found in the cortex, the hippocampus, the olfactory tracts, and the cerebellum. In contrast, activity at the inhibitory GABA-B receptor is complex; it has a lower affinity for GABA-B receptors when compared to GABA-A (1000 times less than GABA), but clinical and experimental evidences demonstrate that GHB has marked GABA-B activity (Schep et al., 2012).

At lower doses (i.e., during recreational use), GHB activates GHB receptors and potentiates dopamine release, accounting for the euphoria and nausea that are common at low doses. At high dose, GHB has a modulatory function at the GABA-B receptor (Koek, Mercer, Coop, & France, 2009) leading to reduced dopamine levels and central nervous system (CNS) depression. There seems to be a limited effect on other transmitters and receptors, although there is evidence that it increases serotonin turnover in the brain and increases total brain acetylcholine (Schep et al., 2012), though the neuropharmacological and clinical sequelae are unclear.

4.2.3 Use, Harmful Use, and Dependence

In an international survey, partying (50%), being alone (20%), sexual enhancement (16%), and body building (6%) were cited as the most common reasons for use (Anderson et al., 2010). Initially, people seek the effects of euphora, sociability, and sexual enhancement. A minority may progress to domestic recreational use (euphoric effects and sexual enhancement) and then lone use (euphoria and sleep enhancement) before the characteristic frequent administration associated with dependence (to abate withdrawal symptoms and induce sleep) (Anderson et al., 2010; Gonzalez & Nutt, 2005; Van Cauter et al., 1997).

Among recreational users, the reward currency of GHB is euphoria and it is regularly used as part of a "party drug cocktail" with alcohol, MDMA, ketamine, and cocaine widely reported as coadministered drugs (Dillon & Degenhardt, 2001; Wood et al., 2009). The average dose among recreational users is in the range of 0.75–2.5 g (Gonzalez & Nutt, 2005). Subjective and clinical effects typically occur between 15 and 45 min following oral administration, though prolonged times to intoxication can occur when 1,4-butanediol is ingested in combination with alcohol. Associated positive effects include sociability, sensory enhancement, increased libido, and euphoria, with associated negative effects such as confusion, blurred vision, aggression, ataxia, nausea, and vomiting (Schep et al., 2012). Drug effects plateau at about 3–4 h following ingestion, disappearing between 4 and 8 h postingestion.

Tolerance, severe dependence, and withdrawal are recognized features of regular GHB misuse, and the withdrawal syndrome is a potentially life-threatening withdrawal state that is associated with high mortality if left untreated. A particular feature of GHB use, due to its short half-life and its ability to induce a rapid alcohol-like physiological tolerance, is the rapid onset of dependence in those who were previously recreational users or new to the drug (Maxwell, 2005). A typical dependent user will pipette the required dose of GHB/GBL every 4–5 h, often in response to feelings of mild agitation or anxiety (Gonzalez & Nutt, 2005). The dose is usually increased by 25–50% to induce sleep, often to counteract the insomnia that is an early feature of the withdrawal syndrome, with sleep usually lasting between 4 and 6 h. People with more severe dependence describe continuing 4–5 h dosing over a 24 h period. Dependence is typically associated with consumption of greater than 18 g in 24 h, and physiological dependence has been reported in between 4% and 21% of GHB users (Carter, Pardi, Gorsline, & Griffiths, 2010; Degenhardt, Darke, & Dillon, 2002; Miotto et al., 2001).

Recreational GHB use is associated with high-risk sexual behaviors, sex with strangers, and increased HIV risk, particularly on the MSM scene and risks of overdose and a dangerous alcohol-like withdrawal syndrome (Maxwell, 2005; Oser & Havens, 2008; Palamar & Halkitis, 2006).

4.2.4 Intoxication and Overdose

The clinical features of GHB intoxication reflect the steep dose–response relationship, though symptoms depend on the level of tolerance. They include short-term anterograde amnesia, hypotonia, nystagmus, euphoria, aggression, and ataxia at doses between 0.75 and 1.5 g (10–20 mg/kg); euphoria, drowsiness, sleep, hallucinations, and myoclonus at doses between 1.5 and 2.5 g (20–30 mg/kg); CNS depression, bradycardia, and respiratory depression at doses between 2.5 and 5 g (40–50 mg/kg); and coma/death at doses in excess of >5 g (50 mg/kg) (Schep et al., 2012).

New users face the risk of a titration trial, with the evidence suggesting that difficulties around titration continue even with regular use, so that users often present on multiple occasions to A&E with symptoms of toxicity (Korf, Nabben, Benschop, Ribbink, & van Amsterdam, 2014; Van Amsterdam et al., 2012). Presentation is more common in clinical units located in high-density urban areas, close to nightclubs, and at music/street festivals (Wood et al., 2011). Overdose is associated with the rapid ingestion of large quantities of GHB or with use of drugs that cause CNS depression including alcohol, ketamine, methadone, and benzodiazepines (Galicia et al., 2011; Korf et al., 2014).

CNS depression can progress quickly in the otherwise stable patient, and particular attention should be paid toward respiratory and cardiovascular support, with management in the ICU environment necessary if intubation and mechanical ventilation are required. Airway management is a particularly important feature of management as the loss of a gag reflex and vomiting can occur early in evolution of GHB overdose. CNS depression typically lasts for between 1 and 3 h with a typical full recovery within 4–8 h (Galicia et al., 2011). Patients should be observed for a minimum of 2 h, with supportive management being the mainstay of treatment.

There are currently no licensed antidotes for GHB, though a GABA-B antagonist SCH 5091 has shown some promise in animal studies, significantly reducing mortality in mice following the administration of fatal doses of GHB or 1,4-butanediol (Schep et al., 2012). Naloxone, flumazenil, and physostigmine have demonstrated limited benefits in GHB toxicity (Anderson et al., 2006; Schep et al., 2012).

4.2.5 The Management of GHB Withdrawal

The recognition of withdrawal states in the A&E or psychiatric ward presents a clinical challenge; in part, this is due to the limited exposure of general psychiatric and medical staff in the United Kingdom to GHB withdrawal. Additionally, patients presenting overdose may rapidly transition from states of intoxication to withdrawal. Moderate to severe withdrawal symptoms usually occur within 24 h of the last dose, though users can present with symptoms up to 4 days following the acute cessation of use. The main differential diagnoses are acute alcohol and overdose of another party drug. The distinct features of GHB withdrawal are the rapid evolution of symptoms, the absence of the physical stigmata of chronic alcohol use, and the presence of psychotic symptoms in clear consciousness. Mild to moderate withdrawal symptoms include anxiety, restlessness, nystagmus, confusion, tachycardia, nausea, and vomiting (Gonzalez & Nutt, 2005) and severe withdrawal symptoms, seizures, delirium, tachypnea, and palpitations (Bearn & Goldin, 2013; Choudhuri, Cross, Dargan, Wood, & Ranjith, 2013).

When managing acute withdrawal, cardiovascular and respiratory support is critical. First-line treatment is oral diazepam or parenteral lorazepam if oral medication is contraindicated, switching to oral diazepam when permissible. Baclofen, a GABA agonist, is helpful for agitation and the prevention of myoclonus. Second-line drugs such as phenobarbital and propofol have been used in cases not responding to high doses of benzodiazepines, and ICU support will be required if the patient requires enhanced levels of sedation or requires continuous cardiac monitoring and ventilator support (Schep et al., 2012).

GHB detoxification can present a challenging clinical entity (Gonzalez & Nutt, 2005). Typically, mildly to moderately dependent users (<3–4 doses and <30 g GHB/15 ml GBL in 24 h, respectively) can be managed as outpatients, with a reducing regime of diazepam starting at 5–10 mg four times daily over 4–5 days (Bearn & Goldin, 2013). Moderately to severely dependent users (>3–4 doses and >30 g GHB/15 ml GBL in 24 h, respectively) and dependent users with comorbid polydrug or alcohol dependence, with a history of withdrawal seizures, epilepsy, and a comorbid psychotic or mood disorder, should be managed in the inpatient environment.

High doses of diazepam between 80 and 150 mg are often required in the first 24 h, which may need to be increased to 200 mg if there is delirium. An agitated delirium and psychiatric symptoms occur in up to 1/3 of people during withdrawal and are more common in severe dependence. Visual and auditory hallucinations, paranoid thoughts, and delusions are the most common presenting psychiatric symptoms; typically, these occur after the first 24 h and antipsychotic medication such as olanzapine or quetiapine may be indicated (Choudhuri et al., 2013).

Clinical planning should be directed toward minimizing the likelihood that a severe withdrawal syndrome emerges and treating neuropsychiatric symptoms. The guiding principles are early treatment and continuous monitoring of withdrawal symptoms. The Alcohol Withdrawal Assessment Scoring Guidelines (CIWA-Ar) can be helpful as an objective measure, as no objective evidence-based measure exists for the GHB withdrawal syndrome (Gonzalez & Nutt, 2005). The course of the withdrawal syndrome runs on average 9 days but can last up to 14 days (Bearn & Goldin, 2013; Fig. 2).

4.3 Ketamine

4.3.1 Administration, Metabolism, and Elimination

Ketamine is an arylcyclohexylamine and as a recreational drug can be administered enterally, parenterally, and intranasally. Euphoriant effects occur rapidly and are dose-dependent, due to high lipid and water solubility and rapid transition across the blood–brain barrier (WHO, 2006). Most commonly encountered on the recreational drug scene as a white powder, it is also available as a liquid. When recreational use began, ketamine was smoked with cannabis, though intramuscular and intravenous use had also been described (Lankenau & Sanders, 2007). On the club scene, ketamine is

The algorithm below shows an example of the management for both GHB and GBL withdrawal.

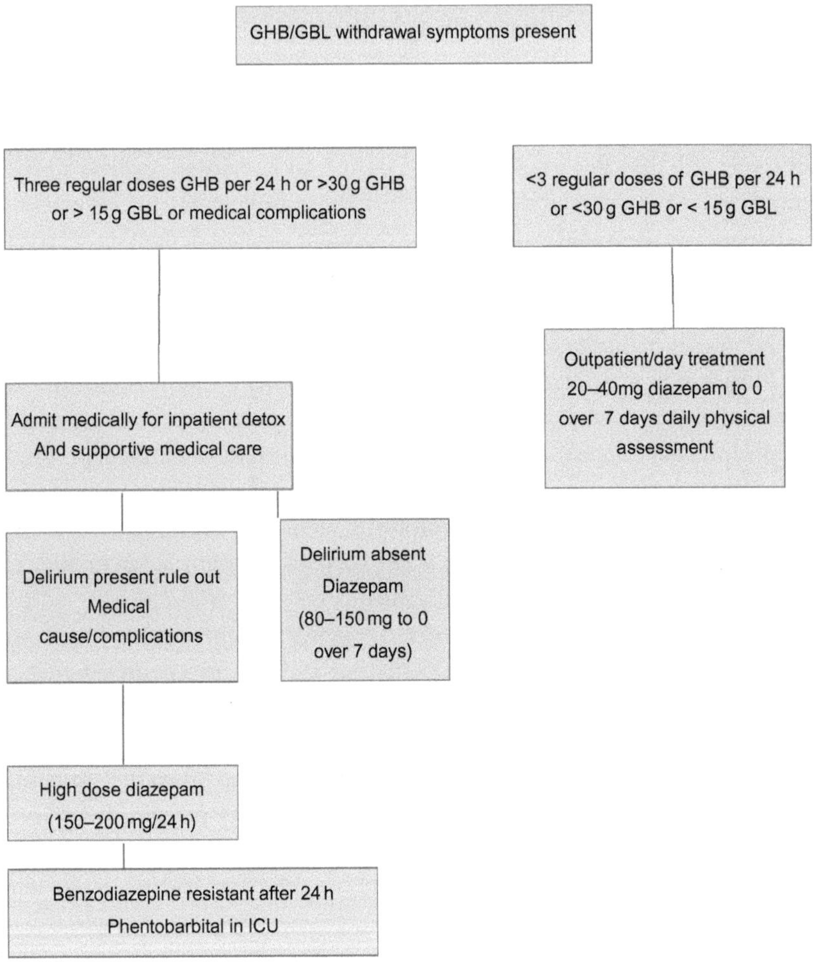

Figure 2 Algorithm for the management of GHB and GBL withdrawal (McDonough, Kennedy, Glasper, & Bearn, 2004). Guidelines for the management of GHB and GBL withdrawal.

primarily snorted, though it can be orally ingested and used rectally (Kalsi et al., 2011). Recreational doses of the drug typically range between 200 and 300 mg when ingested orally and 60–250 mg when snorted (Kalsi et al., 2011). Bioavailability via the nasal route is about 50% (Malinovsky & Servin, 1996). The initial rush occurs after 2–5 min, followed by a trance-like euphoria. When ingested orally, the bioavailability is 17%, and following extensive first-pass metabolism (Clements, Nimmo, & Grant, 1982), the major active metabolite, norketamine, is 1/3 as potent as ketamine (Adamowicz & Kala, 2005) and induces a more sedative experience.

Ketamine has a half-life of between 2 and 16 min and the effects of the drug last about an hour. It is metabolized via N-demethylation by cytochromes CYP3A4, CYPB6, and CYP2C9 to its active metabolite norketamine and inactive metabolite dehydronorketamine (Bokor & Anderson, 2014). Renally excreted mostly as glucuronide conjugates (80%), dehydronorketamine (16.2%), ketamine (2.3%), and norketamine (1.6%) (Wieber, Gugler, Hengstmann, & Dengler, 1975; Wood et al., 2009), ketamine is detectable in urine for up to 48 h following a single dose and norketamine is detectable for between 6 and 14 days (Adamowicz & Kala, 2005).

4.3.2 Neuropharmacology

Ketamine is a noncompetitive receptor antagonist at the *N*-methyl-D-aspartate receptor (NMDA) PCP binding site (Trujillo et al., 2011) and has an R- and S-isomer. While the S-isomer has greater receptor affinity and potency, both isomers demonstrate similar pharmacokinetic profiles (Morgan & Curran, 2012). The NMDA complex is activated by the endogenous agonists glutamic acid, aspartic acid, and glycine and plays a central role in the modulation of synaptic plasticity and memory function (Morgan & Curran, 2006); the receptor is also involved in the processing of sensory inputs at the spinal and thalamic levels (Dougherty & Palecek, 1992). The activity of ketamine at the NMDA receptor has impact on memory, emotion, sensation, and perceptions (Morgan et al., 2013).

Our understanding of mechanisms of action and potential role in the understanding of psychiatric disorders is incomplete. Initially, it was assumed that ketamine inhibited glutamate release, the hypoglutamatergic hypothesis (Trujillo et al., 2011). More recently, it has been suggested that due to its blockade of NMDA receptors on GABAergic neurons, ketamine potentiates glutamate release (Trujillo et al., 2011). This underpins the glutamate hypothesis of schizophrenia and may contribute to psychedelic effects (Deakin et al., 2008).

The analgesic properties of ketamine are likely to occur via its direct and modulatory effect on opioid receptors on spinothalamic pathways. Ketamine has been demonstrated to be a weak agonist at opioid receptors and is able to prevent opiate tolerance in animal models. Ketamine can reduce the amount of opioid medication required (Trujillo et al., 2011) and has been used to treat complex regional pain syndrome (Sigtermans et al., 2009).

Ketamine also activates dopaminergic reward networks. With repeated administration, dopamine supplies are depleted promoting both euphoric effects and the development of tolerance (Ross, 2008). In contrast, repeated administration of ketamine enhances serotonin levels, and a single dose of ketamine has been demonstrated to improve depressive symptoms for up to 1 week (Zarate et al., 2006).

4.3.3 Use, Harmful Use, and Dependence

Ketamine's emergence as a party drug is curious partly owing to the diversity of experience reported by users. Euphoria features high on subjective reporting, though dissociative experiences are also commonly described. The dissociative effects are thought to be a result of an electrophysiological dissociation between the limbic and the thalamoneocortical systems (Kalsi et al., 2011; Mercer, 2008). In one study of the subjective psychological and behavioral effects of ketamine, a range of experiences were described. The absence of time (70%), unusual thought content (60%), psychomotor dissociation (57%), euphoria (55%), derealization (53%), visual hallucinations (49%), weightlessness (47%), and auditory hallucinations (46%) were the seven most commonly reported effects (Dillon, Copeland, & Jansen, 2003). Users have also reported the subjective experience of feeling like they are "flying" or "becoming god" and being "stuck in a K-hole," a zombie-like psychedelic twilight zone particularly associated with intravenous ketamine use (Lankenau & Sanders, 2007). Ketamine use is associated with cognitive dysfunction, particularly difficulties in working and episodic memory (Morgan & Curran, 2006).

Ketamine dependence does occur and reinforcing effects have been demonstrated in both animals and humans. In particular, the short half-life and buzz associated with snorting ketamine can lead to a compulsive binge pattern of use or continuous use in spite of repeated harms. Tolerance is rapid and common among users, with the occasional user doubling their dose in the first year of use and regular users increasing but more (Kalsi et al., 2011). There is limited evidence for a physiological withdrawal syndrome. Anxiety, sweating, and palpitations have been reported on cessation of the drug that may be ameliorated by low doses of benzodiazepines.

4.3.4 *Intoxication and Overdose*

A psychotic-like state or excited delirium can be signs of overdose. Common psychological and behavioral symptoms include agitation, aggression, grandiosity, persecutory and paranoid delusions, and auditory and visual hallucinations (Dillon et al., 2003; Pomarol-Clotet et al., 2006). Dissociative states may present as feelings of impaired somatic or psychic control (passivity phenomena).

Ketamine is a mild respiratory depressant and cardiovascular stimulant inducing increases in heart rate, cardiac output, and blood pressure. Palpitations are sometimes a presenting complaint. Pulmonary edema has been described in ketamine overdose, and this may be related to a combination of increased cardiac output and respiratory depression (Kalsi et al., 2011). The median lethal therapeutic dose in animals is 100 times the average therapeutic dose, and no adverse effects were observed in nine children who had been injected with 100 times the intended dose (Green et al., 1999; Morgan & Curran, 2012). Mortality associated with ketamine is often the result of use within a polydrug cocktail as previously described with MDMA and GHB (Morgan & Curran, 2012). Between 1996 and 2006, only four cases of death associated with ketamine were reported in the United Kingdom (Bokor & Anderson, 2014; Schifano, Corkery, Oyefeso, Tonia, & Ghodse, 2008). Although there was a 10-fold increase in deaths mentioning ketamine as a cofactor between 1999 and 2008 (2–22), this is likely to reflect the increasing use of the drug on the club scene (Morgan & Curran, 2012).

Management of ketamine toxicity is targeted at psychiatric symptoms including auditory and visual hallucinations. As agitation or aggression can also be a feature, benzodiazepines can be used for sedation and the patient should be nursed in a low-stimulus environment. Evidence suggests that both typical and atypical antipsychotic medications may have a role in the treatment of acute ketamine intoxication, haloperidol (Giannini, Underwood, & Condon, 2000), and atypical antipsychotics (Duncan & Miyamoto, 2000) have been used, though low doses are advised as there is a risk of neuroleptic malignant syndrome in the neuroleptic naive patient.

Accidents are a common cause of injury or death in ketamine users, arising in the context of reduced pain perception combined with psychomotor aberration, reduced environmental awareness, grandiosity, perceptual disturbance, and thought disorder. Falls, drowning (Trujillo et al., 2011), jumping off buildings (Kalsi et al., 2011), and car accidents have been recorded as causes of death in ketamine-intoxicated patients. In Hong Kong,

9% of fatal crashes recorded over a 5-year period involved ketamine use (Cheng, Ng, Chan, Mok, & Cheung, 2007; Morgan & Curran, 2006).

Problems with chronic use include ketamine-induced ulcerative cystitis that can present as painful hematuria and suprapubic pain; the course of the condition is variable. Sometimes, this is resolved by abstaining from ketamine use; although up to 1/3 may have long-term difficulties and are at risk of obstructive nephropathy, K-cramps describe a vague abdominal pain associated with the long-term use of ketamine, which again abate following a period of abstinence (Morgan & Curran, 2012).

5. THE FUTURE OF PARTY DRUGS

The use of drugs to induce altered states is interwoven with human history, a history driven by human needs and wants and shaped by social evolution. Timothy Leary's call to "Turn on, tune in, drop out" has become a central ideology of dance or party drug culture, spawning metaphysical association between music, dance, underground culture, and freedom of expression. The emerging pattern is that of an increase in "party drug" use in countries with increasing disposable income and a greater acceptability of party drug use in developed countries. More people are using recreational drugs to induce particular desired feelings or states of mind.

Ecstasy, ketamine, and GHB have a range of pharmacological and physiological effects, abuse potential, clinical uses, and social consequences but have been collected under a label that focuses on the social use and historical and legal classification rather than the properties of the drugs themselves. The three party drugs explored in this chapter are currently being reexplored and investigated, and their potential therapeutic and research value has become a hot topic in psychiatry. In this regard, the history of ecstasy, GHB, and ketamine provides an important narrative for the future of drug use, particularly with the rapid emergence of new designer drugs in the Internet age.

REFERENCES

Abraham, T. T., Barnes, A. J., Lowe, R. H., Kolbrich Spargo, E. A., Milman, G., Pirnay, S. O., et al. (2009). Urinary MDMA, MDA, HMMA and HMA excretion following controlled MDMA administration to humans. *Journal of Analytical Toxicology*, *33*, 439–446.

Adamowicz, P., & Kala, M. (2005). Urinary excretion rates of ketamine and norketamine following therapeutic ketamine administration: Method and detection window considerations. *Journal of Analytical Toxicology*, *28*(August), 31–33.

Alshaikh, M. K., Tricco, A. C., Tashkandi, M., Mamdani, M., Straus, S. E., & BaHammam, A. S. (2012). Sodium oxybate for narcolepsy with cataplexy: Systematic review and meta-analysis. *Journal of Clinical Sleep Medicine: JCSM: Official Publication of the American Academy of Sleep Medicine*, *8*(4), 451–458.

American Psychiatric Pub Inc. (2013). *Diagnostic and statistical manual of mental disorders: DSM5.* Arlington, VA: American Psychiatric Pub Inc.

Anderson, I. B., Kim, S. Y., Dyer, J. E., Burkhardt, C. B., Iknoian, J. C., Walsh, M. J., et al. (2006). Trends in gamma-hydroxybutyrate (GHB) and related drug intoxication: 1999 to 2003. *Annals of Emergency Medicine*, *47*(2), 177–183.

Anderson, I. B., Kim-Katz, S. Y., Dyer, J. E., & Blanc, P. D. (2010). The impact of gamma hydroxybutyrate (GHB) legal restrictions on patterns of use: Results from an international survey. *Drugs: Education, Prevention, and Policy*, *17*(5), 455–469.

Basil, B., Blair, A. M., & Holmes, S. W. (1964). The action of sodium 4-hydroxybutyrate on spinal reflexes. *British Journal of Pharmacology and Chemotherapy*, *22*, 318–328.

Baylen, C. A., & Rosenberg, H. (2006). A review of the acute subjective effects of MDMA/ecstasy. *Addiction*, *101*(7), 933–947.

Bearn, J., & Goldin, M. (2013). *GHB: What psychiatrists need to know.* CPD Online Royal College of Psychiatry, Maney publishing.

Benningfield, M. M., & Cowan, R. L. (2013). Brain serotonin function in MDMA (ecstasy) users: Evidence for persisting neurotoxicity. *Neuropsychopharmacology: Official Publication of the American College of Neuropsychopharmacology*, *38*(1), 253–255.

Berridge, V., & Mars, S. (2004). History of addictions. *Journal of Epidemiology and Community Health*, *58*(9), 747–750.

Blumenfeld, M., Suntay, R. G., & Harmel, M. H. (1962). Sodium gamma-hydroxybutyric acid: A new anesthetic adjuvant. *Anesthesia and Analgesia*, *41*(6), 721–726.

Bokor, G., & Anderson, P. D. (2014). Ketamine: An update on its abuse. *Journal of Pharmacy Practice*, *27*(6), 582–586.

Bonanno, F. G. (2002). Ketamine in war/tropical surgery (a final tribute to the racemic mixture). *Injury*, *33*(4), 323–327.

Carter, L. P., Pardi, D., Gorsline, J., & Griffiths, R. R. (2010). Illicit gamma-hydroxybutyrate (GHB) and pharmaceutical sodium oxybate (Xyrem): Differences in the characteristics of misuse. *Drug and Alcohol Dependence*, *104*(501), 1–10.

Cheng, W.-C., Ng, K.-M., Chan, K.-K., Mok, V. K.-K., & Cheung, B. K.-L. (2007). Roadside detection of impairment under the influence of ketamine—Evaluation of keta mine impairment symptoms with reference to its concentration in oral fluid and urine. *Forensic Science International*, *170*(1), 51–58.

Choudhuri, D., Cross, S., Dargan, P. I., Wood, D. M., & Ranjith, G. (2013). Psychiatric aspects of acute withdrawal from gamma-hydroxybutyrate (GHB) and its analogue gamma-butyrolactone (GBL): Implications for psychiatry services in the general hospital. *International Journal of Psychiatry in Clinical Practice*, *17*(2), 154–156.

Clements, J. A., Nimmo, W. S., & Grant, I. S. (1982). Bioavailability, pharmacokinetics, and analgesic activity of ketamine in humans. *Journal of Pharmaceutical Sciences*, *71*(5), 539–542.

Coyle, J. T. (2001). Reviews and overviews. The emerging role of glutamate in the pathophysiology and treatment of schizophrenia. *The American Journal of Psychiatry*, *158*(9), 1367–1377.

Davison, D., & Parrott, A. C. (1997). Ecstasy (MDMA) in recreational users: Self-reported psychological and physiological effects. *Human Psychopharmacology*, *12*(3), 221–226.

Deakin, J. F. W., Lees, J., McKie, S., Hallak, J. E. C., Williams, S. R., & Dursun, S. M. (2008). Glutamate and the neural basis of the subjective effects of ketamine. *Archives of General Psychiatry*, *65*(2), 154–164.

De La Torre, R., Farré, M., Ortuño, J., Mas, M., Brenneisen, R., Roset, P. N., et al. (2002). Non-linear pharmacokinetics of MDMA ("ecstasy") in humans. *British Journal of Clinical Pharmacology*, *49*(2), 104–109.

Degenhardt, L., Bruno, R., & Topp, L. (2010). Is ecstasy a drug of dependence? *Drug and Alcohol Dependence, 107*(1), 1–10.

Degenhardt, L., Darke, S., & Dillon, P. (2002). GHB use among Australians: Characteristics, use patterns and associated harm. *Drug and Alcohol Dependence, 67*(1), 89–94.

Degenhardt, L., & Hall, W. (Eds.), (2010). *The health and psychological effects of "ecstasy (MDMA) use"*. Sydney: NDARC.

Dillon, P., Copeland, J., & Jansen, K. (2003). Patterns of use and harms associated with non-medical ketamine use. *Drug and Alcohol Dependence, 69*, 23–28.

Dillon, P., & Degenhardt, L. (2001). Ketamine and GHB: New trends in club drug use? *Journal of Substance Use, 6*(1), 11–15.

Domino, E. F., Chodoff, P., & Corssen, G. (1965). Pharmacologic effects of CI-581, a new dissociative anaesthetic, in man. *Clinical Pharmacology and Therapeutics, 6*, 279–291.

Dougherty, P., & Palecek, J. (1992). The role of NMDA and non-NMDA excitatory amino acid receptors in the excitation of primate spinothalamic tract neurons by mechanical, chemical, thermal, and electrical stimuli. *The Journal of Neuroscience, 12*(8), 3025–3041.

Duncan, G., & Miyamoto, S. (2000). Comparison of the effects of clozapine, risperidone, and olanzapine on ketamine-induced alterations in regional brain metabolism. *The Journal of Pharmacology and Experimental Therapeutics, 293*(1), 8–14.

Dyer, J. E. (1991). Gamma-hydroxybutyrate: A health-food product producing coma and seizure like activity. *The American Journal of Emergency Medicine, 9*(4), 321–324.

Edwards, G., & Gross, M. M. (1976). Alcohol dependence: Provisional description of a clinical syndrome. *British Medical Journal, 1*(6017), 1058–1061.

Erowid, E. (2009). *Alexander Shulgin's pharmacology notebooks.* http://www.erowid.org/library/books_online/shulgin_labbooks.

Freudenmann, R. W., Oxler, F., & Bernschneider-Reif, S. (2006). The origin of MDMA (ecstasy) revisited: The true story reconstructed from the original documents. *Addiction, 101*(9), 1241–1245.

Galicia, M., Nogue, S., & Miró, O. (2011). Liquid ecstasy intoxication: Clinical features of 505 consecutive emergency department patients. *Emergency Medicine Journal: EMJ, 28*(6), 462–466.

Giannini, A. J., Underwood, N. A., & Condon, M. (2000). Acute ketamine intoxication treated by haloperidol: A preliminary study. *American Journal of Therapeutics, 7*(6), 389–391.

Giraudon, I., & Bello, P.-Y. (2007). Monitoring ecstasy content in France: Results from the National Surveillance System 1999–2004. *Substance Use & Misuse, 42*(10), 1567–1578.

Gonzalez, A., & Nutt, D. J. (2005). Gamma hydroxy butyrate abuse and dependency. *Journal of Psychopharmacology, 19*(2), 195–204.

Green, S. M., Clark, R., Hostetler, M. A., Cohen, M., Carlson, D., & Rothrock, S. G. (1999). Inadvertent ketamine overdose in children: Clinical manifestations and outcome. *Annals of Emergency Medicine, 34*(4 Pt 1), 492–497.

Green, A. R., Mechan, A. O., Elliott, J. M., O'Shea, E., & Colado, M. I. (2003). The pharmacology and clinical pharmacology of 3,4-methylenedioxymethamphetamine (MDMA, "ecstasy"). *Pharmacological Reviews, 55*(3), 463–508.

Greer, G. (1985). Using MDMA in psychotherapy. *Advances, 2*, 57–59.

Greer, G., & Tolbert, R. (1986). Subjective reports of the Effects of MDMA in a clinical setting. *Journal of Psychoactive Drugs, 18*, 319–327.

Hall, A. P., & Henry, J. A. (2006). Acute toxic effects of "Ecstasy" (MDMA) and related compounds: Overview of pathophysiology and clinical management. *British Journal of Anaesthesia, 96*(6), 678–685.

Hardman, H. F., Haavik, C. O., & Seevers, M. H. (1973). Relationship of the structure of mescaline and seven analogs to toxicity and behaviour in five species of laboratory animals. *Toxicology and Applied Pharmacology, 25*(2), 299–309.

Hashimoto, K. (2014). Targeting of NMDA receptors in new treatments for schizophrenia. *Expert Opinion on Therapeutic Targets, 18*, 1049–1063, 1–15.

Hasin, D. S., O'Brien, C. P., Auriacombe, M., Borges, G., Bucholz, K., Budney, A., et al. (2013). DSM-5 criteria for substance use disorders: Recommendations and rationale. *The American Journal of Psychiatry, 170*(8), 834–851.

Jansen, K. (2001). *Ketamine: Dreams and realities.* Sarasota, FL: Multidisciplinary Association for Psychedelic Studies.

Kalsi, S. S., Wood, D. M., & Dargan, P. I. (2011). The epidemiology and patterns of acute and chronic toxicity associated with recreational ketamine use. *Emerging Health Threats Journal, 4*, 7107.

Koek, W., Mercer, S. L., Coop, A., & France, C. P. (2009). Behavioural effects of gamma-hydroxybutyrate, its precursor gamma-butyrolactone, and GABA(B) receptor agonists: Time course and differential antagonism by the GABA(B) receptor antagonist 3-aminopropyl(diethoxymethyl)phosphinic acid (CGP35348). *The Journal of Pharmacology and Experimental Therapeutics, 330*(3), 876–883.

Korf, D. J., Nabben, T., Benschop, A., Ribbink, K., & van Amsterdam, J. G. C. (2014). Risk factors of γ-hydroxybutyrate overdosing. *European Addiction Research, 20*(2), 66–74.

Laborit, H., Buchard, F., Laborit, G., Kind, A., & Weber, B. (1960). Use of sodium 4-hydroxybutyrate in anesthesia and resuscitation. *Agressologie: Revue Internationale de Physio-Biologie et de Pharmacologie Appliquées aux Effets de L'agression, 1*, 549–560.

Lahti, A., Weiler, M., & Tamara, M. (2001). Effects of ketamine in normal and schizophrenic volunteers. *Neuropsychopharmacology, 25*(4), 455–467.

Lankenau, S. E., & Sanders, B. (2007). Patterns of ketamine use among young injection drug users. *Journal of Psychoactive Drugs, 39*(1), 21–29.

Large, C. H. (2007). Do NMDA receptor antagonist models of schizophrenia predict the clinical efficacy of antipsychotic drugs? *Journal of Psychopharmacology (Oxford, England), 21*(3), 283–301.

Leone, M. A., Vigna-Taglianti, F., Avanzi, G., Brambilla, R., & Faggiano, F. (2010). Gamma-hydroxybutyrate (GHB) for treatment of alcohol withdrawal and prevention of relapses. *The Cochrane Database of Systematic Reviews.*

Malinovsky, J., & Servin, F. (1996). Ketamine and norketamine plasma concentrations after i.v., nasal and rectal administration in children. *British Journal of Anaesthesia, 77*, 203–207.

Maxwell, J. C. (2005). Party drugs: Properties, prevalence, patterns, and problems. *Substance Use & Misuse, 40*(9–10), 1203–1240.

McCambridge, J., Winstock, A., Hunt, N., & Mitcheson, L. (2007). 5-Year trends in use of hallucinogens and other adjunct drugs among UK dance drug users. *European Addiction Research, 13*(1), 57–64.

McDonough, M., Kennedy, N., Glasper, A., & Bearn, J. (2004). Clinical features and management of gamma-hydroxybutyrate (GHB) withdrawal: A review. *Drug and Alcohol Dependence, 75*, 3–9.

Mercer, S. (2008). "The Drug of War"—A historical review of the use of Ketamine in military conflicts. *Journal of the Royal Naval Medical Service, 95*, 145–150, September 1970.

Miotto, K., Darakjian, J., Basch, J., Murray, S., Zogg, J., & Rawson, R. (2001). Gamma-hydroxybutyric acid: Patterns of use, effects and withdrawal. *The American Journal on Addictions/American Academy of Psychiatrists in Alcoholism and Addictions, 10*(3), 232–241.

Moore, K., & Miles, S. (2004). Young people, dance and the sub-cultural consumption of drugs. *Addiction Research & Theory, 12*(6), 507–523.

Morgan, C. J. A., & Curran, H. V. (2006). Acute and chronic effects of ketamine upon human memory: A review. *Psychopharmacology, 188*(4), 408–424.

Morgan, C. J. A., & Curran, H. V. (2012). Ketamine use: A review. *Addiction, 107*(1), 27–38.

Morgan, C. J. A., Noronha, L. A., Muetzelfeldt, M., Fielding, A., & Curran, H. V. (2013). Harms and benefits associated with psychoactive drugs: Findings of an international survey of active drug users. *Journal of Psychopharmacology (Oxford, England)*, *27*(6), 497–506.

Nutt, D., King, L. A., Saulsbury, W., & Blakemore, C. (2007). Development of a rational scale to assess the harm of drugs of potential misuse. *Lancet*, *369*(9566), 1047–1053.

Oser, C., & Havens, J. (2008). HIV sexual risk behaviours among ketamine and non-ketamine using criminal offenders prior to prison entry. *Addiction Research & Theory*, *16*(3), 289–302.

Pai, A., & Heining, M. (2007). Ketamine. *Continuing Education in Anaesthesia, Critical Care & Pain*, 7(2), 59–63.

Palamar, J. J., & Halkitis, P. N. (2006). A qualitative analysis of GHB use among gay men: Reasons for use despite potential adverse outcomes. *The International Journal on Drug Policy*, *17*(1), 23–28.

Parrott, A. C. (2002). Recreational Ecstasy/MDMA, the serotonin syndrome, and serotonergic neurotoxicity. *Pharmacology, Biochemistry, and Behavior*, *71*(4), 837–844.

Parrott, A. C. (2013). Human psychobiology of MDMA or "Ecstasy": An overview of 25 years of empirical research. *Human Psychopharmacology*, *28*(4), 289–307.

Parviza, M., Vogelb, K., Gibsonb, K. M., & Pearl, P. L. (2014). Disorders of GABA metabolism: SSADH and GABA-transaminase deficiencies. *Journal of Pediatric Epilepsy*, *3*(4), 217–227.

Pomarol-Clotet, E., Honey, G. D., Murray, G. K., Corlett, P. R., Absalom, A. R., Lee, M., et al. (2006). Psychological effects of ketamine in healthy volunteers. Phenomenological study. *The British Journal of Psychiatry: The Journal of Mental Science*, *189*, 173–179.

Ross, S. (2008). Ketamine and addiction. *Primary Psychiatry*, *15*, 61–69.

Rugani, F., Bacciardi, S., Rovai, L., Pacini, M., Maremmani, A. G. I., Deltito, J., et al. (2012). Symptomatological features of patients with and without Ecstasy use during their first psychotic episode. *International Journal of Environmental Research and Public Health*, *9*(7), 2283–2292.

Ryan, J. M., & Stell, I. (1997). Gamma hydroxybutyrate—A coma inducing recreational drug. *Journal of Accident & Emergency Medicine*, *14*(4), 259–261.

Saunders, N. (1993). *E for Ecstasy*. London: W.B. Saunders.

Schep, L. J., Knudsen, K., Slaughter, R. J., Vale, J. A., & Mégarbane, B. (2012). The clinical toxicology of γ-hydroxybutyrate, γ-butyrolactone and 1,4-butanediol. *Clinical Toxicology (Philadelphia, Pa.)*, *50*(6), 458–470.

Schifano, F. (2004). A bitter pill. Overview of ecstasy (MDMA, MDA) related fatalities. *Psychopharmacology*, *173*(3–4), 242–248.

Schifano, F., Corkery, J., Oyefeso, A., Tonia, T., & Ghodse, A. H. (2008). Trapped in the "K-hole": Overview of deaths associated with ketamine misuse in the UK (1993–2006). *Journal of Clinical Psychopharmacology*, *28*(1), 114–116.

Sewell, R. (2007). Ketamine: Peril and promise. *MAPS Bulletin*, *17*(1), 23–27.

Shulgin, A. T. (1986). The background and chemistry of MDMA. *Journal of Psychoactive Drugs*, *18*(4), 291–304.

Shulgin, A. (1989). History of MDMA. In S. Peroutka (Ed.), *Ecstasy: The clinical, pharmacological and neurotoxicological effects of the drug MDMA* (pp. 1–20). Boston: Kluwer, Springer Science & Business Media (p. 244).

Shulgin, A., & Nichols, D. (1978). Characterization of three new psychotomimetics. In R. C. Stillman, & R. E. Willette (Eds.), *The psychopharmacology of hallucinogens* (pp. 1–9). New York: Pergamon Press.

Sigtermans, M. J., van Hilten, J. J., Bauer, M. C. R., Arbous, M. S., Marinus, J., Sarton, E. Y., et al. (2009). Ketamine produces effective and long-term pain relief in patients with Complex Regional Pain Syndrome Type 1. *Pain*, *145*(3), 304–311.

Steele, M. T., & Watson, W. A. (1995). Acute poisoning from gamma hydroxybutyrate (GHB). *Missouri Medicine, 92*(7), 354–357.
Tanner-Smith, E. E. (2006). Pharmacological content of tablets sold as "ecstasy": Results from an online testing service. *Drug and Alcohol Dependence, 83*(3), 247–254.
Teltzrow, R., & Bosch, O. (2012). Ecstatic anaesthesia: Ketamine and GHB between medical use and self-experimentation. *Applied Cardiopulmonary Pathophysiology, 16,* 309–321.
Torre, R. D. la, & Farré, M. (2004). Human pharmacology of MDMA: Pharmacokinetics, metabolism, and disposition. *Therapeutic Drug Monitoring, 26*(2), 137–144.
Trujillo, K. A., Smith, M. L., Sullivan, B., Heller, C. Y., Garcia, C., & Bates, M. (2011). The neurobehavioral pharmacology of ketamine: Implications for drug abuse, addiction, and psychiatric disorders. *ILAR Journal/National Research Council, Institute of Laboratory Animal Resources, 52,* 366–378.
Van Amsterdam, J. G. C., Brunt, T. M., McMaster, M. T. B., Niesink, R., van Noorden, M. S., & van den Brink, W. (2012). Cognitive impairment due to intensive use and overdoses of gammahydroxybutyric acid (GHB). *Tijdschrift voor Psychiatrie, 54*(12), 1001–1010.
Van Cauter, E., Plat, L., Scharf, M. B., Leproult, R., Cespedes, S., L'Hermite-Balériaux, M., et al. (1997). Simultaneous stimulation of slow-wave sleep and growth hormone secretion by gamma-hydroxybutyrate in normal young Men. *The Journal of Clinical Investigation, 100*(3), 745–753.
Verrico, C. D., Miller, G. M., & Madras, B. K. (2007). MDMA (Ecstasy) and human dopamine, norepinephrine, and serotonin transporters: Implications for MDMA-induced neurotoxicity and treatment. *Psychopharmacology, 189*(4), 489–503.
WHO (1964). *WHO expert committee on addiction-producing drugs: Thirteenth report.*
WHO (2006). *Critical review of ketamine.* (September 2002, pp. 1–30).
WHO (2012). *Gamma-hydroxybutyric acid (GHB) critical review report* (June, pp. 4–8).
Wieber, J., Gugler, R., Hengstmann, J. H., & Dengler, H. J. (1975). Pharmacokinetics of ketamine in man. *Der Anaesthesist, 24*(6), 260–263.
Wolff, K., Hay, A. M., Sherlock, K., & Conner, M. (1995). Contents of "ecstasy" *The Lancet, 346*(8982), 1100–1101.
Wong, C. G. T., Gibson, K. M., & Snead, O. C. (2004). From the street to the brain: Neurobiology of the recreational drug γ-hydroxybutyric acid. *Trends in Pharmacological Sciences, 25*(1), 29–34.
Wood, D., & Beaumont, P. (2010). Recreational drug use presentations during a large outdoor festival event: Reduction in hospital emergency department transfer where medical physicians are present. *Journal of Substance Use, 15*(6), 434–441.
Wood, D. M., Brailsford, A. D., & Dargan, P. I. (2011). Acute toxicity and withdrawal syndromes related to γ-hydroxybutyrate (GHB) and its analogues γ-butyrolactone (GBL) and 1,4-butanediol (1,4-BD). *Drug Testing and Analysis, 3*(7–8), 417–425.
Wood, D., Nicolaou, M., & Dargan, P. (2009). Epidemiology of recreational drug toxicity in a nightclub environment. *Substance Use & Misuse, 44*(11), 1495–1502.
World drug report. (1997). *Trends in Organized Crime, 3,* 11–14.
Zarate, C. A., Singh, J. B., Carlson, P. J., Brutsche, N. E., Ameli, R., Luckenbaugh, D. A., et al. (2006). A randomized trial of an N-methyl-D-aspartate antagonist in treatment-resistant major depression. *Archives of General Psychiatry, 63*(8), 856–864.

CHAPTER ELEVEN

"Natural Amphetamine" Khat: A Cultural Tradition or a Drug of Abuse?

Nilesh B. Patel[1]
Department of Medical Physiology, College of Health Sciences, University of Nairobi, Nairobi, Kenya
[1]Corresponding author: e-mail address: npatel@uonbi.ac.ke

Contents

Abstract

Khat, *Catha edulis* Forsk, is among the most widely used plant-based psychoactive substance in the world. Grown in Eastern Africa, Horn of Africa, and southwestern part of the Arabian Peninsula, its fresh young leaves and twigs are used daily by over 20 million people for the psychostimulatory effects it produces in the user, a practice deeply rooted in the history, tradition, and culture of the indigenous population. Once hardly known outside the regions where it is grown and used, khat use has now spread to other countries. This review will cover the, phytochemistry, pharmacokinetics of the active ingredients—cathinone, cathine, norephedrine, neurochemistry, effects on cognitive and executive functions as well as its ability to produce dependency in the user. Whether it is an innocuous cultural practice or a drug of abuse is debatable as the preclinical and clinical data needed to arrive at an authoritative conclusion is lacking.

International Review of Neurobiology, Volume 120
ISSN 0074-7742
http://dx.doi.org/10.1016/bs.irn.2015.02.006

On 24 June 2014, the United Kingdom (UK) joined the list of countries that have banned the use, possession, and trade in khat (*Catha edulis* Forsk). In the preceding years, the UK government had tasked the Advisory Council on the Misuse of Drugs (ACMD) to give its recommendation on whether khat should be banned. The ACMD (2013) reported that, it "... considers that the evidence of harm associated with the use of khat is insufficient to justify control and it would be inappropriate and disproportionate to classify khat under the Misuse of Drugs Act 1971. In summary, the ACMD considers that the harms of khat do not reach the level required for classification." The UK government ignored these recommendations and justified its decision to ban khat use on the basis that it did not wish Great Britain to become a hub for the smuggling of khat into those European countries and North America where khat use had been prohibited.

1. INTRODUCTION

"Khat" refers to the fresh young leaves and twigs of the shrub, *C. edulis* Forsk, (Fig. 1) which is consumed for its psychostimulant effects by over 20 million people worldwide on a daily basis (Al-Motarreb, Al-Kebsi, Al-Adhi, & Broadley, 2002; Magdum, 2011; Saha & Dollery, 2006).

In recent years, khat use has spread well beyond its traditional strongholds in Africa as a consequence of its use among Yemeni, Somali, and Ethiopian emigrant communities in Europe and America.

The shrub of the moonseed family Celatraceae that is the source of khat was given its scientific name, *C. edulis*, by Peter Forsskål, and later renamed *C. edulis* Forsk, by Carsten Niebuhr, in memory of his friend, Peter Forsskål, who died during the 1761 Arabian Peninsula expedition. They, as other travelers to the Arabian Peninsula, could not help but notice and comment on the widespread habit of the people there to chew on green leaves and twigs that carried different local names: qat and gat in Yemen, qaat or jaad in Somalia, chat and jimma in Ethiopia, and miraa and veve in Kenya. Other popular names still in use are kaht, tchat, qaad, Kus es, Salahin, Tchaad, Tochat, and Tohai. Regular khat users classify the leaves based on type, taste, and potency, and the particular variety of khat used by a person can reflect their social and financial status: for example, white leaves are rarer and more expensive than red leaves; Harai in Ethiopia is considered the best and, in Kenya, Giza is the preferred type.

The distribution of *C. edulis* Forsk stretches from Yemen to Madagascar growing wild at high altitudes, 1500–2000 m above sea level. Production is

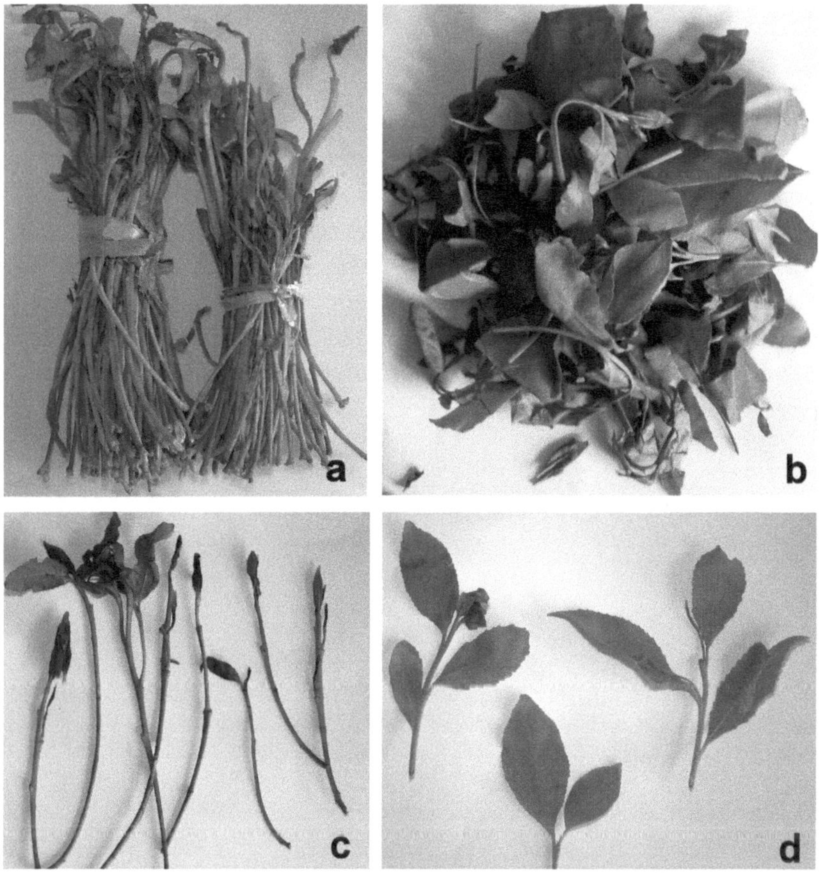

Figure 1 Bundles of khat (A) and the fresh leaves and twigs (B). Three to four bundles or more are consumed during a khat session. Muguka (C and D) another plant becoming popular for its psychostimulatory effect and cheaper than khat.

carried out on a large commercial scale in khat plantations, especially in the Harar province of Ethiopia, Jebel Sabr Mountains of Yemen, and Nyambene area of Meru, County of Kenya. It is also cultivated to a lesser extent in South Africa, Uganda, Tanzania, Zimbabwe, Rwanda, and Indonesia. In many regions, khat cultivation has displaced other commercial crops, such as coffee, and makes a sizeable contribution to both individual income and national economies. In Ethiopia, 85–90% of the khat produced is exported, contributing significantly to the country's foreign exchange earnings (Lemessa, 2001). The harvesting and rapid distribution to local and international markets is organized through cartels, and khat availability is now widely advertised on the Internet. It is hard to obtain figures for the value of the global khat trade, but from khat seizures, it is possible to get a feel for the size of the operation. United Nations Office on Drug and Crime (UNODC, 2013) reported khat to be the most frequent plant-based substance seized. The highest seizures in 2010 were made in Saudi Arabia with 374 metric-tons (mt), followed by the United States with 90 mt and Germany with 30.4 mt with khat seizures also reported by Denmark (2010: 5 mt), Sweden (2010: 14 mt), and the United Republic of Tanzania (2010: 10 mt). Several countries experienced significant increases in seizures of khat between 2009 and 2010 such as Saudi Arabia (182 kg–374 mt), Ireland (50–218 kg), and Norway (3–7 mt). Figure 2 (UNODC, 2008–2012) shows the main sources of khat and its flow to Europe and North America.

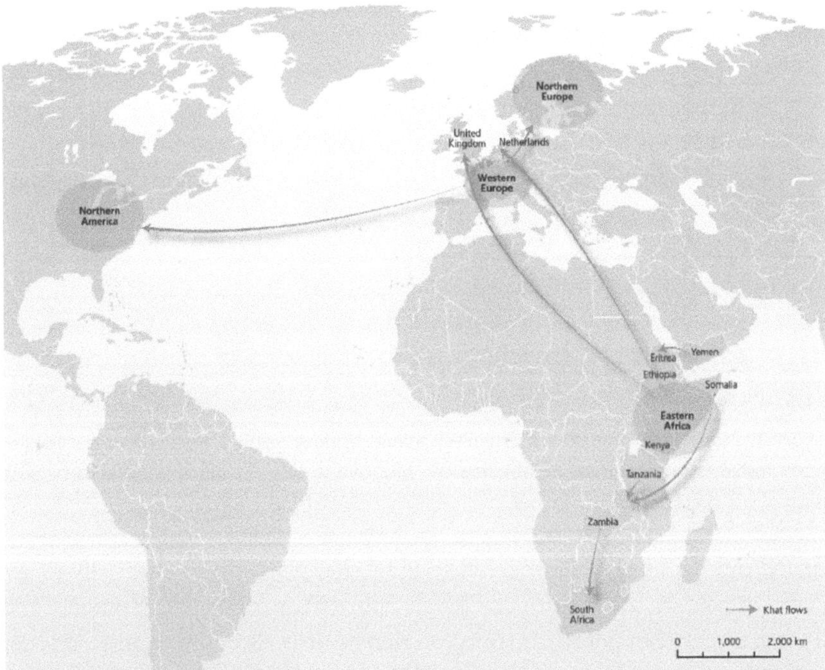

Figure 2 Global trade in khat. Main regions of commercial khat production are Harar province of Ethiopia, Nyambene area of Meru County of Kenya, and Jebel Sabr Mountains of Yemen. *Note*: The origin of the flow arrows does not necessarily indicate the source/manufacture of khat. These arrows represent the flows as perceived by recipient countries. The boundaries shown on this map do not imply official endorsement or acceptance by the United Nations. Dashed lines represent undetermined boundaries. Dotted lines represent approximately the Line of Control in Jammu and Kashmir agreed by India and Pakistan. The final status of Jammu and Kashmir has not yet been agreed upon by the parties. The final boundary between the Sudan and South Sudan has not yet been determined. *UNODC (2008–2012).*

Khat is consumed by chewing the fresh young leaves and bark of twigs which are stored as a bundle in the cheek of the mouth, called a quid. The exudate is swallowed and the residue spit out. Chewing gum is often used to bind the material and sweet drinks taken to reduce the quid's astringent taste. In a typical session, 100–300 g may be consumed over a 3–4-h period. In Scotland, khat was blended, filtered, and served as a drink—"Herbal Ecstasy" (Brown, Jarvie, & Simpson, 1995).

The pattern and amount of khat consumption varies from those who use it as a pick me up in the morning similar to a cup of coffee, to students, shift workers, and long haul lorry drivers who use it more often during the day to ward off sleep and fatigue. Some consumers take large amounts in a single sitting and others partake in binge sessions lasting 24 h or more (Klein & Beckerleg, 2007; Nabuzoka & Badhadhe, 2000; Odenwald et al., 2007a, 2007b; Patel, Wright, & Gammampila, 2005; Widmann et al., 2014). The reasons given for khat use are similar to those for coca leaves use by the Andean people of South America. Khat leads to euphoria, alertness, and improved vigilance. Adverse events with high doses and abrupt withdrawal in chronic users are also well recognized (Table 1).

Table 1 Some Acute and Chronic Effects of Khat Use

Acute Effects	**Chronic Effects**
Euphoria	*Liver toxicity*
Alertness	*Reproductive*
Loquacity	Impaired sexual function
Relief from fatigue	Spermatorrhoea
Insomnia	Low birth weight
Anorexia	*Oral*
Hyperthermia	Periodontal disease
Tachycardia	Mucosal lesions
Hypertension	*Gastrointestinal Tract*
Mydriasis	Gastritis
After effects of acute khat use	Enteritis
Depressive mood	Constipation
Poor sleep quality	*Cardiovascular*
Nightmares	Arrhythmias
Lethargy	Infraction
Irritability	Palpitations
	Central Nervous System
	Psychotic episodes
	Possible cognitive and executive function impairment

Note: Tolerance to the sympathomimetic effects does develop.

Until relatively recently, khat use was hardly known outside Eastern Africa, the Horn of Africa, and the southwestern parts of the Arabian Peninsula where it has been used for centuries and has deep historical roots in the culture and tradition of the people as well as entheogenic connotations. There is a poetic reference to its use in ancient Egypt: "The ancient Egyptians considered *C. edulis* to be a most sacred plant, a "divine food" like royal jelly to bees, capable of releasing humanity's nascent divinity. The Egyptians did not ingest khat merely to "get high", they used it to "trigger and impel the metamorphic process leading to a theurgic transmutation of human nature into apotheosis". Allowing the lowly mortal being to be made God-like." (The Lycaeum, 2015).

Khat came to the attention of law enforcement and regulatory authorities following the increasing enforced emigration of Yemenis, Ethiopians, and Somalis to other parts of the world and, as a result of improved transportation allowing khat to be shifted rapidly after harvest to consumers all over the world. Some of these refugees brought with them the practice of khat chewing, eventually leading to publicity, commentary, and debate both in national newspapers and international journals (Butters, 2009). It was questioned whether the khat use was an innocuous cultural habit and left at that or a more insidious practice that warranted government regulation on its use to protect society. For some countries, the matter was straightforward, the main active ingredient in khat, cathinone, had been shown to be an addictive substance and its natural source should therefore be put under some category of control. For other nations, the question was to distinguish between khat use and the use of cathinone and its derivatives, such as methcathinone, 3,4-methylenedioxypyrovalerone, and mephedrone, which arrived on the "legal high" drug scene around 2007 and are now widely used as "rave drugs" competing with ecstasy, cocaine, and other psychostimulants (Watterson & Olive, 2014).

This use of synthetic cathinones also raised the profile of khat as a potential natural source of cathinone and the question remained, as with coca leaves, whether its consumption is detrimental to mental and physical health as are synthetic cathinones and cocaine.

The sharp rise in use of synthetic cathinones and their adverse effects are covered in the chapters "Home-made methcathinone and permanent neurological damage" by Sikk and Taba and "'Legal highs' – an emerging epidemic of novel psychoactive substances" by Zawilska. This chapter will focus on the use of khat and its effects on brain function and health. How khat use remained for so long low on the global drug of abuse radar, the isolation, and structural elucidation of its main active ingredient, cathinone, and research done to provide evidence that cathinone has addictive potential has been previously discussed by the author in an earlier article (Patel, 2014).

2. THE PREVALENCE OF KHAT USE

The estimate of 20 million people using khat on a daily basis (Al-Motarreb et al., 2002; Magdum, 2011; Saha & Dollery, 2006) is now likely to be an underestimate. In nations where khat use is legal, there are no laws regulating its use as also for alcohol and tobacco. Today, the age to start the use of khat has declined to as young as 12 years (World Health Organization, 2008) and, while previously, khat was used predominantly by men, it is now increasingly used by women (Alem, Kebede, & Kullgren, 1999; Nabuzoka & Badhadhe, 2000; Patel et al., 2005) including pregnant and breastfeeding women (Belew, Kebede, Kassaye, & Enquoselassie, 2000; Eriksson, Ghani, & Kristiansson, 1991; Khawaja, Al-Nsour, & Saad, 2008).

In particular, tribal, ethnic, or community groups, the prevalence of khat use can be extremely high. It is estimated that up to 90% of adult males chew khat 3–4 h daily in Yemen. A recent study for the World Bank also estimated that as many as 73% of women in Yemen chew the khat leaf more or less frequently. A staggering 15–20% of children under the age of 12 are also daily consumers in the same community (Bulletin of the World Health Organization, 2008).

Table 2 summarizes some prevalence data, which shows that where khat use is an acceptable cultural practice, the percentage prevalence is high. As commented in the World Drug Report (UNODC, 2012), a general population survey among people aged 16 and above in Yemen, where khat is not under national control and is being cultivated, showed a lifetime prevalence of 52%, which is the highest lifetime prevalence rate recorded for any psychoactive substance in any country in the world after alcohol, tobacco, and caffeine.

3. PHYTOCHEMISTRY OF *CATHA EDULIS* FORSK

Studies of *C. edulis* Forsk have provided fascinating insight into its remarkable phytochemistry. It contains more than 40 alkaloids, glycosides, tannins, amino acids, vitamins, and minerals (Halbach, 1972), but its stimulant effect derives from two phenylalkylamines—cathinone and cathine—which are structurally related to amphetamine (Nencini, Ahmed, Aminconi, & Elmi, 1984). In 1975, cathinone was isolated and

Table 2 Prevalence of Khat Use

Country/ Region	% Lifetime Use (Male/ Female)[a]	% Regular/ Daily Use (Male/ Female)[a]	Notes	Reference
Yemen	82/43	32/9		Numan (2004)
Yemen	80–85/50–60			Kennedy (1987)
Yemen	73/34			World Bank Report (2007)
Yemen/Sanaa	29.6		Females only	Ali AL-abed, Sutan, Al-Dubai, and Aljunid (2014)
Ethiopia/ Butajiru		75/7–10		Alem et al. (1999)
Ethiopia Rural homes	40/18	5.7		Belew et al. (2000)
Ethiopia	24	12.7		Gebrehanna, Berhane, and Worku (2014)
Ethiopia/ Harar Town	71.5/28.5		15–25 year students	Reda, Moges, Biadgilign, and Wondmagegn (2013)
Ethiopia/ Southwestern	64.9		15–22 year students	Adugna, Jira, and Molla (1994)
Somalia/ North		64	Males	Elmi (1983)
Somalia/South		21	Males	Elmi (1983)
Somalia		31	Males	Odenwald et al. (2005)
Kenya/ Northeastern	68	34		Njuguna, Olieva, Muruka, and Owek (2013)
Kenya/ Northeastern	88			Aden, Dimba, Ndolo, and Chindia (2006)

Table 2 Prevalence of Khat Use—cont'd

Country/ Region	% Lifetime Use (Male/ Female)	% Regular/ Daily Use (Male/ Female)	Notes	Reference
Uganda/ Southwestern	32	20		Ihunwo, Kayanja, and Amadi-Ihunwo (2004)
UK Somali	63/17			Bhui et al. (2003)
UK/London Somali	79/76	6		Griffiths et al. (1997) and Griffiths (1998)
Kingdom of Saudi Arabia/ Jazan Region	33.1/4.3		10–19-year-old students; Khat banned in Saudi Arabia	Alsanosy, Mohamed Salih Mahfouz, and Gaffar (2013)

[a]Single figure represents both genders.

identified by the United Nations' Narcotics Laboratory (UNODC, 1980) and its absolute configuration determined by Schorno and Steinegger (1978). These molecules are substituted phenethylamines many members of which have potent psychostimulant effects (e.g., amphetamine) and bioactive effects (e.g., dopamine (DA) and epinephrine). In addition, khat contains 62 types of cathedulins (Kite, Ismail, Simmonds, & Houghton, 2003) most of which have not yet been studied for their biological effects. The tannin content has been proposed as the cause of the frequently observed constipation. Cathinone is a biosynthetic precursor in the synthesis of cathine (norpseudoephedrine) and norephedrine from L-phenylalanine involving 8–10 biochemical reactions, with the last step catalyzed by the enzyme, cathinone reductase (Hagel et al., 2011; Krizevski, Dudai, Bar, & Lewinsohn, 2007).

Khat has been referred to as a "natural amphetamine" due the presence of cathinone, the main molecule producing its psychostimulatory effects, which is structurally related to and produces similar effects as amphetamine (Kalix, 1996). In young fresh leaves, cathinone can represent nearly 70% of the alkaloid content which declines on its conversion to cathine and norephedrine (Schorno, Brenneisen, & Steinegger, 1982; Schorno & Steinegger, 1979; United Nations, 1978). Furthermore, the cathinone content varies depending on the country of origin (Geisshusler & Brenneisen, 1987). The conversion of cathinone to cathine in a few days after harvesting is one reason given for the traditional geographical restriction of khat use as ancient modes of transport could not deliver fresh khat with a sufficiently high cathinone content to geographical regions far afield. However, assessing cathinone content in seized khat for judicial process, Chappell and Lee (2010) reported that, drying the plant material preserved some cathinone and found khat alkaloids to be relatively stable over 3 years, with some cathinone still detectable in 10-year-old khat samples. The preference for fresh khat usually attributed largely to its higher cathinone content may therefore also stem from the fact that dried khat due to its lack of taste and unpalatability is less agreeable to chew. Khat traditionally was also transported wrapped in banana leaves to keep it moist, which might have allowed, the enzyme, cathinone reductase, to reduce cathinone to the lesser stimulant cathine.

4. THE PHARMACOKINETICS OF KHAT

Once Szendrei (1980) had isolated the alkaloid cathinone, (*S*-(−)-aminopropiophenone), and it could be synthesized, studies of the effect in humans and animals were performed. Brenneisen et al. administered cathinone orally in a gelatin capsule (0.5 mg/kg body weight) to six healthy adult male volunteers to assess its pharmacological effects (Brenneisen, Fisch, Koelbing, Geisshusler, & Kalix, 1990). Plasma cathinone levels peaked in an hour and declined to control levels by 6 h while norephedrine levels reached a peak in an hour and maintained that level over the 8-h study period. This increase in plasma norephedrine was due to the liver metabolism of cathinone to norephedrine. Within 0.5 h after ingestion, the participants reported stimulation/euphoria effects that lasted 7 h. Widler et al. gave as a single dose khat (0.8 mg/kg body weight) and alkaloid-free khat to six drug-naïve volunteers (Widler, Mathys, Brenneisen, Kalix, & Fisch, 1994). Plasma cathinone levels peaked 127 ± 30 min (mean $\pm$ SD) at 127 ± 53 ng/ml. The half-life of cathinone was calculated as 260 ± 102 min.

Halket et al. had five healthy adults (two females, three males) chewing 60 g of khat leaves which had a cathinone content of 0.9 mg/g giving a cathinone dose of around 54 mg per volunteer assuming all the cathinone was extracted and absorbed (Halket, Karasu, & Murray-Lyon, 1995). The range of cathinone absorbed was 0.8–1 mg/kg body weight for the subjects. Peak plasma cathinone levels were reached 1.5–3.5 h with the peak range of 41–141 ng/ml (mean 83 ng/ml). The peak occurred an hour later than seen by Brenneisen et al., reflecting the delay introduced in cathinone absorption by chewing of the khat leaves (Brenneisen et al., 1990; Halket, Karasa, & Murry-Lyon, 1995). The plasma cathinone levels declined over the next

7.5 h and were undetectable 24 h later. No evaluation of the psychological effect of the khat use was reported in this study.

Toennes et al. studied the absorption mechanism by measuring the plasma cathinone and its metabolites cathine and norephedrine in four healthy volunteers (two males, two females) over a period of 54 h following chewing of fresh khat leaves for 1 h (0.6 g/kg body weight; range 36.1–59.2 g). From the analysis of khat residue, the volunteers had ingested (mean $\pm$ SD) 0.63 ± 0.04 mg of cathinone, 0.45 mg cathine, and 0.26 ± 0.01 mg norephedrine per kg body weight. Maximum plasma concentration was reached by 2.3 h for cathinone, 2.6 h cathine, and 2.8 h for norephedrine, and the time profile is shown in Fig. 3 (Toennes et al., 2003). The mean half-life was 1.5 ± 0.8 h for cathinone and 5.2 ± 3.4 h for cathine, respectively. As found by Brenneisen et al. (1990), sympathomimetic effects were observed, in particular, elevation of blood pressure for 3 h following the chewing of khat (Brenneisen et al., 1990). However, no impairment of physical or mental condition was found, though all the participants reported personal feeling of being alert and "energetic." In conclusion, khat absorption involved a two-compartment model with the first compartment being the buccal or oral cavity and the second delayed absorption from the stomach (Toennes et al., 2003).

Measurements of plasma cathinone levels and metabolites in regular khat users are still largely lacking despite the opportunities available to fill this gap in the literature without fear of prosecution in Africa. Toennes et al. (2003) reported in their article drivers suspected of driving under the influence of khat, the following cathine levels: 109, 154, and 229 μg/l from analysis report from the Centre of Legal Medicine, Frankfurt/Main, Germany, which are higher than those measured their volunteers.

5. THE NEUROCHEMISTRY OF KHAT

There are a number of studies showing that cathinone increases DA levels and probably also has similar effects on the catecholamines serotonin and noradrenaline reviewed by Feyissa and Kelly (2008) and Patel (2014). However, for khat itself, there are no *in vitro* studies. Banjaw and Schmidt (2005) after giving khat extract to rats for 9 days to test for behavioral sensitization, found on postmortem analysis of the brain 2 weeks later, only at the highest khat extract dose (200 mg/kg) a decrease in the DA, 3,4-dihydrophenylacetic acid, and homovanilic acid levels in the caudate and putamen.

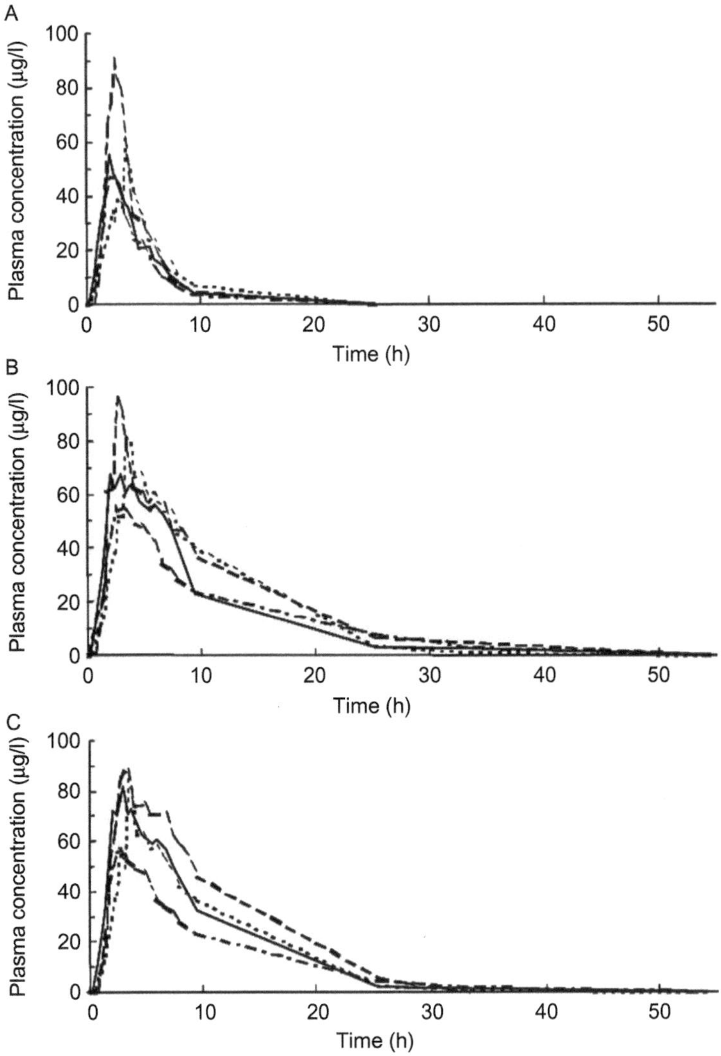

Figure 3 Time profile of plasma cathinone (A), cathine (B), and norephedrine (C) levels in four healthy naïve drugs users following chewing of khat leaves for 1 h (0.6 g/kg body weight) (Toennes, Harder, Schramm, Niess, & Kauert, 2003). *Permission obtained from Blackwell Publishing © 2003 Blackwell Publishing Ltd.*

6. EFFECTS ON NEONATAL DEVELOPMENT

Neonatal exposure to psychostimulants is associated with morphological and functional changes in the CNS producing motor dysfunction, cognitive impairment, altered stress response, and effects on learning and memory. Psychoactive drugs easily cross the blood–brain barrier, and even more easily, the placental barrier (Šlamberová, 2012).

In healthy full-term, single babies, born after uneventful pregnancies and deliveries, the average birth weight was reported significantly lower for mothers who were khat chewers, either habitually or occasionally (Abdul Ghani, Eriksson, Kristiansson, & Qirbi, 1987). A larger study covering 1141 consecutive deliveries in Yemen, occasional and regular khat using mothers had significantly higher number of low-birth-weight babies (less than 2500 g) with no differences in the rate of stillbirth or congenital malformations (Eriksson et al., 1991). As low birth weight is a well-established risk factor for both perinatal and young infant death, khat chewing during pregnancy may contribute adversely to normal child development and increase infant mortality.

To determine if khat has an effect on the placental blood flow, Jansson, Kristiansson, and Qirbi (1988a, 1988b) fed guinea pigs khat leaves and found a reduction in placental blood flow by a quarter 180 min later. There was also a reduction in a birth weight but not litter size or gestational period. The urinary concentrations of (+)-norpseudoephedrine was of a similar magnitude to that reported for women who use khat suggesting that khat chewing during pregnancy may reduce placental blood flow and impair fetal growth. To investigate whether khat use during pregnancy would have a cognitive and behavioral effect on the offspring, Bedada and Engidawork (2010) tested the offspring of mice exposed to khat and found that khat exposed mice had significant motor in-coordination and emotional instability at the highest khat dose used and poor Y-maze performance. In addition, liver and kidney function tests were abnormal, which may have either contributed to the results or had a role in alteration of CNS development or performance. In Wistar rats given khat extract orally, a dose-dependent embryotoxic as well as teratogenic toxicity were found (Islam, al-Shabanah, al-Harbi, & al-Gharably, 1994).

These studies of khat on development are important, as khat chewing during pregnancy has been reported to be highly prevalent in Yemen (40.7% in a 1997 survey) especially among the socio-economically disadvantaged women (Khawaja et al., 2008). Furthermore, anemia and restrictive dietary habit among khat users are also high, which could also have detrimental effects on fetal development (Kedir, Berhane, & Worku, 2013).

7. EFFECT ON COGNITIVE AND EXECUTIVE FUNCTION IN HUMANS AFTER KHAT EXPOSURE

Studies on the cognitive effects of khat use in humans are limited. In a Federal Aviation Authority (FAA) medical examination, regular (daily) khat-chewing flight attendants and occasional (recreational) khat users scored significantly lower in memory function test compared to non-khat-chewing staff, and the results correlated significantly negatively with both the duration and quantity of khat abuse in both khat-chewing groups. The EEG analysis revealed a statistically significant shift toward fast frequency bands in regular users but this did not significantly correlate with, or influence, any of the tested memory functions (Khattab & Amer, 1995). Colzato et al. compared khat users (average use for 10.5 ± 6.5 years, 3.1 ± 1.8 times a week, consuming 3.0 ± 1.2 bundles) to non-khat users from Leiden and The Hague, Netherlands, and found that while users and non-users were comparable in terms of response execution, users needed significantly more time to inhibit responses to stop signals than non-users, reflecting impaired inhibitory control (Colzato, Ruiz, van den Wildenberg, Bajo, & Hommel, 2011). For this study, the khat users were requested to refrain from khat use or alcohol 24 h preceding the test day and thus it is possible that the difference in results between khat users and non-users could be due to the withdrawal effect of previous chronic khat consumption, although the study provided some indication that chronic khat use could lead to impairment of cognitive function. In a similar set of subjects, working memory performance and cognitive flexibility were significantly worse in chronic khat users assessed using the N-back task and Global–local task (Colzato, Ruiz, van den Wildenberg, & Hommel, 2011). Hoffman and al'Absi (2013) confirmed these negative effects on cognitive function in chronic khat users using the forward and backward digit span test for working memory, and Digit Symbol Substitution Test for speed of information processing.

As khat has amphetamine-like effects, the question of its emotional regulation was investigated, using a mental arithmetic task by Bongarda, al'Absib, Khalil, and Al Haboric (2011), who found that regular khat chewers scored higher on trait anger than occasional or non-khat chewers. The participants were not asked to abstain from khat use and it was assumed that the participants' last khat session was a day or so earlier. In a more controlled study, Colzato, Ruiz, van den Wildenberg, and Hommel (2012) found khat users who had abstained for 24 h performed significantly slower and were more strongly affected by stimulus-induced response conflict on the Simon task then non-khat users. When the same task was done by subjects allowed to chew khat during the task (Colzato, Sellaro, Ruiz, Sikora, & Hommel, 2013), chronic users were better than controls in resolving stimulus-induced response. These results indicate that short- and long-term abstinence in chronic khat users could be confounding variables. However, the study does provide support for increase in concentration or alertness reported by khat users. Irritability, irascibility, and disrupted sleep can occur in khat users after the effects of khat had worn off.

Khat parties can number up to 20 participants or so and during traditional or ceremonial occasions, the number can be much larger, yet there are no reports of frequent unpleasant verbal or physical altercations during these séances.

8. KHAT USE AND PSYCHOSIS

There are many case reports of reversible khat-induced psychosis similar to those reported with amphetamine (Carothers, 1945; Critchlow & Seifert, 1987; Dhadphale, Mengech, & Chege, 1981; Giannini & Castellani, 1982; Gough & Cookson, 1984; Pantelis, Hindler, & Taylor, 1989). In a comprehensive study of the relationship between khat and psychosis involving 8723 personnel of armed groups in Somalia, a positive relationship between khat use, posttraumatic stress disorder (PTSD) and paranoia was found, with those suffering from PTSD using more khat in an attempt to forget or dull their war-time memories (Odenwald et al., 2009). However, the results of the study did not help to elucidate whether people already predisposed or susceptible to psychosis, were at greater risk of mental illness after khat exposure (Odenwald, 2014).

9. DEPENDENCE

That long-term khat use can result in deterioration of general health is well known but it remains uncertain whether it can lead to true addiction and physical dependence. Psychological evaluation using the Addiction Research Center Inventory (ARCI) and visual analogue scale by Widler et al. found in drug–naïve volunteers given khat to chew, a significant effect in the abuse potential, motor stimulation, amphetamine-like effects, and stimulation euphoria categories as well as in excitation–calm and energetic–lethargic category (Widler et al., 1994). After the appropriate validation of the Severity of Dependence Scale (Gossop et al., 1995) for assessing psychological dependence in khat users, a significant correlation was found between khat-chewing dependency and the levels of cathinone, norephedrine, and norpseudoephedrine measured in the saliva in 30 UK-resident Somali khat users (Kassim, Hawash, Johnston, & Croucher, 2012; Kassim, Islam, & Croucher, 2010). Using the same instrument, male khat chewers showed more khat dependence symptoms compared to females and a significant positive correlation between age and khat dependence in women only (Nakajima et al., 2014).

Using the substance dependence syndrome (DSM-IV, 1994), a third of the 204 khat chewers interviewed reported symptoms consistent with dependence syndrome and 38% reported continued khat chewing despite of an impact on their health, while 17% reported withdrawal symptoms (depression, increase in appetite, and sleep pattern disruption) (Kassim, Croucher, & al'Absi, 2013). A recent study, using also the DSM-IV instrument, found among khat using subjects tolerance (66.7%), withdrawal (94.0%), more used than intended (72.7%), wish to reduce or stop (78.8%), reduced social life (97.0%), and continued consumption despite health problems (93.9%) (Widmann et al., 2014). The subjects of this study were Somali refugees living in Nairobi, Kenya, thus the results may not be applicable to all khat users but are suggestive that khat use can lead to dependence, which in time may progress to addiction. However, in comparison with 19 other legal and illegal drugs of abuse, including cocaine, alcohol, amphetamines, tobacco, and ecstasy, khat is ranked as the lowest in dependency risk (Nutt, King, Saulsbury, & Blakemore, 2007).

10. CULTURAL TRADITION OR DRUG OF ABUSE?

Information on the mechanisms of action of khat and its short- and long-term effects is not as detailed as that for other amphetamine type stimulants. The tools for assessing dependence and addiction to address the impact of khat use have been used only recently. But, as with other drugs of abuse, those who have susceptibility to drugs of abuse could develop addiction to khat. There are no long-term follow up studies of khat users but the following questions have addressed by Widmann et al.: (1) attempts to stop using of khat that has not been in successful despite knowing the negative effect on health, job, and family; (2) number of abusers who stopped using of khat but then relapsed; and (3) use of khat in inappropriate situations (Widmann et al., 2014).

Khat use raises a challenging issue: can daily exposures of psychostimulant to the brain tissue starting at a young age lead to changes that will have subsequently negative effects on mental function? The amount and rate of khat consumption is self-regulated by the method of consumption of low doses over hours. There is no data on the plasma cathinone or cathine levels achieved during a regular or extended khat sessions. Thus, simulating the effect of khat doses in animals similarly to those used by humans by monitoring plasma cathinone levels is not possible, and it may be khat extract dosing causing toxic khat effects maybe cited in published work on animals.

While the question "is khat a drug of abuse?" remains to be clearly answered, given the currently available reports on its adverse effect on the individual, family, and society, it might be advisable to have some regulatory control of its use such as is in place for alcohol and tobacco use. To paraphrase Nutt (2011), banning a substance does not prevent the harm the drug causes and may even lead to a widening of its sphere of damage.

ACKNOWLEDGMENT

The author thanks Diana Patel and Brian Maiyo for valuable comments on this chapter.

REFERENCES

Abdul Ghani, N., Eriksson, M., Kristiansson, B., & Qirbi, A. (1987). The influence of khat-chewing on birth-weight in full-term infants. *Social Science and Medicine, 24*, 625–627.

Aden, A., Dimba, E. A., Ndolo, U. M., & Chindia, M. L. (2006). Socio-economic effects of khat chewing in northeastern Kenya. *East African Medical Journal, 83*, 69–73.

Adugna, F., Jira, C., & Molla, T. (1994). Khat chewing among Agaro secondary school students, Agaro, southwestern Ethiopia. *Ethiopian Medical Journal, 32*, 161–166.

Advisory Council on the Misuse of Drugs (ACMD). (2013). *Khat: A review of its potential harms to the individual and communities in the UK.*

Alem, A., Kebede, D., & Kullgren, G. (1999). The prevalence and socio-demographic correlates of khat chewing in Butajira, Ethiopia. *Acta Psychiatrica Scandinavica. Supplementum, 100*, 84–91.

Ali AL-abed, AL-abed, Sutan, R., Al-Dubai, S. A. R., & Aljunid, S. M. (2014). Family context and khat chewing among adult Yemeni women: A cross-sectional study. *BioMed Research International, 2014*, 505474. http://dx.doi.org/10.1155/2014/505474.

Al-Motarreb, A., Al-Kebsi, M., Al-Adhi, B., & Broadley, K. J. (2002). Khat chewing and acute myocardial infarction. *Heart, 87*, 279–280.

Alsanosy, R. M., Mohamed Salih Mahfouz, M. S., & Gaffar, A. M. (2013). Khat chewing habit among school students of Jazan region, Saudi Arabia. *PLoS one, 8*(6), e65504.

Banjaw, M. Y., & Schmidt, W. J. (2005). Behavioral sensitization following repeated intermittent oral administration of *Catha edulis* in rats. *Behavioral Brain Research, 156*, 181–189.

Bedada, W., & Engidawork, E. (2010). The neuropsychopharmacological effects of Catha edulis in mice offspring born to mothers exposed during pregnancy and lactation. *Phytotherapy Research*, *24*, 268–276.

Belew, M., Kebede, D., Kassaye, M., & Enquoselassie, F. (2000). The magnitude of khat use and its association with health, nutrition and socio-economic status. *Ethiopian Medical Journal*, *38*, 11–26.

Bhui, K., Abdi, A., Abdi, M., Pereira, S., Dualeh, M., Robertson, D., et al. (2003). Traumatic events, migration characteristics and psychiatric symptoms among Somali refugees—Preliminary communication. *Social Psychiatry and Psychiatric Epidemiology*, *38*, 35–43.

Bongarda, S., al'Absib, M., Khalil, N. S., & Al Haboric, M, M. (2011). Khat use and trait anger: Effects on affect regulation during an acute stressful challenge. *European Addiction Research*, 7, 285–291.

Brenneisen, R., Fisch, H. U., Koelbing, U., Geisshusler, S., & Kalix, P. (1990). Amphetamine-like effects in humans of the khat alkaloid cathinone. *British Journal of Clinical Pharmacology*, *30*, 825–828.

Brown, E. R., Jarvie, D. R., & Simpson, D. (1995). Use of drugs at 'raves'. *Scottish Medical Journal*, *40*, 168–171.

Butters, A. L. (2009). Is Yemen chewing itself to death? *Time*, (25th August 2009). http://content.time.com/time/world/article/0,8599,1917685,00.html.

Carothers, J. (1945). Miraa as a cause of insanity. *East African Medical Journal*, *22*, 4–6.

Chappell, J. S., & Lee, M. M. (2010). Cathinone preservation in khat evidence via drying. *Forensic Science International*, *195*, 108–120.

Colzato, L. S., Ruiz, M. J., van den Wildenberg, W. P., & Hommel, B. (2011). Khat use is associated with impaired working memory and cognitive flexibility. *PLoS One*, *6*, e20602.

Colzato, L. S., Ruiz, M. J., van den Wildenberg, W. P., & Hommel, B. (2012). Khat use is associated with increased response conflict in humans. *Human Psychopharmacology*, *27*, 315–321.

Colzato, L. S., Ruiz, M. J., van den Wildenberg, W. P., Bajo, M. T., & Hommel, B. (2011). Long-term effects of chronic khat use: Impaired inhibitory control. *Frontiers in Psychology*, *1*, 219. http://dx.doi.org/10.3389/fpsyg.2010.00219.

Colzato, L. S., Sellaro, R., Ruiz, M. J., Sikora, K., & Hommel, B. (2013). Acute khat use reduces response conflict in habitual users. *Frontiers in Human Neuroscience*, 7, 285, 19.

Critchlow, S., & Seifert, R. (1987). Khat-induced paranoid psychosis. *British Journal of Psychiatry*, *150*, 247–249.

Dhadphale, M., Mengech, A., & Chege, S. (1981). Miraa (Catha edulis) as a cause of psychosis. *East African Medical Journal*, *58*, 130–135.

Elmi, A. S. (1983). The chewing of khat in Somalia. *Journal of Ethnopharmacology*, *8*, 163–176.

Eriksson, M., Ghani, N. A., & Kristiansson, B. (1991). Khat-chewing during pregnancy effect upon the off-spring and some characteristics of the chewers. *East African Medical Journal*, *68*, 106–111.

Feyissa, A. M., & Kelly, J. P. (2008). A review of the neuropharmacological properties of khat. *Progress in Neuro-Psychopharmacology & Biological Psychiatry*, *32*, 1147–1166.

Gebrehanna, E., Berhane, Y., & Worku, A. (2014). Khat chewing among Ethiopian University Students—A growing concern. *BioMed Central Public Health*, *14*, 1198.

Geisshusler, S., & Brenneisen, R. (1987). The content of psychoactive phenylpropyl and phenylpentenyl khatamines in *Catha edulis* Forsk of different origin. *Journal of Ethnopharmacology*, *19*, 269–277.

Giannini, A., & Castellani, S. (1982). A manic-like psychosis due to khat (Catha edulis Forsk). *Journal of Toxicology. Clinical Toxicology*, *19*, 455–459.

Gossop, M., Darke, S., Griffiths, P., Hando, J., Powis, B., Hall, W., et al. (1995). The Severity of Dependence Scale (SDS): Psychometric properties of the SDS in English and Australian samples of heroin, cocaine and amphetamine users. *Addiction, 90*, 607–614.
Gough, S., & Cookson, I. (1984). Khat-induced schizophreniform psychosis in UK. *Lancet, 1*, 455, i.
Griffiths, P. (1998). *Qat use in London: A study of khat use among a sample of Somalis living in London*. London: Stationery Office (Home Office Paper 26).
Griffiths, P., Gossop, M., Wickenden, S., Dunworth, J., Harris, K., & Lloyd, C. A. (1997). Transcultural pattern of drug use: Qat (khat) in the UK. *British Journal of Psychiatry, 170*, 281–284.
Hagel, J. M., Krizevski, R., Kilpatrick, K., Sitrit, Y., Marsolais, F., Lewinsohn, E., et al. (2011). Expressed sequence tag analysis of khat (Catha edulis) provides a putative molecular biochemical basis for the biosynthesis of phenylpropylamino alkaloids. *Genetics and Molecular Biology, 34*, 640–646.
Halbach, H. (1972). Medical aspects of the chewing of khat leaves. *Bulletin of the World Health Organization, 47*, 21–29.
Halket, J. M., Karasu, Z., & Murray-Lyon, I. M. (1995). Plasma cathinone levels following chewing of khat leaves (*Catha edulis* Forsk). *Journal of Ethnopharmacology, 49*, 111–113.
Hoffman, R., & al'Absi, M. (2013). Working memory and speed of information processing in chronic khat users: Preliminary findings. *European Addiction Research, 19*, 1–6.
Ihunwo, A. O., Kayanja, F. I., & Amadi-Ihunwo, U. B. (2004). Use and perception of the psychostimulant, khat (*Catha edulis*) among three occupational groups in south western Uganda. *East African Medical Journal, 81*, 468–473.
Islam, M. W., al-Shabanah, O. A., al-Harbi, M. M., & al-Gharably, N. M. (1994). Evaluation of teratogenic potential of khat (*Catha edulis* Forsk.) in rats. *Drug and Chemical Toxicology, 17*, 51–68.
Jansson, T., Kristiansson, B., & Qirbi, A. (1988a). Effect of khat on maternal food intake, maternal weight gain and fetal growth in the late-pregnant guinea pig. *Journal of Ethnopharmacology, 23*, 11–17.
Jansson, T., Kristiansson, B., & Qirbi, A. (1988b). Effect of khat on uteroplacental blood flow in awake, chronically catheterized, late-pregnant guinea pigs. *Journal of Ethnopharmacology, 23*, 19–26.
Kalix, P. (1996). *Catha edulis*, a plant that has amphetamine effects. *Pharmacy World and Science, 18*, 69–73.
Kassim, S., Croucher, R., & al'Absi, M. (2013). Khat dependence syndrome: A cross sectional preliminary evaluation amongst UK-resident Yemeni khat chewers. *Journal of Ethnopharmacology, 146*, 835–841.
Kassim, S., Hawash, A., Johnston, A., & Croucher, R. (2012). Validation of self-reported khat chewing amongst khat chewers: An exploratory study. *Journal of Ethnopharmacology, 140*, 193–196.
Kassim, S., Islam, S., & Croucher, R. (2010). Validity and reliability of a Severity of Dependence Scale for khat (SDS-khat). *Journal of Ethnopharmacology, 132*, 570–577.
Kedir, H., Berhane, Y., & Worku, A. (2013). Khat chewing and restrictive dietary behaviors are associated with anemia among pregnant women in high prevalence rural communities in eastern Ethiopia. *PLoS One, 8*, e78601.
Kennedy, J. G. (1987). *The flower of paradise. The institutionalized use of the drug (Qat) in North Yemen*. Dordrecht: D. Reidel.
Khattab, N. Y., & Amer, G. (1995). Undetected neuropsychophysiological sequelae of khat chewing in standard aviation medical examination. *Aviation, Space and Environmental Medicine, 66*, 739–744.

Khawaja, M., Al-Nsour, M., & Saad, G. (2008). Khat (*Catha edulis*) chewing during pregnancy in Yemen: Findings from a national population survey. *Maternal and Child Health Journal, 12*, 308–312.
Kite, G. C., Ismail, M., Simmonds, M. S., & Houghton, P. J. (2003). Use of doubly protonated molecules in the analysis of cathedulins in crude extracts of khat (Catha edulis) by liquid chromatography/serial mass spectrometry. *Rapid Communications in Mass Spectrometry, 17*, 1553–1564.
Klein, A., & Beckerleg, S. (2007). Building castles of spit—The role of khat chewing in worship, work and leisure. In J. Goodman, P. Lovejoy, & A. Sherrat (Eds.), *Consuming habits: Global and historical perspective on how cultures define drug use*. London: Routledge.
Krizevski, R., Dudai, N., Bar, E., & Lewinsohn, E. (2007). Developmental patterns of phenylpropylamino alkaloids accumulation in khat (Catha edulis, Forsk.). *Journal of Ethnopharmacology, 114*, 432–438.
Lemessa, D. (2001). *Khat (Catha edulis): Botany, distribution, cultivation, usage and economics in Ethiopia* (p. 10). Addis Ababa: UN Emergencies Unit for Ethiopia.
Magdum, S. S. (2011). An overview of khat. *Addictive Disorders and Their Treatments, 10*, 72–83.
Nabuzoka, D., & Badhadhe, F. A. (2000). Use and perception of khat among young Somalis in a UK city. *Addiction Research, 8*, 5–26.
Nakajima, M., Dokam, A., Alsameai, A., AlSoofi, M., Khalil, N., & al'Absi, M. (2014). Severity of khat dependence among adult khat chewers: The moderating influence of gender and age. *Journal of Ethnopharmacology, 155*, 1467–1472.
Nencini, P., Ahmed, A. M., Aminconi, G., & Elmi, A. S. (1984). Tolerance develops to sympathetic effects of khat in humans. *Pharmacology, 28*, 150–154.
Njuguna, J., Olieva, S., Muruka, C., & Owek, C. (2013). Khat consumption in Masalani town, northeastern Kenya. *Journal of Psychoactive Drugs, 45*(4), 355–359.
Numan, N. (2004). Exploration of adverse psychological symptoms in Yemeni khat users by the Symptoms Checklist-90 (SCL-90). *Addiction, 199*, 61–65.
Nutt, D. (2011). Perverse effects of the precautionary principle: How banning mephedrone has unexpected implication for pharmaceutical discovery. *Therapeutic Advances in Psychopharmacology, 1*, 35–36.
Nutt, D., King, L. A., Saulsbury, W., & Blakemore, C. (2007). Development of rational scale to assess the harm of drugs of potential misuse. *The Lancet, 369*, 1047–1053.
Odenwald, M. (2014). Mental health problems associated with the use and abuse of khat (Catha edulis). In M. Bentivoglio, E. A. Cavalheiro, K. Kristensson, & N. Patel (Eds.), *Neglected tropical diseases and conditions of the nervous system* (pp. 293–305). New York: Springer.
Odenwald, M., Hinkel, H., Schauer, E., Neuner, F., Schauer, M., Elbert, T. R., et al. (2007). The consumption of khat and other drugs in Somali combatants: A cross-sectional study. *PLoS One, 4*, e341.
Odenwald, M., Hinkel, H., Schauer, E., Schauer, M., Elbert, T., Neuner, F., et al. (2009). Use of khat and posttraumatic stress disorder as risk factors for psychoti Dudai N c symptoms: A study of Somali combatants. *Social Science and Medicine, 69*, 1040–1048.
Odenwald, M., Lingenfelder, B., Schauer, M., Neuner, F., Rockstroh, B., Hinkel, H., et al. (2007). Screening for posttraumatic stress disorder among Somali ex-combatants: A validation study. *Conflict and Health, 1*, 10.
Odenwald, M., Neuner, F., Schauer, M., Elbert, T., Catani, C., & Lingenfelder, B. (2005). Khat use as risk factor for psychotic disorders: A cross- sectional and case–control study in Somalia. *BioMed Central Medicine, 3*, 5, 12.
Pantelis, C., Hindler, C., & Taylor, J. (1989). Use and abuse of khat (Catha edulis): A review of the distribution, pharmacology, side effects and a description of psychosis attributed to khat chewing. *Psychological Medicine, 19*, 657–668.

Patel, N. B. (2014). Neurobiology of khat (Catha edulis Forsk). In M. Bentivoglio, E. A. Cavalheiro, K. Kristensson, & N. Patel (Eds.), *Neglected tropical diseases and conditions of the nervous system* (pp. 307–319). New York: Springer.

Patel, S. L., Wright, S., & Gammampila, A. (2005). *Khat use among Somalis in four English cities: Home Office Online Report 47/05*. London: Home Office.

Reda, A. A., Moges, A., Biadgilign, S., & Wondmagegn, B. Y. (2013). Prevalence and determinants of khat (Catha edulis) chewing among high school students in Eastern Ethiopia: A cross-sectional study. *PLoS One*, 7(3), e33946.

Saha, S., & Dollery, C. (2006). Severe ischaemic cardiomyopathy associated with khat chewing. *Journal of the Royal Society of Medicine*, *99*, 316–318.

Schorno, X., Brenneisen, R., & Steinegger, E. (1982). Qualitative und quantitative Untersuchungen uber das Vorkommen ZNS-aktiver Phenylpropylamine in Handelsdrogen und uber deren Verteilung in verschiedenen Organen von Catha edulis. *Pharmaceutica Acta Helvetiae*, *57*, 168–176.

Schorno, X., & Steinegger, E. (1978). *The phyenylalkylamines of Catha edulis forsk: The absolute configuration of cathinone*, United Nations Document MNAR/7/1978.

Schorno, X., & Steinegger, E. (1979). CNS-active phenylpropylamines of Catha edulis of Kenyan origin. *Experientia (Basel)*, *35*, 572–574.

Šlamberová, R. (2012). Drugs in pregnancy: The effects on mother and her progeny. *Physiological Research*, *61*(Suppl. 1), S123–S135.

Szendrei, K. (1980). The chemistry of khat. *UNODC Bulletin on Narcotics*, *32*(3), 5–35.

The Lycaeum. (2015). http://www.lycaeum.org/leda/Documents/Catha_Edulis%253A_Sacred_Plant_of_the_Ancient_Egyptians.8645.shtml.

Toennes, S. W., Harder, S., Schramm, M., Niess, C., & Kauert, G. F. (2003). Pharmacokinetics of cathinone, cathine and norephedrine after chewing khat leaves. *British Journal of Clinical Pharmacology*, *56*, 125–130.

United Nations Document. (1978). *Etudes sur la composition chimique du khat; la configuration absolue de la cathinone*, MNAR/7/1978.

United Nations Office on Drug and Crime. (2013). *The challenge of new psychoactive substances: A report from the Global SMART Program*.

United Nations Office on Drugs and Crime. (UNODC). (2008–2012). *Khat use in Europe: Implications for European policy: Annual Report Questionnaire 2008–2012*, Drugs in focus of the European Monitoring Centre for Drugs and Drug Addiction (EMCDDA), Luxembourg, 2011.

United Nations Office on Drugs and Crime (UNODC). (2012). World Drug Report.

United Nations Office on Drugs and Crime (UNDOC). (1980). Bulletin Narcotics (3).

Watterson, L. R., & Olive, M. F. (2014). Synthetic cathinones and their rewarding and reinforcing effects in rodents. *Advances in Neuroscience (Hindawi)*, *2014*, 209875.

Widler, P., Mathys, K., Brenneisen, R., Kalix, P., & Fisch, H. U. (1994). Pharmacodynamics and pharmacokinetics of khat: A controlled study. *Clinical Pharmacology and Therapeutics*, *55*, 556–562.

Widmann, M., Warsame, A. H., Mikulica, J., von Beust, J., Isse, M. M., Ndetei, D., et al. (2014). Khat use, PTSD and psychotic symptoms among Somali refugees in Nairobi—A pilot study. *Frontiers in Public Health*, *2*, 71, 30.

World Bank Report. (2007). *Yemen-towards qat demand reduction: Report No., pp: 39738-YE.* New York: United Nations Office on Drugs and Crime (UNODC).

World Health Organization. (2008). *Bulletin of the World Health Organization*, *86*(10), 737.

CHAPTER TWELVE

Methcathinone "Kitchen Chemistry" and Permanent Neurological Damage

Katrin Sikk*, Pille Taba†,1
*Department of Neurology, North-Estonian Regional Hospital, Tallinn, Estonia
†Department of Neurology and Neurosurgery, University of Tartu, Tartu, Estonia
[1]Corresponding author: e-mail address: pille.taba@kliinikum.ee

Contents

Abstract

Methcathinone abuse is a significant cause of parkinsonism among young patients in the Eastern European countries. The drug is synthesized from over-the-counter cold remedies containing ephedrine or pseudoephedrine. The final mixture contains a high concentration of manganese if potassium permanganate is used as the oxidant agent. Though manganese is an essential trace element and its homeostasis is well maintained, exposure to a high level of manganese is neurotoxic. The use of manganese-contaminated methcathinone may cause permanent neurological damage and severe disability. Drug users develop a distinctive extrapyramidal syndrome that resembles classic manganese intoxication. Methcathinone could have additive neurotoxic effect to the progression of parkinsonism. The most prevalent symptoms are symmetrical

International Review of Neurobiology, Volume 120
ISSN 0074-7742
http://dx.doi.org/10.1016/bs.irn.2015.02.002

bradykinesia, dystonias, and early postural, gait, and speech impairment. After cessation of exposure, the syndrome is generally irreversible and can even progress.

1. INTRODUCTION

Methcathinone (ephedrone) is a synthetic cathinone with an amphetamine-like chemical structure and pharmacological properties. Cathinone, a naturally occurring phenylalkylamine found in the leaves of the khat bush (*Catha edulis*), can be considered the prototype from which a range of synthetic cathinones have been developed. Typically, synthetic cathinones have an amphetamine-type analogue, i.e., cathinone, methcathinone, and methylone are structurally related to amphetamine, methamphetamine, and 3,4-methylenedioxy-methamphetamine, respectively (Kelly, 2011).

Methcathinone was first synthesized by the Germans and the French in the late 1920s as an intermediate in the synthesis of ephedrine. It was originally used in the Soviet Union during the 1930s and 1940s as an antidepressant and went on to be used recreationally (especially during the 1970s and 1980s). Methcathinone is known in Russia as ephedrone and is also called by the street names "jeff" or "mulka" (Glennon, Young, Martin, & Dal Cason, 1995).

In the 1950s, the US pharmaceutical company Parke-Davis considered marketing methcathinone as an appetite suppressant and an antidepressant, and in 1957 a US patent was granted on the production process. Due to the adverse reactions, the drug never went into human testing. In 1989, a student from the University of Michigan, who was interning at Parke-Davis, found documentation of the manufacturing process and started to synthesize and sell the product. It was sold as "cat," probably named after the shrub khat (Bailey, 1995). Soon its use spread from Michigan to the rest of the States (Emerson & Cisek, 1993). In 1992, the Drug Enforcement Administration placed methcathinone into Schedule I of the United Nations Controlled Substance Act.

Neurologic and psychopathologic disturbances in methcathinone abusers were described in Russian literature almost 30 years ago (Lukacher, Vrublevskii, Laskova, Rokhlina, & Marsakova, 1987). This topic has gained international attention in 2007, when several cases of parkinsonian syndrome in methcathinone users from Estonia (Sikk et al., 2007), Canada (de Bie, Gladstone, Strafella, Ko, & Lang, 2007), Ukraine

(Sanotsky et al., 2007), and Turkey (Meral, Kutukcu, Atmaca, Ozer, & Hamamcioglu, 2007) were reported.

2. SYNTHESIS OF METHCATHINONE

Ephedrine or pseudoephedrine available in over-the-counter drugs is commonly used to synthesize methcathinone. Ephedrine can be oxidized to methcathinone and reduced to methamphetamine, but the reductive route is much more complicated. In Russia and the Eastern Europe, potassium permanganate is used as the oxidant agent, followed by almost no refinement, while in the United States dichromates are mainly used followed by several cleanup steps.

2.1 Oxidation with Potassium Permanganate

According to the information gained from the patients in Estonia, the following recipe is regularly used in the preparation of methcathinone: a package (12 tablets) of the nasal decongestant Sudafed, containing 60 mg pseudoephedrine hydrochloride, 1–2 mL 30% acetic acid, and "a point of the knife" of potassium permanganate are poured into 60–100 mL of boiling water. The mixture is left to cool down for about 10 min, filtered through a cotton pad, and injected intravenously several times per day. Methcathinone yield in the reaction was approximately 44% and manganese concentration was 595 ppm (0.6 g/L) (Sikk et al., 2007).

2.2 Oxidation with Sodium Dichromate

A chilled solution of sodium dichromate in dilute sulfuric acid is added in a dropwise manner over 45 min to dilute sulfuric acid solutions of ephedrine. The reaction mixtures are washed with cold chloroform made basic with a saturated sodium carbonate solution, extracted (four times) with chloroform, and dried with anhydrous sodium sulfate. The hydrochloride salt is formed by addition of a solution of hydrogen chloride in isopropanol diluted 10-fold with diethyl ether. Additional diethyl ether is added to produce turbidity, with subsequent precipitation of the hydrochloride salts. Methcathinone is collected by filtration and allowed to air dry. Methcathinone hydrochloride salt is a white crystalline powder, usually snorted, less commonly smoked, or taken orally mixed in drinks (Glennon et al., 1995).

3. EFFECTS OF METHCATHINONE INTOXICATION

Similar to amphetamines, methcathinone can increase the release of dopamine and noradrenaline (Gygi, Fleckenstein, Gibb, & Hanson, 1997; Rothman et al., 2003).

Methcathinone abuse produces enhanced energy, feelings of toughness and invincibility, and increased sexual desire. Unwanted effects are tachycardia, sweating, fever, anxiety, insomnia, muscle twitching, headaches, and abdominal cramps. Paranoid psychosis may develop after chronic use (Emerson & Cisek, 1993).

Parkinsonian syndrome has been described only in methcathinone users preparing the drug with potassium permanganate.

4. ROLE OF MANGANESE IN METHCATHINONE INTOXICATION

Using potassium permanganate as an oxidant in methcathinone synthesis, the final mixture contains high residual manganese. Compared to recommended daily manganese supplementation in long-term total parenteral nutrition, methcathinone users are exposed to approximately 2000 times higher loads (Sikk et al., 2007).

Manganese is an essential trace metal. It is necessary for a multitude of functions, including skeletal system development, energy metabolism, activation of certain enzymes, nervous system function, and reproductive hormone function, and is an antioxidant that protects cells from damage due to free radicals (Santamaria & Sulsky, 2010). Under normal dietary consumption, systemic homeostasis of manganese is maintained via tight homeostatic control of both gastrointestinal absorption and biliary excretion. Exposure to high oral, parenteral, or ambient air concentrations of manganese can result in elevations in tissue manganese levels (Aschner & Aschner, 2005).

Chronic manganese poisoning was first reported by James Couper in 1837 in five men who worked in a manganese ore-crushing plant in France (Couper, 1837). Manganese neurotoxicity was subsequently reported in miners (Cotzias, Horiuchi, Fuenzalida, & Mena, 1968; Mena, Marin, Fuenzalida, & Cotzias, 1967; Rodier, 1955), smelters (Huang et al., 1989), welders (Tanaka & Lieben, 1969), and workers involved in the manufacture of dry-cell batteries (Emara, El-Ghawabi, Madkour, & El-Samra, 1971). Manganese toxicity has been described in patients receiving long-term parental nutrition (Ejima et al., 1992), drinking contaminated water (Kondakis, Makris, Leotsinidis, Prinou, & Papapetropoulos, 1989), and following potassium permanganate ingestion (Holzgraefe, Poser, Kijewski, & Beuche, 1986). Manganism also may be associated with chronic liver disease (Spahr et al., 1996), due to markedly impaired excretion of manganese, with subsequent accumulation in the brain. Recently, inherited syndrome of hepatic cirrhosis, dystonia, polycythemia, and hypermanganesemia in cases without environmental manganese exposure has been reported (Tuschl et al., 2008) with an autosomal recessive mutation in *SLC30A10* gene (Tuschl et al., 2012).

Manganism is characterized by symmetric bradykinesia, rigidity, postural instability, gait disturbance, difficulties in walking backward, micrographia, masked face, hypophonia, and dysphonia. Dystonia is a common and early feature and usually presents as facial grimacing, hand dystonia, and/or a peculiar "cock gait." Tremor is less common and tends to be action or postural. In early stages of manganese intoxication, psychiatric symptoms including irritability, mania, uncontrollable laughter, compulsive or aggressive behavior, hallucinations, and cognitive disorder have been described (Cersosimo & Koller, 2006; Guilarte, 2010). Serial follow-up studies of previous chronic manganese intoxication patients were conducted in a small group of Taiwanese ferromanganese smelters. Their parkinsonian symptoms showed a rapid progression during the initial 10 years, followed by a plateau during the following 10 years (Huang, Chu, Lu, Chen, & Calne, 1998; Huang et al., 2007, 1993).

Levodopa therapy in patients with manganese-induced parkinsonism is ineffective (Lu, Huang, Chu, & Calne, 1994). Chelating treatment with ethylenediaminetetraacetic acid (EDTA) reduced blood manganese levels in acutely poisoned patients and had therapeutic benefit if patients were removed from exposure at early stages of the disease (Herrero Hernandez et al., 2006).

A limited number of autopsy studies have been performed on patients with chronic manganese intoxication. They demonstrate a consistent pattern characterized by neuronal loss and reactive gliosis in the globus pallidus (particularly the internal segment) and substantia nigra pars reticulata with sparing of the substantia nigra pars compacta and an absence of Lewy bodies (Perl & Olanow, 2007; Yamada et al., 1986).

Brain magnetic resonance imaging (MRI) in manganese-exposed subjects shows symmetrical signal intensity increase in the basal ganglia, especially in the globus pallidus on T1-weighted images (Nelson et al., 1993).

5. PREVALENCE OF PARKINSONISM IN METHCATHINONE ABUSERS

There is little epidemiological data regarding methcathinone use. In Estonia, 11% of intravenous drug users reported methcathinone use in their history: 1.3% were current users, and in 0.9% it was the main drug of abuse (Lõhmus et al., 2008). Methcathinone abuse is a common cause of parkinsonism among Estonian patients younger than 40 years of age. Methcathinone-induced parkinsonism has been reported mainly in the Eastern European countries, including Estonia, Latvia, Georgia, Poland, Ukraine, Russia, and Turkey, and a few immigrant cases have been described in Canada, Italy, and Ireland (Sikk, Haldre, Aquilonius, & Taba, 2011).

6. CLINICAL SYMPTOMATOLOGY

Methcathinone abusers are young adults, on average 30 years old (Selikhova et al., 2008; Sikk et al., 2010; Stepens et al., 2008). The first neurological symptoms usually appear a few years after the beginning of injections, but can occur after only a few months (Sanotsky et al., 2007) or up to 17 years later (Stepens et al., 2008). The main presenting features reported by subjects were gait and speech impairment and loss of balance (Sikk et al., 2010).

The most common neurological findings were postural instability, gait and speech disturbance, symmetric bradykinesia, and dystonias. Most often, dystonia was seen in feet, presenting as a cock-like gait. Some patients had dystonic smile, dystonic hand postures, or severe generalized dystonia (Sikk et al., 2010). A quantitative analysis of 15 speech dimensions in 28 patients with history of methcathinone abuse revealed a distinct variant of mixed hyperkinetic–hypokinetic dysarthria that was related to dystonia and bradykinesia (Rusz et al., 2014). Less frequently described symptoms included limb and axial rigidity, gait freezing, postural and resting tremor, micrographia, apraxia of eyelid opening, pathological laughter, palilalia, and primitive reflexes. Although hyperactive deep tendon reflexes were commonly found, pathological reflexes were mentioned only in one case

(Colosimo & Guidi, 2009). A few cases had oromandibular dyskinesia, blepharospasm (Varlibas et al., 2009), myoclonus (Levin, 2005), or restriction of vertical saccadic eye movements (de Bie et al., 2007). Video-oculography in 28 patients showed slow and hypometric horizontal saccades, long latencies of vertical antisaccades, increased occurrence of square wave jerks, and a high error rate in antisaccade task (Bonnet et al., 2014).

Neuropsychological testing showed mild executive cognitive impairment, including bradyphrenia, attenuated attention, reduced working capacity, and decreased phonetic verbal fluency (Colosimo & Guidi, 2009; Levin, 2005; Selikhova et al., 2008; Yildirim et al., 2009). Compared to healthy controls, increased reflection impulsivity has been demonstrated in methcathinone users (Djamshidian et al., 2012). Differences in calculation and verbal and nonverbal memory have been also noted and the cognitive dysfunction did not recover in repeated testing 2 years later (Koksal et al., 2014).

The outcome of the neurological deficit after the cessation of methcathinone abuse is individual. Mild to moderate improvements have been observed in some cases (Levin, 2005; Sanotsky et al., 2007), but in several cases progression after withdrawal has been described (Colosimo & Guidi, 2009; Selikhova et al., 2008; Yildirim et al., 2009).

No improvement was noted in former methcathinone users in two large follow-up studies, and some assessment scales indicated statistically significant worsening (Sikk et al., 2010; Stepens et al., 2014). These findings indicate the possibility that methcathinone–manganese exposure may trigger a chronic neurodegenerative process.

There is a lack of neuropathological studies in methcathinone users. Stereotactic brain biopsy from the globus pallidus in a former user contained only white matter tissue, with abnormalities of mitochondria in the axons of neurons and oligodendrocytes and astrocytes in electron microscopy. Myelin sheaths were focally decompacted, demonstrating widely varying thickness. Osmiophilic bodies were observed adjacent to the myelin sheath in oligodendroglia (Stepens et al., 2014).

7. NEUROIMAGING AND BIOMARKERS OF EXPOSURE

7.1 Magnetic Resonance Imaging

MRI in the brain in active methcathinone users shows symmetrical hyperintensities on T1-weighted images in the globus pallidus and substantia nigra pars reticulata (Fig. 1). Less frequently involved structures are the

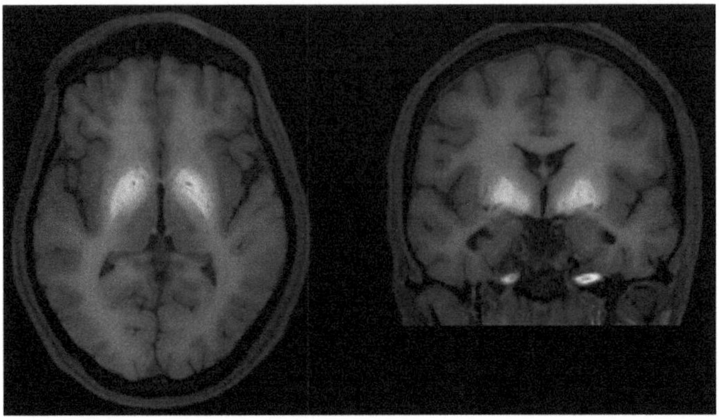

Figure 1 Brain MRI T1-weighted axial and coronal image of an active methcathinone user. Increased signal in the globus pallidus.

subthalamic nucleus, substantia innominata, putamen, caudate, anterior midbrain, pontine tegmentum, dentate nucleus, pituitary gland, and white matter (Poniatowska et al., 2014; Selikhova et al., 2008; Sikk et al., 2010). Widespread white matter abnormalities in methcathinone users are demonstrated with diffusion tensor imaging (Stepens et al., 2010). Despite the neurological damage, normal MRI findings have been described in patients who have stopped methcathinone abuse 0.5–2 years before (Iqbal, Monaghan, & Redmond, 2012; Yildirim et al., 2009). However, in some cases, a visible MRI signal change has been demonstrated up to 5 years after the cessation of methcathinone use (Selikhova et al., 2008; Stepens et al., 2008).

T1 relaxation time measurements show shortened T1 relaxation in some of the former users with normal conventional MRI signals. Measuring of T1 relaxation time could be more sensitive for detecting low manganese level in the brain and former exposure (Sikk et al., 2010).

High MRI signal intensities on T1-weighted images reflect recent exposure to manganese, but normal findings do not exclude former exposure. High signal intensities several years after cessation of exposure should awake a suspicion of active abuse, unless other susceptibility factors like chronic liver disease are present.

7.2 Transcranial Sonography

Transcranial sonography in a patient with methcathinone-induced parkinsonism revealed hyperechogenicity in the lenticular nucleus and substantia nigra. In follow-up imaging 6 months later, hyperechogenicity in sonography was still present in the lenticular nucleus, but MRI hyperintensity in the globus pallidus was lower. Transcranial sonography could be at least as sensitive as MRI in detecting manganese accumulation in brain in methcathinone users (Skowronska, Dziezyc, & Czlonkowska, 2013).

7.3 Imaging of the Pre- and Postsynaptic Dopaminergic System

Lasting reduction of dopamine transporter (DAT) density has been shown in abstinent methcathinone and methamphetamine abusers without overt neurological or psychiatric illness by means of positron emission tomography (PET) (McCann et al., 1998). However, later studies in former methamphetamine abusers revealed significant recovery of DAT levels with protracted abstinence, suggesting that the changes were adaptive rather than neurotoxic (Volkow et al., 2001b).

DAT single-photon emission computed tomography (SPECT) studies in manganese-contaminated methcathinone users have been normal, indicating that the presynaptic neurons in the nigrostriatal pathway are intact in methcathinone abusers after prolonged abstinence (Colosimo & Guidi, 2009; Selikhova et al., 2008; Sikk et al., 2010). Instead, there could be an impairment of dopamine release as shown in studies with nonhuman primates chronically exposed to manganese (Guilarte et al., 2008, 2006). This theory might explain why patients reported a progressively weaker psychostimulatory effect of methcathinone, acting as a dopamine releaser. Occupationally exposed workers with manganese-induced parkinsonism and patients with chronic liver disease also had normal DAT levels in the striatum, whereas there is asymmetric loss of DAT in Parkinson's disease (Kim et al., 2007).

Untreated Parkinson's disease patients have normal or elevated levels of D2 receptors in the striatum (Brooks et al., 1992). In atypical parkinsonian syndromes, D2 receptor bindings are usually decreased (Koch, Hamann, Radau, & Tatsch, 2007; Vlaar et al., 2008). Iodobenzamide SPECT in methcathinone users showed normal symmetric tracer uptake in the striatum, indicating preserved striatal dopamine D2 receptors (Sikk et al., 2010).

7.4 Imaging of Brain Metabolism

In typical idiopathic Parkinson's disease, glucose metabolism in the putamen and globus pallidus is preserved or raised, whereas it is reduced in most atypical parkinsonian cases (Brooks, 2010). Detoxified methamphetamine abusers had a higher metabolism in the parietal cortex and lower metabolism in the striatum and thalamus (Volkow et al., 2001a). With protracted abstinence, there was significant recovery of the thalamic, but no improvement in striatal, metabolism (Wang et al., 2004). A single study in humans with mild manganism showed decrease of cortical metabolism (Wolters et al., 1989). PET study in former manganese-contaminated methcathinone users showed a widespread nonuniform pathological subcortical affection of FDG uptake (Sikk et al., 2010). These changes could be induced by manganese toxicity or by long-term methcathinone abuse.

7.5 Manganese Concentration

There is limited information about the pharmacokinetics of methcathinone. The half-life of cathinone after the chewing of khat leaves was only 1.5 h (Toennes, Harder, Schramm, Niess, & Kauert, 2003). Methcathinone was present in urine only in 8.3% of subjects, while an elevated level of manganese in urine was detected in 29.2% of abusers (Golasik, Wodowski, Gomolka, Herman, & Piekoszewski, 2014). Manganese is rapidly eliminated from plasma (Sikk et al., 2010) and urine (Golasik et al., 2014). Hair level remains higher for a longer period. In a Ukrainian study, patients who had been off methcathinone for over 2.5 years had some elevation in pubic hair manganese levels (Selikhova et al., 2008). There is a large variability in mean levels of hair manganese. At an individual level, manganese concentrations are not reliable biomarkers of exposure due to fast elimination from plasma and urine and large variability in hair.

8. TREATMENT

Levodopa therapy up to the maximum tolerated doses showed no improvement (Poniatowska et al., 2014; Selikhova et al., 2008). Dopamine agonists were ineffective as well (Colosimo & Guidi, 2009; de Bie et al., 2007). Some patients reported a subjective short-term improvement with amantadine (Selikhova et al., 2008). In an open crossover trial of biperiden and trihexyphenidyl, there was some decrease in dystonia and increase in quality of life (Levin & Datieva, 2013).

Chelating treatment with EDTA reduced blood manganese levels but had no effect on clinical symptoms (Stepens et al., 2008; Varlibas et al., 2009) or led to a mild improvement probably related to abstinence (Sanotsky et al., 2007; Selikhova et al., 2008). *para*-Aminosalicylic acid, another medication with chelating properties, did not change clinical findings (Varlibas et al., 2009).

Generally, the syndrome is unresponsive to levodopa, the mainstay treatment for Parkinson's disease, and to other antiparkinsonian medications. Treatment with chelating agents has not proven to be effective and is often not suitable, because former users with parkinsonian syndrome have normal manganese levels in tissues, and many active subjects continue methcathinone use despite undergoing substance abuse counseling. Caution should be taken in treating HIV-positive subjects with levodopa, because dopamine-enhancing drugs could induce viral replication in the central nervous system (Gaskill et al., 2009).

9. CONCLUSIONS

Methcathinone is a rather widespread recreational drug because it is relatively cheap and easy to prepare. Manganese-contaminated methcathinone users develop a distinctive extrapyramidal syndrome that is similar to classical manganism. Methcathinone addiction is an alarming new cause of toxic parkinsonism. The prognosis of the parkinsonian syndrome in methcathinone users is poor as there is no curative therapy. Biomarkers of exposure are characteristic only of recent abuse. The diagnosis in former users is based on the clinical picture and history of methcathinone abuse.

REFERENCES

Aschner, J. L., & Aschner, M. (2005). Nutritional aspects of manganese homeostasis. *Molecular Aspects of Medicine*, *26*(4–5), 353–362.

Bailey, W. J. (1995). Indiana Prevention Resource Center.

Bonnet, C., Rusz, J., Megrelishvili, M., Sieger, T., Matouskova, O., Okujava, M., et al. (2014). Eye movements in ephedrone-induced parkinsonism. *PLoS One*, *9*(8), e104784.

Brooks, D. J. (2010). Imaging approaches to Parkinson disease. *Journal of Nuclear Medicine*, *51*(4), 596–609.

Brooks, D. J., Ibanez, V., Sawle, G. V., Playford, E. D., Quinn, N., Mathias, C. J., et al. (1992). Striatal D2 receptor status in patients with Parkinson's disease, striatonigral degeneration, and progressive supranuclear palsy, measured with 11C-raclopride and positron emission tomography. *Annals of Neurology*, *31*(2), 184–192.

Cersosimo, M. G., & Koller, W. C. (2006). The diagnosis of manganese-induced parkinsonism. *Neurotoxicology*, *27*(3), 340–346.

Colosimo, C., & Guidi, M. (2009). Parkinsonism due to ephedrone neurotoxicity: A case report. *European Journal of Neurology*, *16*(6), e114–e115.

Cotzias, G. C., Horiuchi, K., Fuenzalida, S., & Mena, I. (1968). Chronic manganese poisoning. Clearance of tissue manganese concentrations with persistance of the neurological picture. *Neurology*, *18*(4), 376–382.

Couper, J. (1837). On the effects of black oxide of manganese when inhaled into the lungs. *British Annals of Medicine Pharmacy*, *1*, 41–42.

de Bie, R. M., Gladstone, R. M., Strafella, A. P., Ko, J. H., & Lang, A. E. (2007). Manganese-induced parkinsonism associated with methcathinone (ephedrone) abuse. *Archives of Neurology*, *64*(6), 886–889.

Djamshidian, A., Sanotsky, Y., Matviyenko, Y., O'Sullivan, S. S., Sharman, S., Selikhova, M., et al. (2012). Increased reflection impulsivity in patients with ephedrone-induced parkinsonism. *Addiction*, *108*(4), 771–779.

Ejima, A., Imamura, T., Nakamura, S., Saito, H., Matsumoto, K., & Momono, S. (1992). Manganese intoxication during total parenteral nutrition. *Lancet*, *339*(8790), 426.

Emara, A. M., El-Ghawabi, S. H., Madkour, O. I., & El-Samra, G. H. (1971). Chronic manganese poisoning in the dry battery industry. *British Journal of Industrial Medicine*, *28*(1), 78–82.

Emerson, T. S., & Cisek, J. E. (1993). Methcathinone: A Russian designer amphetamine infiltrates the rural midwest. *Annals of Emergency Medicine*, *22*(12), 1897–1903.

Gaskill, P. J., Calderon, T. M., Luers, A. J., Eugenin, E. A., Javitch, J. A., & Berman, J. W. (2009). Human immunodeficiency virus (HIV) infection of human macrophages is increased by dopamine: A bridge between HIV-associated neurologic disorders and drug abuse. *The American Journal of Pathology*, *175*(3), 1148–1159.

Glennon, R. A., Young, R., Martin, B. R., & Dal Cason, T. A. (1995). Methcathinone ("cat"): An enantiomeric potency comparison. *Pharmacology, Biochemistry, and Behavior*, *50*(4), 601–606.

Golasik, M., Wodowski, G., Gomolka, E., Herman, M., & Piekoszewski, W. (2014). Urine as a material for evaluation of exposure to manganese in methcathinone users. *Journal of Trace Elements in Medicine and Biology*, *28*(3), 338–343.

Guilarte, T. R. (2010). Manganese and Parkinson's disease: A critical review and new findings. *Environmental Health Perspectives*, *118*(8), 1071–1080.

Guilarte, T. R., Burton, N. C., McGlothan, J. L., Verina, T., Zhou, Y., Alexander, M., et al. (2008). Impairment of nigrostriatal dopamine neurotransmission by manganese is mediated by pre-synaptic mechanism(s): Implications to manganese-induced parkinsonism. *Journal of Neurochemistry*, *107*(5), 1236–1247.

Guilarte, T. R., Chen, M. K., McGlothan, J. L., Verina, T., Wong, D. F., Zhou, Y., et al. (2006). Nigrostriatal dopamine system dysfunction and subtle motor deficits in manganese-exposed non-human primates. *Experimental Neurology*, *202*(2), 381–390.

Gygi, M. P., Fleckenstein, A. E., Gibb, J. W., & Hanson, G. R. (1997). Role of endogenous dopamine in the neurochemical deficits induced by methcathinone. *Journal of Pharmacology and Experimental Therapeutics*, *283*(3), 1350–1355.

Herrero Hernandez, E., Discalzi, G., Valentini, C., Venturi, F., Chiò, A., Carmellino, C., et al. (2006). Follow-up of patients affected by manganese-induced parkinsonism after treatment with CaNa2EDTA. *Neurotoxicology*, *27*, 333–339.

Holzgraefe, M., Poser, W., Kijewski, H., & Beuche, W. (1986). Chronic enteral poisoning caused by potassium permanganate: A case report. *Journal of Toxicology Clinical Toxicology*, *24*(3), 235–244.

Huang, C. C., Chu, N. S., Lu, C. S., Chen, R. S., & Calne, D. B. (1998). Long-term progression in chronic manganism: Ten years of follow-up. *Neurology*, *50*(3), 698–700.

Huang, C. C., Chu, N. S., Lu, C. S., Chen, R. S., Schulzer, M., & Calne, D. B. (2007). The natural history of neurological manganism over 18 years. *Parkinsonism & Related Disorders*, *13*(3), 143–145.

Huang, C. C., Chu, N. S., Lu, C. S., Wang, J. D., Tsai, J. L., Tzeng, J. L., et al. (1989). Chronic manganese intoxication. *Archives of Neurology*, *46*(10), 1104–1106.

Huang, C. C., Lu, C. S., Chu, N. S., Hochberg, F., Lilienfeld, D., Olanow, W., et al. (1993). Progression after chronic manganese exposure. *Neurology*, *43*(8), 1479–1483.

Iqbal, M., Monaghan, T., & Redmond, J. (2012). Manganese toxicity with ephedrone abuse manifesting as parkinsonism: A case report. *Journal of Medical Case Reports*, *6*(1), 52.

Kelly, J. P. (2011). Cathinone derivatives: A review of their chemistry, pharmacology and toxicology. *Drug Testing and Analysis*, *3*(7–8), 439–453.
Kim, C. H., Cheon, K. A., Koo, M. S., Ryu, Y. H., Lee, J. D., Chang, J. W., et al. (2007). Dopamine transporter density in the basal ganglia in obsessive-compulsive disorder, measured with [123I]IPT SPECT before and after treatment with serotonin reuptake inhibitors. *Neuropsychobiology*, *55*(3–4), 156–162.
Koch, W., Hamann, C., Radau, P. E., & Tatsch, K. (2007). Does combined imaging of the pre- and postsynaptic dopaminergic system increase the diagnostic accuracy in the differential diagnosis of parkinsonism? *European Journal of Nuclear Medicine and Molecular Imaging*, *34*(8), 1265–1273.
Koksal, A., Keskinkilic, C., Sozmen, M. V., Dirican, A. C., Aysal, F., Altunkaynak, Y., et al. (2014). Evaluation of cognitive characteristics of patients developing manifestations of parkinsonism secondary to long-term ephedrone use. *European Neurology*, *71*(3–4), 208–212.
Kondakis, X. G., Makris, N., Leotsinidis, M., Prinou, M., & Papapetropoulos, T. (1989). Possible health effects of high manganese concentration in drinking water. *Archives of Environmental Health*, *44*(3), 175–178.
Levin, O. S. (2005). "Ephedron" encephalopathy. *Zhurnal Nevrologii i Psikhiatrii Imeni S.S. Korsakova*, *105*(7), 12–20.
Levin, O. S., & Datieva, V. K. (2013). The use of biperiden (akineton) in patients with ephedrone encephalopathy. *Zhurnal Nevrologii i Psikhiatrii Imeni S.S. Korsakova*, *113*(8), 33–37.
Lõhmus, L., Rüütel, K., Abel-Ollo, K., Loit, H.-M., Talu, A., & Uusküla, A. (2008). *HIV-nakkuse ning teiste infektsioonide ja riskikäitumise levimus süstivate narkomaanide seas Tallinnas ja Kohtla-Järvel*. Tervise Arengu Instituut, Tartu Ülikooli Tervishoiu Instituut.
Lu, C. S., Huang, C. C., Chu, N. S., & Calne, D. B. (1994). Levodopa failure in chronic manganism. *Neurology*, *44*(9), 1600–1602.
Lukacher, G., Vrublevskii, A. G., Laskova, N. B., Rokhlina, M. L., & Marsakova, G. D. (1987). Ephedrine addiction. *Zhurnal Nevropatologii i Psikhiatrii Imeni S.S. Korsakova*, *87*(5), 751–757.
McCann, U. D., Wong, D. F., Yokoi, F., Villemagne, V., Dannals, R. F., & Ricaurte, G. A. (1998). Reduced striatal dopamine transporter density in abstinent methamphetamine and methcathinone users: Evidence from positron emission tomography studies with [11C]WIN-35,428. *Journal of Neuroscience*, *18*(20), 8417–8422.
Mena, I., Marin, O., Fuenzalida, S., & Cotzias, G. C. (1967). Chronic manganese poisoning. Clinical picture and manganese turnover. *Neurology*, *17*(2), 128–136.
Meral, H., Kutukcu, Y., Atmaca, B., Ozer, F., & Hamamcioglu, K. (2007). Parkinsonism caused by chronic usage of intravenous potassium permanganate. *The Neurologist*, *13*(2), 92–94.
Nelson, R. C., Chezmar, J. L., Thompson, G. H., Webber, J. B., Garrison, M. H., Spencer, H. B., et al. (1993). Magnetic resonance imaging after arterial portography with manganese dipyridoxal diphosphate. *Investigative Radiology*, *28*(4), 335–340.
Perl, D. P., & Olanow, C. W. (2007). The neuropathology of manganese-induced parkinsonism. *Journal of Neuropathology and Experimental Neurology*, *66*(8), 675–682.
Poniatowska, R., Lusawa, M., Skierczynska, A., Makowicz, G., Habrat, B., & Sienkiewicz-Jarosz, H. (2014). MRI brain findings in ephedrone encephalopathy associated with manganese abuse: Single-center perspective. *Polish Journal of Radiology*, *79*, 150–155.
Rodier, J. (1955). Manganese poisoning in Moroccan miners. *British Journal of Industrial Medicine*, *12*(1), 21–35.
Rothman, R. B., Vu, N., Partilla, J. S., Roth, B. L., Hufeisen, S. J., Compton-Toth, B. A., et al. (2003). In vitro characterization of ephedrine-related stereoisomers at biogenic amine transporters and the receptorome reveals selective actions as norepinephrine transporter substrates. *Journal of Pharmacology and Experimental Therapeutics*, *307*(1), 138–145.

Rusz, J., Megrelishvili, M., Bonnet, C., Okujava, M., Brozova, H., Khatiashvili, I., et al. (2014). A distinct variant of mixed dysarthria reflects parkinsonism and dystonia due to ephedrone abuse. *Journal of Neural Transmission, 121*(6), 655–664.

Sanotsky, Y., Lesyk, R., Fedoryshyn, L., Komnatska, I., Matviyenko, Y., & Fahn, S. (2007). Manganic encephalopathy due to "ephedrone" abuse. *Movement Disorders, 22*(9), 1337–1343.

Santamaria, A. B., & Sulsky, S. I. (2010). Risk assessment of an essential element: Manganese. *Journal of Toxicology and Environmental Health. Part A, 73*(2), 128–155.

Selikhova, M., Fedoryshyn, L., Matviyenko, Y., Komnatska, I., Kyrylchuk, M., Krolicki, L., et al. (2008). Parkinsonism and dystonia caused by the illicit use of ephedrone—A longitudinal study. *Movement Disorders, 23*(15), 2224–2231.

Sikk, K., Haldre, S., Aquilonius, S. M., & Taba, P. (2011). Manganese-induced parkinsonism due to ephedrone abuse. *Parkinson's Disease, 17*, 865319.

Sikk, K., Taba, P., Haldre, S., Bergquist, J., Nyholm, D., Askmark, H., et al. (2010). Clinical, neuroimaging and neurophysiological features in addicts with manganese-ephedrone exposure. *Acta Neurologica Scandinavica, 121*(4), 237–243.

Sikk, K., Taba, P., Haldre, S., Bergquist, J., Nyholm, D., Zjablov, G., et al. (2007). Irreversible motor impairment in young addicts—Ephedrone, manganism or both? *Acta Neurologica Scandinavica, 115*(6), 385–389.

Skowronska, M., Dziezyc, K., & Czlonkowska, A. (2013). Transcranial sonography in manganese-induced parkinsonism caused by drug abuse. *Clinical Neuroradiology, 24*(4), 385–387.

Spahr, L., Butterworth, R. F., Fontaine, S., Bui, L., Therrien, G., Milette, P. C., et al. (1996). Increased blood manganese in cirrhotic patients: Relationship to pallidal magnetic resonance signal hyperintensity and neurological symptoms. *Hepatology, 24*(5), 1116–1120.

Stepens, A., Groma, V., Skuja, S., Platkajis, A., Aldins, P., Eksteina, I., et al. (2014). The outcome of the movement disorder in methcathinone abusers: Clinical, MRI and manganesemia changes, and neuropathology. *European Journal of Neurology, 21*(2), 199–205.

Stepens, A., Logina, I., Liguts, V., Aldins, P., Eksteina, I., Platkajis, A., et al. (2008). A parkinsonian syndrome in methcathinone users and the role of manganese. *The New England Journal of Medicine, 358*(10), 1009–1017.

Stepens, A., Stagg, C. J., Platkajis, A., Boudrias, M. H., Johansen-Berg, H., & Donaghy, M. (2010). White matter abnormalities in methcathinone abusers with an extrapyramidal syndrome. *Brain, 133*(Pt. 12), 3676–3684.

Tanaka, S., & Lieben, J. (1969). Manganese poisoning and exposure in Pennsylvania. *Archives of Environmental Health, 19*(5), 674–684.

Toennes, S. W., Harder, S., Schramm, M., Niess, C., & Kauert, G. F. (2003). Pharmacokinetics of cathinone, cathine and norephedrine after the chewing of khat leaves. *British Journal of Clinical Pharmacology, 56*(1), 125–130.

Tuschl, K., Clayton, P. T., Gospe, S. M., Jr., Gulab, S., Ibrahim, S., Singhi, P., et al. (2012). Syndrome of hepatic cirrhosis, dystonia, polycythemia, and hypermanganesemia caused by mutations in SLC30A10, a manganese transporter in man. *The American Journal of Human Genetics, 90*(3), 457–466.

Tuschl, K., Mills, P. B., Parsons, H., Malone, M., Fowler, D., Bitner-Glindzicz, M., et al. (2008). Hepatic cirrhosis, dystonia, polycythaemia and hypermanganesaemia—A new metabolic disorder. *Journal of Inherited Metabolic Disease, 31*(2), 151–163.

Varlibas, F., Delipoyraz, I., Yuksel, G., Filiz, G., Tireli, H., & Gecim, N. O. (2009). Neurotoxicity following chronic intravenous use of "Russian cocktail" *Clinical Toxicology (Philadelphia, Pa.), 47*(2), 157–160.

Vlaar, A. M., de Nijs, T., Kessels, A. G., Vreeling, F. W., Winogrodzka, A., Mess, W. H., et al. (2008). Diagnostic value of 123I-ioflupane and 123I-iodobenzamide SPECT scans in 248 patients with parkinsonian syndromes. *European Neurology, 59*(5), 258–266.

Volkow, N. D., Chang, L., Wang, G. J., Fowler, J. S., Franceschi, D., Sedler, M., et al. (2001a). Loss of dopamine transporters in methamphetamine abusers recovers with protracted abstinence. *Journal of Neuroscience*, *21*(23), 9414–9418.

Volkow, N. D., Chang, L., Wang, G. J., Fowler, J. S., Franceschi, D., Sedler, M. J., et al. (2001b). Higher cortical and lower subcortical metabolism in detoxified methamphetamine abusers. *The American Journal of Psychiatry*, *158*(3), 383–389.

Wang, G. J., Volkow, N. D., Chang, L., Miller, E., Sedler, M., Hitzemann, R., et al. (2004). Partial recovery of brain metabolism in methamphetamine abusers after protracted abstinence. *The American Journal of Psychiatry*, *161*(2), 242–248.

Wolters, E. C., Huang, C. C., Clark, C., Peppard, R. F., Okada, J., Chu, N. S., et al. (1989). Positron emission tomography in manganese intoxication. *Annals of Neurology*, *26*(5), 647–651.

Yamada, M., Ohno, S., Okayasu, I., Okeda, R., Hatakeyama, S., Watanabe, H., et al. (1986). Chronic manganese poisoning: A neuropathological study with determination of manganese distribution in the brain. *Acta Neuropathologica*, *70*(3–4), 273–278.

Yildirim, E. A., Essizoglu, A., Koksal, A., Dogu, B., Baybas, S., & Gokalp, P. (2009). Chronic manganese intoxication due to methcathinone (ephedron) abuse: A case report. *Türk Psikiyatri Dergisi*, *20*(3), 294–298.

CHAPTER THIRTEEN

"Legal Highs" – An Emerging Epidemic of Novel Psychoactive Substances

Jolanta B. Zawilska*,†,1
*Department of Pharmacodynamics, Medical University of Lodz, Lodz, Poland
†Institute of Medical Biology, Polish Academy of Sciences, Lodz, Poland
1Corresponding author: e-mail address: jolanta.zawilska@umed.lodz.pl

Contents

Abstract

During the last decade, there has been an increase in the availability and use of novel psychoactive substances (NPS), also known as "legal highs," across the world. They include a wide range of products, from natural plant-originated substances to synthetic compounds, that can be purchased both online and from high street retailers. "Legal highs" mimic psychoactive effects of illicit drugs of abuse. However, they are claimed to consist of compounds that are legal to sell, possess, and use, often labeled as "not for human consumption" to circumvent drug abuse legislation. Based on the spectrum of their actions on cognitive processes, mood, and behavior, "legal highs" can be classified into four basis categories: amphetamine- and ecstasy-like stimulants, synthetic cannabinoids (SCs), hallucinogenic/dissociative, and opioid-like compounds. NPS may, however, exhibit a combination of these actions due to their designed chemical structure. Although the prevalence and pattern of NPS use differ between various countries, the most popular groups are SCs and psychostimulants, described in this chapter. Currently, there is limited information available on the potential acute toxicity (harms) associated with the use of these substances. However, the number of intoxicated

International Review of Neurobiology, Volume 120
ISSN 0074-7742
http://dx.doi.org/10.1016/bs.irn.2015.02.009

people presenting with emergencies is constantly increasing, providing evidence that negative health and social consequences may indeed seriously affect recreational and chronic users.

1. INTRODUCTION

Recently, a new class of psychoactive substances, known as "legal highs," "herbal highs," "designer drugs," or "party pills," has emerged on the drug use market. They are frequently advertised as "plant fertilizers/food," "air fresheners," "herbal incenses," "spice," "bath salts," "research chemicals." "Legal highs" include a wide range of products from natural, plant-originated substances to semisynthetic and synthetic compounds (EMCDDA, 2013; Gibbons, 2012; Johnson, Johnson, & Portier, 2013; Papaseit, Farré, Schifano, & Torrens, 2014; Winstock & Barratt, 2013; Zawilska, 2011). The European Union (EU) warning system operated by the European Monitoring Centre for Drugs and Drug Addition (EMCDDA) notified the appearance of 236 new psychoactive substances during the period of May 2005–December 2012 (EMCDDA, 2013), and 81 in 2013 (EMCDDA, 2014a; Fig. 1). The EU drug market report emphasizes that "... while the appearance of new drugs is not a new phenomenon, over the last few years there has been an unprecedented growth in their number, type, and availability" (EMCDDA, 2013). Specialists alarmed that

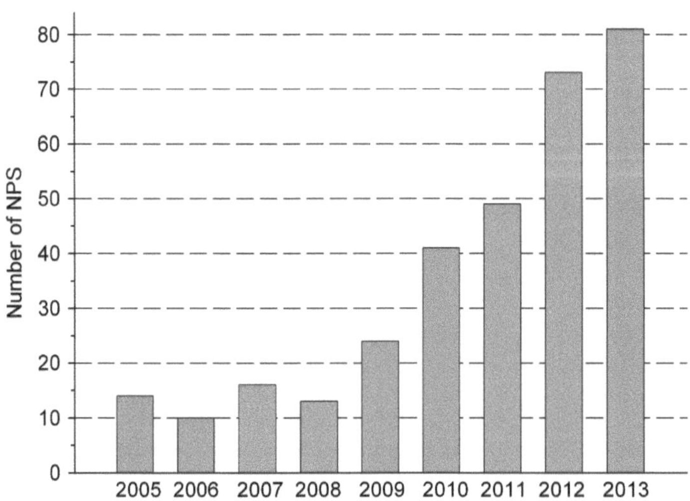

Figure 1 Number of novel psychoactive compounds notified for the first time to the European Early Warning System since May 2005. *Data by EMCDDA (2013, 2014a).*

"... the term "legal highs," besides being inaccurate from a scientific point of view, carries the risk of advertisement because of its emphasis on positive, enjoyable effects that are available without any legal consequences ..." (Corazza, Demetrovics, van den Brink, & Schifano, 2013). Hence, the term novel psychoactive substances (NPS), defined as "new narcotic or psychotropic drugs, in pure form or in preparation, that are not controlled by the 1961 United Nations Single Convention on Narcotic Drugs or the 1971 United Nations Convention on Psychotropic Substance, but which may pose a public health threat comparable to that posed by substances listed in these conventions," has been introduced by the EMCDDA (EMCDDA, 2012) and is now widely used (UNODC, 2013). NPS have been reported in a number of countries. A recent World Drug Report revealed in a worldwide survey of 80 countries that 70 of them had reported the emergence of NPS in recent years (UNODC, 2013). It has been estimated that 2.9 million people aged 15–24 (around 5% of the total) in the EU have already tried NPS (Corazza et al., 2014).

NPS products can be purchased both online and from high street retailers in a variety of formulation, including powders, crystals, tablets, capsules, liquids, prerolled joints, smoking blends, herbal mixtures, and blotters (Deluca et al., 2012; Johnson et al., 2013; Papaseit et al., 2014; UNODC, 2013; Zawilska, 2011). Although various products are labeled with warnings "not for human consumption," "not tested for hazards or toxicity," or "technical use only," they are intended to mimic psychoactive effects of illicit drugs of abuse. Usually, the product names refer directly to controlled substances (e.g., "Coco Power," "Crack Inside," "EXTC," "Fake marijuana," "Xtacy," "Speedway," "Snow Blow," "White Ice Resins," "X Pillz") or to expected/desired effects (e.g., "Bliss," "Chill out," "Dynamite," "Euphoria," "Explosion," "Loved Up," "Mister Feel Good," "Rocket Fuel," "Sextasy," "Torpedo") (Corazza et al., 2014; McGraw & McGraw, 2012; Zawilska, 2011; Zawilska & Wojcieszak, 2013, 2014; Zuba & Byrska, 2013). A comprehensive analysis of 1074 brand names used to advertise NPS has shown that in order to attract consumers, especially teenagers, the names often refer to popular movies (e.g., "Black Mamba," "Clockwork orange," "Vanilla Sky," "Scarface"), cartoons (e.g., "Scooby snax," "Kryptonite," "He-Man"), animals (e.g., "Magic Dragon," "Dragonfly," "Meow Meow"), or landscapes (e.g., "Yukatan fire," "K2," "Ocean snow," "Rainbows") (Corazza et al., 2014). The names of commercial products containing NPS lack consistency, with many vendors making similarly named products with different chemical compositions.

The active components of the products can vary markedly, both quantitatively and qualitatively, even within the same name-brand (EMCDDA, 2013; Zuba & Byrska, 2013). Furthermore, the list of ingredients gives no indication of the presence of psychoactive compounds, and no or little safety information is provided. As some products can contain illicit substances, consumers might unknowingly purchase and use them. Importantly, the vast majority of NPS has not been tested on humans or animals, and the potential health implications of their use are largely unknown. It should be emphasized that after a ban of the particular substance, novel compounds usually quickly appear on the market in order to satisfy demands from consumers and at the same time to avoid criminalization, and are advertised as being better than the previous ones (EMCDDA, 2013, 2014a). Altogether, these factors pose a serious threat for consumers and increase the risk of acute harm and toxicity associated with the use of NPS-containing products.

Based on the spectrum of exerted psychoactive effects, NPS can be classified into four basic categories: synthetic cannabinoids (SCs), stimulants, opioid-like compounds, and hallucinogenic/dissociative (psychodysleptic); however, they may have a combination of these effects due to their designed chemical structure. Although the prevalence and pattern of NPS use differ between various countries, the most popular groups are SCs and psychostimulants (Araújo et al., 2014; Deluca et al., 2012; EMCDDA, 2013, 2014a; Helander, Bäckberg, Hultén, Al-Saffar, & Beck, 2014; Maxwell, 2014; UNODC, 2013). Both groups are described in this chapter.

2. PSYCHOSTIMULANTS

The main classes of the stimulant NPS are listed in Table 1.

At present, the most popular group is that of synthetic cathinones (Maxwell, 2014; Papaseit et al., 2014; Zawilska, 2014). They represent a large family of β-keto phenethylamine (2-amino-1-phenylpropan-1-one) derivatives chemically related to the parent compound cathinone, one of the psychoactive alkaloids present in the khat plant (*Catha edulis*). Cathinones can be substituted on the ring (i.e., methylenedioxy substituted), position 3′ and/or amine group (*N*-alkyl substituted, pyrrolidinyl substituted) (Fig. 2). All synthetic cathinones are chiral and can exist in two stereoisomer forms.

Table 1 The Most Common NPS ("Legal Highs"): Psychostimulants

Chemical Group	Representatives
I. Piperazines	1-Benzylpiperazine (BZP) 1-(3-Trifluoromethylphenyl)piperazine (TFMPP) 1-(4-Methoxyphenyl)piperazine (MeOPP) 1-(4-Chlorophenyl)piperazine (*m*CPP) 1-(4-Fluorophenyl)piperazine (*p*FPP)
II. Synthetic cathinones, so-called beta-keto (bk) amphetamines	Butylone Ephedone (methcathinone) Ethylone Flephedrone(4-fluoromethcathinone, 4-FMC) Mephedrone (4-methylmethcathinone, 4-MMC) 4-Methylethcathinone (4-MEC) Methylone (MDMC) 3,4-Methylenodioxypyrovalerone (MDPV) Naphyrone Pyrovalerone
III. 2,5-Dimethoxyamphetamines	4-Bromo-2,5-dimethoxyamphetamine (DOB) 4-Iodo-2,5-dimethoxyamphetamine (DOI) 2,5-Dimethoxy-4-methylamphetamine (DOM) 2,4,5-Trimethoxyamphetamine (TMA-2)
IV. 2-Aminoindanes	5-Iodo-2-aminoindane (5-IAI) 5,6-Methylenedioxy-2-aminoindane (MDAI) 5,6-Methylenedioxy-*N*-methyl-2-aminoindane (MMDAI)
V. Derivatives of pipradole	2-(Diphenylmethyl)-piperidine (desoxypipradrol, 2-DPMP) Diphenyl-2-pyrrolidinyl-methanol (diphenylprolinol; D2PM)
VI. Tryptamines	5-(2-Aminopropyl)indole (5-IT, 5-API)
VII. 2C Agents—substituted phenylethylamines (2C-X)	2C-B, 2C-C, 2C-D, 2C-E, 2C-G, 2C-I, 2C-T

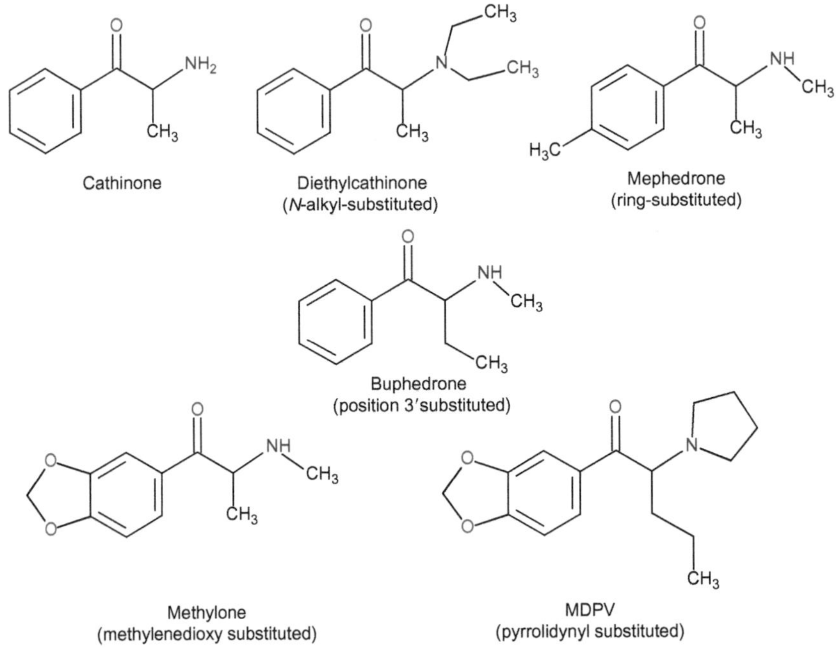

Figure 2 Major chemical classes of synthetic derivatives of cathinone.

In Europe and the USA, the most commonly used cathinones were: 4-methylmethcathinone (mephedrone; "Meow/Miaow Miaow," "4-MMC," "MMCat," "Meph," "Rush," "Crab"), methylone, 4-methylethcathinone (4-MEC), 3,4-methylenedioxypyrovalerone (MDPV; "Cherry Coke," "Doves Red," "Hurricane Charlie," "Sextasy," "Stardust," "Xtacy"), pentedrone, α-pyrovalerone (Araújo et al., 2014; EMCDDA, 2014b, Helander et al., 2014; Maxwell, 2014; Zawilska & Wojcieszak, 2013; Zuba & Byrska, 2013). Detailed information on chemical structures and the analytical methods for cathinones detection is provided by Paillet-Loilier, Cesbon, Le Boisselier, Jourgine, and Debruyene (2014). In contrast to cathinones and piperazines, such as 1-benzylpiperazine (BZP, "A2," "Legal X," "Bliss," "Flying Angel," "Mitsubishi," "Smiley Face") and 1-(3-trifluoromethylphenyl)piperazine (TFMPP, "X4," "Molly"), very little is known about analogues of pipradol, 2-DPMP ("Ivory Wave," "Pippy") and D2PM ("Head Candy"), a tryptamine derivative, 5-IT ("Benzofury"), and 2-aminoindanes, such as 5-IAI, MDAI, and MMDAI ("Sparcle," "Mindy," "Blow").

The so-called 2C drugs constitute another group of psychoactive phenethylamine derivatives. The name "2C," originally created by Alexander Shulgin, refers to their chemical structure, where two carbon atoms separate the amine from the phenyl ring. The substituted phenylethylamines (2C-X) contain methoxy groups on 2 and 5 positions of the phenyl ring and a variety of substituents at position 4. They exert stimulating, hallucinogenic, and psychedelic effects, depending on the structure and dose (ACMD, 2013; Dean, Stellpflug, Burnett, & Engebretsen, 2013; King, 2014). The first compound from this group was 2C-B (4-bromo-2,5-dimethoxyphenethylamine), sold under names such as "Nexus," "Erox," "Bromo," or "Venus" in the 1980s and early 1990s. Since the scheduling of 2C-B by Drug Enforcement Agency in 1995, several new 2C compounds have been synthesized and introduced on the drug market (Dean et al., 2013).

Psychostimulant NPS mimic the action of scheduled stimulants, namely, amphetamine, methamphetamine, 3,4-dimethoxymethamphetamine (MDMA, ecstasy), and cocaine, albeit to varying degrees. It was originally thought that the rapid growth in interest and use of these drugs, especially mephedrone, notified at the end of the last decade, was in part due to the potent decrease in purity of ecstasy and cocaine, and instability of the ecstasy market (Brunt, Poortman, Niesink, & van den Brink, 2011; McElrath & O'Neill, 2011). However, recent studies suggest that this was not the case. Instead of replacing or displacing ecstasy and cocaine, mephedrone, and most likely other NPS from this group, appears to have been added to the established repertoires of psychostimulant narcotics (Chen, Kostakis, Irvine, & White, 2013; Moore, Dargan, Wood, & Measham, 2013).

2.1 Pharmacology and Metabolism

There is little information on the pharmacology and pharmacokinetics of stimulatory NPS, and the available data are mainly limited to synthetic cathinones and BZP. It is postulated that, by analogy to their narcotic counterparts, these compounds, with the exception of the 2C drugs, exert their action via increasing synaptic levels of monoamines: noradrenaline (NA), dopamine (DA), and serotonin (5-HT). The drugs interact with the plasma membrane monoamine transporter proteins, namely, NAT, DAT, and SERT, inhibiting reuptake of NA, DA, and 5-HT, respectively, but their selectivity for these transporters varies considerably. Some drugs can also promote the release of DA (e.g., BZP, mephedrone, cathinone, methcathinone, flephedrone, 5-IAI, D2PM, 2-DPMP), NA (e.g., BZP, MDAI, D2PM, 2-DPMP), and 5-HT (e.g., *m*CPP, TFMPP, mephedrone, methylone, ethylone, butylone, 5-IAI, MDAI) (Corkery, Elliott, Schifano, Corazza, & Ghodse, 2012; Gallagher et al., 2012; Simmler et al., 2013, Simmler, Rickli, Schramm, Hoener, & Liechti, 2014, Zawilska & Wojcieszak, 2013).

Synthetic cathinones could be classified into four main groups based on their relative potency to act as SERT, NAT, and DAT inhibitors and their action as substrate releasers (Simmler et al., 2013, 2014):

1. *Cocaine-MDMA-mixed cathinones*, e.g., mephedrone, methylone, ethylone, butylone, and naphyrone. They act as relatively nonselective monoamine uptake inhibitors, similar to cocaine, with an affinity for DAT up to five times higher than the affinity for SERT. In addition, these compounds, with the exception of naphyrone, induce the release of 5-HT, similar to MDMA, and mephedrone also enhances the release of DA.
2. *Methamphetamine-like cathinones*, e.g., cathinone, methcathinone, flephedrone, ethcathinone, and 3-fluoromethcathinone. By analogy to amphetamine and methamphetamine, they act as preferential catecholamine (DA and NA) uptake inhibitors and, with an exception of ethcathinone, DA releasers.
3. *MDMA-like cathinones*, e.g., methedrone and 4-trifluoromethylmethcathinone. They are potent NAT and SERT inhibitors with low potency at DAT. These compounds also release NA and 5-HT.
4. *Pyrovalerone-cathinones*: pyrovalerone and MDPV. They are very potent and selective catecholamine uptake inhibitors, but do not evoke the release of monoamines. A similar profile of action is characteristic for pentedrone and *N,N*-dimethylcathinone. Importantly, when compared to cocaine, MDPV is 50 times more potent at interacting with DAT and 10 times more potent with NAT (Baumann et al., 2013).

Some synthetic cathinones can additionally act as agonists or antagonists of different subtypes of 5-HT_2 receptors (Simmler et al., 2013). Similarly, the 2C drugs bind to 5-HT_2, and additionally to α-adrenergic receptors, and act as either agonist or antagonists, depending on the compound and the receptor type (Dean et al., 2013),

At the cellular level, mephedrone has been shown to increase Fos expression in the cortex, striatum, and ventral tegmental area of the rat brain, resembling the action of methamphetamine and MDMA, and in the supraoptic nucleus, which is characteristic of MDMA (Motbey, Hunt, Bowen, Artissm, & McGregor, 2012).

Studies on animals have revealed that BZP and cathinones, such as methylone, mephedrone, and MDPV, exert powerful locomotor stimulant effects in a dose- and compound-dependent manner (Gregg & Rawls, 2014; Monteiro et al., 2013). In a similar way to psychostimulant drugs of abuse, prolonged administration of BZP, mephedrone, and cathinone leads to the development of sensitization to their actions (Brennan, Johnstone, Fitzmaurice, Lea, & Schenk, 2007; Shortall et al., 2013). The results of behavioral experiments suggest that synthetic cathinones and BZP could have abuse and addiction potential in humans. Thus, it was found that MDPV, mephedrone, and methylone were self-administrated in rats; the same action was exerted by BZP in rhesus monkeys (Aarde, Angrish, et al., 2013, Aarde, Huang, Creehan, Dickerson, & Taffe, 2013; Fantegrossi, Winger, Woods, Woolverton, & Coop, 2005; Watterson, Watterson, & Olive, 2013). Mephedrone produced conditioned place preference in various species and lowered intracranial self-stimulation thresholds in mice (Gregg & Rawls, 2014). Another important observation indicating the abuse potential of BZP and cathinones is the capability of animals to discriminate them from saline and other substances. Interestingly, BZP possesses discriminative responses similar to that of amphetamine and MDMA (Fantegrossi et al., 2005; Yarosh, Katz, Coop, & Fantegrossi, 2007), discriminative effects of mephedrone are similar to MDMA, cocaine, and methamphetamine. MDPV discriminates from saline and fully substitutes for MDMA and methamphetamine, while methylone substitutes for methamphetamine (Gregg & Rawls, 2014).

There is little available information about pharmacokinetic properties of stimulant NPS. Metabolism of the 2C compounds involves O-demethylation at 2 and 5 positions, deamination, and oxidation either to the corresponding acid or base (Meyer & Maurer, 2010). Studies on metabolism of cathinone derivatives in rats and humans indicate that they undergo complex transformation: N-demethylation to the primary amine, reduction of the keto group to the hydroxyl group, and oxidation of the tolyl moiety to the corresponding alcohol and carboxylic acid (Meyer, Vollmar, Schwaninger, Wolf, & Maurer, 2012; Meyer, Wilhelm, Peters, & Maurer, 2010). Six phase I metabolites of mephedrone were detected in rat urine and seven in human urine (Meyer, Wilhelm, et al., 2010). Cytochrome P450 2D6 (CYP2D6) is the main enzyme responsible for the *in vitro* phase I metabolism of mephedrone and methylone (Pedersen, Petersen, &

Linnet, 2013; Pedersen, Reitzel, Johansen, & Linnet, 2013); CYP2D6, CYP2C19, and COMT are involved in metabolism of MDPV (Meyer, Du, Schuster, & Maurer, 2010; Strano-Rossi, Cadwallader, de la Torre, & Botrè, 2010); CYP1A2, CY3A4, and CYP2D6 catalyze dealkylation and hydroxylation of BZP and TFMPP (Antia, Lee, Kydd, Tingle, & Russell, 2009; Antia, Tingle, & Russell, 2009). Phase I metabolites are eliminated with urine as glucuronide conjugates and sulfate conjugates. Demonstration of the important role of CYP2D6 in metabolism of cathinones and piperazines is of clinical importance. As CYP2D6 is involved in metabolism of numerous drugs and xenobiotics, pharmacokinetic interactions between psychostimulants and other compounds are likely to occur. Furthermore, the rate of metabolism and toxicity of NPS may depend on the genetic polymorphism of CYPP2D6. The effects of specific metabolites of stimulant NPS on the brain function need to be elucidated in order to better understand the complexity of their action.

2.2 Users, Routes of Administration, Dosages

By analogy to other drugs of abuse, the prevalence of stimulant NPS use is difficult to measure. Users of these drugs tended to be males and either youth or young adults (Buttler & Sheridan, 2007; EMCDDA, 2014b; Maxwell, 2014; Zawilska & Wojcieszak, 2013). Due to potent stimulant and entactogenic properties, compounds such as BZP or cathinones have been frequently used on weekend nights at night clubs, discos, and dance/rave parties or other forms of social activity; daytime use was less common. A very popular combination of BZP with TFMPP, present in party pills, was used in an attempt to mimic the effects of MDMA (Helander et al., 2014; Monteiro, Bastos, Guedes de Pinho, & Carvalho, 2013). In addition, BZP has been reported to be used to increase alertness and overcome sleepiness by shift workers, truck drivers, and by students (Monteiro et al., 2013). Of clinical and epidemiological importance is a very recent observation of the increased popularity of mephedrone among men who have sex with men (MSM), who use the drug solely to facilitate sex. Alarmingly, an increased spread of HIV and other sexually transmitted infections has been notified in this subpopulation (Hunter, Dargan, Benzie, White, & Wood, 2014; Stuart, 2013).

The most common administration routes of psychostimulatory NPS are insufflation (snorting), with the exception of 5-IAI (Coppola & Mondola,

2013), and oral ingestion of capsules or tablets: the substance being diluted with water/juice drink or taken as a powder wrapped in a cigarette paper and swallowed (the so-called bombing or hammer method used to consume high doses). Rectal insertion, intravenous and intramuscular injections, and smoking were also reported (Buttler & Sheridan, 2007; Corkery, Elliott, et al., 2012; Corkery, Elliott, Schifano, Corazza, & Ghodse, 2013; Corkery, Schifano, & Ghodse, 2012; Dean et al., 2013; EMCDDA, 2011, 2013, 2014b,c; Katselou, Papoutsis, Nikolaou, Spiliopoulou, & Athanaselis, 2014; Monteiro et al., 2013; Wood & Dargan, 2012; Zawilska & Wojcieszak, 2013). The intravenous administration of BZP was reported as being painful due to alkalinity of the solution (Gee, Richardson, Woltersdorf, & Moore, 2005), whereas that of mephedrone produces an intense burning sensation on injection. Continued attempts to inject mephedrone resulted in vein blockages, with development of skin erosion, localized infections, blisters, spots, abscesses, scabs, lumps, gangrenous tissue, blood clots, and large holes at overused injecting sites, thus limiting a number of injections to maximally three per site (Van Hout & Bingham, 2012).

Dosages and duration of action depend on the route of administration; they vary markedly among different compounds (Table 2). Drugs are often taken in a binge-like fashion, and several consumers mix routes of administration, for example, nasal and oral, in a single session in order to achieve both rapid and long-lasting effects (Monteiro et al., 2013; Zawilska & Wojcieszak, 2013).

Accumulating evidence indicates that stimulant NPS, in addition of being uses as mixtures of compounds from the same chemical class (Zuba & Byrska, 2013), are frequently used in conjunction with other substances, particularly with alcohol, cannabinoids, ecstasy, amphetamines, benzodiazepines, β-blockers, opiates (morphine or tramadol to create "speedball"-like effects), γ-hydroxybutyric acid (as an aphrodisiac), in order to (1) increase or extend the stimulant effects and improve mood, (2) allow a greater intake of alcohol, (3) reduce negative effects (Buttler & Sheridan, 2007; EMCDDA, 2014b; Monteiro et al., 2013; Schifano et al., 2011; Tekulve, Alexander, & Tormoehlen, 2014; Zawilska & Wojcieszak, 2013). It has been demonstrated that synthetic cathinone products often contain various concentrations (<2–96%) of caffeine, a psychostimulant (Zuba & Byrska, 2013), and less frequently, lidocaine or benzocaine (Spiller, Ryan, Weston, & Jansen, 2011; Zuba & Byrska, 2013), local anesthetics that cause a stronger numbness of gums than cocaine, giving the user the impression of a high quality cocaine-like product.

Table 2 Dosage, Onset, and Duration of Action of Psychostimulatory NPS

Compound	Doses	Onset and Duration of Effects	Comments	References
Benzylpiperazine, TFMPP	100–500 mg orally		Due to high alkalinity of BZP solution ($pH > 12$), its i.v. administration is painful	Monteiro et al. (2013)
Mephedrone	25–75 mg intranasally 150–250 orally	Onset: within minutes Duration: less than an hour Onset: 45 min—2 h Duration: 2–4 h	Several consumers first snort and then ingest the drug in order to achieve both fast and long-lasting effects When taken intranasally could have a potential for abuse comparable to that of cocaine	Zawilska & Wojcieszak (2013)
MDPV (3,4-methylenedioxypyrovalerone)	3–15 mg (typical 5–10 mg)	Onset: 5–20 min (nasal); 15-30 min (oral) Duration: 30 min–2.5 h (nasal); up to 7 h (oral)	High risk of overdose due to the fact that packages usually contain as much as 500 mg and some labels suggests escalating the dose to more than 50 mg Intravenous administration is strongly discouraged due to vasoconstriction and increased potential for vein damage	
Naphyrone	10–50 mg (typical 20–30 mg)	Onset: 5–10 min (nasal); 30–60 min (oral) Duration: 30–120 min (nasal); up to 4 h (oral)	Intravenous administration is strongly discouraged due to vasoconstriction and increased potential for vein damage	

2-DPMP	1–10 mg orally	Onset: within 1 h (oral) Duration: up to 24–48 h		Corkery, Elliott, et al. (2012)
D2PM	2–5 mg orally 35–50 mg orally	Onset: 15 min (oral) Duration: 10 h	Typical dose Dose suggested in users self-reports	Corkery, Elliott, et al. (2012)
MDAI	70–300 mg	Onset: 10–12 min (cral)		Corkery et al. (2013)

2.3 Desired and Adverse Effects

The consumption of psychostimulatory NPS results in typical stimulant-related subjective effects. Users frequently compare their effects to those exerted by cocaine, amphetamine, and MDMA: heightened alertness and awareness, increased energy and motivation, euphoria, excitement, improved mood, mild empathogenic effects, openness in communication, sociability and talkativeness, intensification of sensory experiences, reduced appetite and insomnia (Buttler & Sheridan, 2007; Corkery, Elliott, et al., 2012, Corkery et al., 2013; Gallagher et al., 2012; Katselou et al., 2014; Schifano et al., 2011; Wood & Dargan, 2012; Zawilska & Wojcieszak, 2013). The use of cathinones was also reported to be associated with increased sexual desire and sexual HIV risk behavior (Hunter et al., 2014; Johnson & Johnson, 2014; Stuart, 2013). The majority of users, who had taken MDMA and cocaine before, estimated the effects of mephedrone to be more similar to those of MDMA as compared to those of cocaine. Some users described strong craving to repeat or increase doses after taking mephedrone (EMCDDA, 2011). Mephedrone induces stronger feeling of craving in comparison to MDMA (Brunt et al., 2011), and users who snort mephedrone rate it more addictive than cocaine (EMCDDA, 2011).

The adverse effects, at present best known to be associated with the use of synthetic cathinones and BZP, include a vast array of symptoms (Buttler & Sheridan, 2007; Coppola & Mondola, 2013; Corkery, Elliott, et al., 2012; EMCDDA, 2014b,c; Gallagher et al., 2012; Katselou et al., 2014; Monteiro et al., 2013; Wood et al., 2008; Wood & Dargan, 2012; Wood, Puchnarewicz, Johnston, & Dargan, 2012; Zawilska & Wojcieszak, 2013), which can be divided into the following main groups:

- *Cardiovascular*—sinus tachycardia, heart palpitations, chest pain, hypertension, S-T segmental changes, cardiac arrest.
- *Cognitive*—confusion, cognitive impairment, mental fatigue, disorientation to name, place, and time, loosening of association.
- *Psychiatric*—irritability, anxiety, panic attacks, lack of motivation, anhedonia, depression, agitation, dysphoria, aggression that progressed sometimes to violent or even criminal behavior, and self-destructive behavior. There were also cases of suicidal ideation and self-mutilation.
- *Neurological*—disturbed sleep patterns and nightmares, insomnia, tremors, seizures, hyperthermia, mydriasis, blurred vision, paresthesias, bruxism, motor automatisms, headache, and dizziness. Of note, a distinctive extrapyramidal syndrome has been observed in intravenous methcathinone (ephedrone) users in Eastern Europe and Russia (see Chapter

"Home-made methcathinone and permanent neurological damage"). The very recent study of a large pediatric group with cathinones intoxications has documented that seizures occur in 5.5% of cases, with almost 40% of those patients experiencing multiple seizures. The seizure activity was associated with acidosis and fever (Tekulve et al., 2014).

- *Perceptual*—paranoid delusion, visual, and auditory hallucinations.
- *Hematologic*—disseminated intravascular coagulation, thrombocytopenia, anemia.
- *Gastrointestinal*—nausea/vomiting, anorexia, abdominal pain.
- *Miscellaneous*—profuse sweating leading to diaphoresis, dry mouth, sore mouth/throat, hyponatremia, hyperkalemia, hyperuricemia, increased serum levels of creatinine and creatinine kinase, metabolic and respiratory acidosis, weight loss after prolonged use (Buttler & Sheridan, 2007; Coppola & Mondola, 2013; Corkery, Elliott, et al., 2012; Monteiro et al., 2013; Wood et al., 2012; Zawilska & Wojcieszak, 2013). In some cases, intoxication with synthetic cathinones resulted in kidney and liver failure (Zawilska & Wojcieszak, 2013). Recently, cases of local injury with necrotizing fasciitis following intravenous or intramuscular cathinones' injection have been reported (Dorairaj, Healy, McMenamin, & Eadie, 2012; Russo et al., 2012).

Clinical effects of 2C drugs are dose dependent. At low doses, they generally act as stimulants and produce euphoria, increased empathy, sociability, acceleration of thoughts, conceptual thinking, agitation, as well as increased visual, auditory, olfactory, and tactile sensations. At moderate doses, hallucinations and life-changing spiritual experiences occur. Higher doses lead to psychedelic effects, such as depersonalization, derealization and time distortion, extreme unpleasant hallucinations, anxiety, panic and fear, acute psychosis, insomnia, and seizures, as well as sympatomimetic signs such as dilated pupils, tachycardia, hypertension, and hyperthermia (Bosak, LoVecchio, & Levine, 2013; Dean et al., 2013). Common adverse effects of 2C drugs include nausea, vomiting, headache, sweating, and temporary dysuria (Dean et al., 2013). Massive ventricular hemorrhage (Drees, Stone, & Wu, 2009) and fatal toxic leukoencephalopathy (Sacks, Ray, Williams, & Opatowsky, 2012) were reported after consumption of 2C-I and 2C-E, respectively.

2.4 Deaths Related to the Recreational Use of Psychostimulant NPS

The highest number of fatal intoxications have been reported for mephedrone (Corkery, Schifano, et al., 2012; Cosbey, Peters, Quinn, &

Bentley, 2013; Elliott & Evans, 2014) and MDPV (Elliott & Evans, 2014; EMCDDA, 2014b). In the majority of those cases, the drugs were identified postmortem. Most of the victims were young males with a previous history of drug abuse. In the case of mephedrone, there was a notable number of deaths that involved self-harm, mainly from suicidal hanging (Corkery, Schifano, et al., 2012; Cosbey et al., 2013). Other reported and analytically confirmed fatalities involved BZP (Monteiro et al., 2013), cathinones such as methylone, butylone, 2-methylamino-1-(3,4-methylenedioxyphenyl) butan-1-one (bk-MBDB), methcathinone (ephedrone), and 4-methylethcathinone (Rojek, Kłys, Maciów-Głąb, Kula, & Strona, 2014; Zawilska & Wojcieszak, 2013), 5-IT (EMCDDA, 2014c; Kronstrand et al., 2013; Seetohul & Pounder, 2013), 2-DPMP (Corkery, Elliott, et al., 2012), and MDAI (Corkery et al., 2013). The victims usually died due to cardiac arrest and respiratory failure, and less frequently from multiorgan failure, disseminated intravascular coagulation, hemorrhages, and fatal wounds.

3. SYNTHETIC CANNABINOIDS

Smokeable herbal mixtures containing SCs appeared in Europe in the early 2000s and became popular around 2008. They are sold under a variety of brand names; the most common are "Spice" in Europe, "K2" in the United States, "Kronic" in Australia and New Zealand. As advertisements describe SCs containing products as "harmless incense herbal blends," some consumers infer that these products are safe (Fattore & Fratta, 2011). Since the first identification of a SC in the herbal mixture "Spice Gold" at the end of 2008 (Auwärter et al., 2009), their market has grown continuously. At present, over 150 SCs are known (Presley, Jansen-Varnum, & Logan, 2013). They are classified into different chemical groups (Table 3; Hudson & Ramsey, 2011). Compounds from so-called JWH series, designed by the medicinal chemist J.W. Huffman (Clemenson University, Clemenson, USA), represent the dominant SCs detected in the "Spice" products (Carroll, Lewin, Mascarella, Seltzman, & Reddy, 2012; Hudson & Ramsey, 2011). Although SCs vary markedly in terms of the chemical structure, all are lipid soluble, nonpolar, and typically consist of 20–26 carbon atoms, which explains why they volatilize readily when smoked (Castaneto et al., 2014; Wiley, Marusich, & Huffman, 2014).

In addition to SCs, several other substances have been identified in "Spice"-type products, such as amides of fatty acids (oleamide, palmitamide,

Table 3 The Most Common NPS ("Legal Highs"): Synthetic Cannabinoids

Chemical Group	Representatives
I. JWH compounds:	
Naphthoylindoles	JWH-015, JWH-018, JWH-073, JWH-210, JWH-387
Naphthylmethylindoles	JWH-175
Naphthoylpyrroles	JWH-147
Naphthylmethylindenes	JWH-176
Phenacetylindoles	JWH-203, JWH-250, JWH-253
II. Cyclohexylphenols	CP 47,497 and its homologues
III. Benzoylindoles	AM-694, AM-2201, AM-679, RCS-4
IV. Classical cannabinoids	HU-210
V. TMCP compounds	TMCP-H, TMCP-018, TMCP-2201, TMCP-200, TMCP-1220
VI. Other	WIN 55,212-2, UR-144, PB-22

and stearamide, which could mimic the action of natural cannabinoids), substances presumably originating from plants (e.g., eugenol, eucalyptol, phytosterole, thymol, squalene, persicol), ethyl linoleate, linoleic acid, palmitic acid, flavors (ethyl vanillin, acetyl vanillin), and preservatives—benzophenone, benzyl benzoate, hydroxybenzoic acid. Moreover, "Spice"-type products have been found to contain large amounts of vitamin E, added to hamper the analysis of the active cannabinoids (Dresen et al., 2010; Zuba, Byrska, & Maciow, 2011).

To produce "Spice"-type products, SCs are first dissolved in an organic solvent, acetone, or alcohol. The solution is then spayed onto dried plant material. After drying, the final product is packed and sold. The plant material itself is sometimes green or brown, but may be colored in a similar manner to the packaging, or as suggested by the name of the material. To increase its attractiveness, the material is often perfumed with vanilla, fruit, or "bubblegum" scents (Presley et al., 2013).

3.1 Pharmacology and Metabolism

Cannabinoids exert their biological effects primarily by interacting with specific membrane-bound G protein-coupled cannabinoid receptors termed CB_1 and CB_2. CB_1 receptors are abundantly expressed in the central nervous system, namely, in the cerebral cortex, hippocampus, basal ganglia, cerebellum, and hypothalamus. In addition, they are expressed in the peripheral nervous system, both on sensory nerve fibers and in the autonomic nervous system. CB_2 receptors are located predominantly in cells and tissues of the immune system (Pertwee, 2005).

At present, little is known about the detailed pharmacology and toxicology of SCs, and no systematic studies on humans have been published. Ironically, many of these compounds have been developed as research tools to study the endocannabinoid system, or for use as potential therapeutics. SCs elicit effects similar but not identical to Δ^9-tetrahydrocannabinol (Δ^9-THC), the main psychoactive constituent of cannabis. *In vitro* tests have shown that, in contrast to the partial agonist activity of Δ^9-THC, SCs are high-affinity full agonist of CB_1 and CB_2 receptors, acting in low nanomolar range, thus demonstrating cannabimimetic activity (e.g., Castaneto et al., 2014; Fantegrossi, Moran, Radominska-Pandya, & Prather, 2014; Wiley et al., 2014). Of note, some of them, such as JWH-015, JWH-365, JWH-372, and (+)WIN 55,212-2, exhibit higher affinity for CB_2 than CB_1 receptors (Aung et al., 2000; Wiley et al., 2014). Studies on animals have revealed that SCs elicit a characteristic cannabinoid tetrad of effects: hypothermia, analgesia, catalepsy, and suppression of locomotor activity (Brents et al., 2012; Wiebelhaus et al., 2012; Zawilska & Wojcieszak, 2014). In a drug discrimination stimulus test, JWH-015, JWH-073, and (+)WIN 55,212-2 substituted for Δ^9-THC (Ginsburg, Schulze, Hruba, & McMahon, 2012; Vann et al., 2009). Furthermore, like Δ^9-THC, JWH-018 and JWH-073 dose-dependently attenuated the withdrawal symptoms produced by rimonabant, a CB_1 receptor antagonist (Ginsburg et al., 2012). It is well documented that CB_2 receptors are involved in modulation of immune system function (Pertwee, 2005). Whether SCs, especially those with high affinity for CB_2 receptors, are endowed with immunosuppressive activity remains to be elucidated.

It is suggested that both phase I (oxidation, and to a lesser extent, carboxylation) and phase II (conjugation with glucuronic acid) processes are involved in metabolism of SCs. Unlike Δ^9-THC, metabolites of SCs retain varying amounts of biologic activity and can act as full agonists, partial agonists, neutral antagonists, or inverse agonists of cannabinoid receptors (reviewed by Fantegrossi et al., 2014).

3.2 Users, Routes of Administration, Dosages

"Spice"-type products are usually sold in metal-foil sachets, typically containing 1–3 g of dried vegetable matter (leaves, flowers, resin) to which one or more SCs has been added (Barratt, Cakic, & Lenton, 2013; Johnson et al., 2013). Although the products are mostly purchased online, they can also be obtained from retail vendors, from friends, or relatives. Users of "Spice"-type products are primarily male adolescents and young adults (Barratt et al., 2013; Papanti et al., 2013; Vandrey, Dunn, Fry, & Girling, 2012; Zawilska & Wojcieszak, 2014). In this age group, ever SC use was first reported to be around 10% (e.g., Barratt et al., 2013; Forrester, Kleinschmidt, Schwarz, & Young, 2012; Gunderson, Haughey, Ait-Daoud, Joshi, & Hart, 2014; Hu, Primack, Barnett, & Cook, 2011; Vandrey et al., 2012), but the recently published results of a self-reported study, including almost 15,000 participants from different countries, revealed lifetime use to be more prevalent: 16.8% (Winstock & Barratt, 2013). Accumulating evidence demonstrates the increasing popularity of SCs amongst soldiers (Bebarta, Ramirez, & Varney, 2012; Loeffler, Hurst, Penn, & Yung, 2012) and athletes (Heltsley et al., 2012; Möller et al., 2011).

Common reasons reported for use of SCs included: curiosity, seeking a new "high" similar to that produced by marijuana, belief in the safety of use, relaxation, and enjoyment of effects, and a desire to achieve marijuana-like psychoactive effects while avoiding detection in drug tests. Less frequently, SCs are taken in order to reduce or cease cannabis use (Bebarta et al., 2012; Bonar, Ashrafioun, & Illgen, 2014; Fattore & Fratta, 2011; Vandrey et al., 2012). SCs use was found to occur predominantly at a private residence, with the users being alone or in small groups (Forrester et al., 2012; Vandrey et al., 2012). The most common mode of administration is by smoking as a joint or in water-pipe ("bong"), while oral consumption or inhalation using a vaporizer is uncommon (Barratt et al., 2013; Vandrey et al., 2012).

During an average episode, approximately 1 g of SCs containing product or 4.5 "hits" was consumed, and the maximum amount consumed in a single episode was reported to be 1.5 g or 7.6 "hits." It has been reported that the action of JWH-018 in humans lasted for 1–2 h, whist that of CP 47,497 for 6–8 h (Auwärter et al., 2009; Barratt et al., 2013). According to recent self-reports by users, SCs have a shorter time until peak and shorter duration of action when compared with natural cannabis (Barratt et al., 2013; Winstock & Barratt, 2013).

Surveys of SCs consumption revealed it to be a common practice among current marijuana users (Barratt et al., 2013; Gunderson et al., 2014; Winstock & Barratt, 2013). The vast majority of those who reported to use SCs also consumed alcohol and smoked cigarettes. In addition, some of them used other psychoactive compounds, namely, MDMA, benzodiazepines, cocaine, LSD, and hallucinogenic mushrooms (Barratt et al., 2013; Winstock & Barratt, 2013).

3.3 Desired and Adverse Effects

Human users of "Spice"-type products reported that they share some but not all of the subjective effects of cannabis (Vardakou, Pistos, & Spiliopoulou, 2010; Zawilska & Wojcieszak, 2014). The intended effects include euphoria, increased empathy, and social interactions. After smoking a cigarette containing CP 47,497 (Auwärter et al., 2009) or JWH-018 (Teske et al., 2010), healthy volunteers reported sickness, sedation, xerostomia, hot flushes, burning eyes, and deterioration of mood and perception. There are currently few published case reports on clinical features of acute intoxication with SCs. Additional information on the toxicity related to SCs use mainly comes from web-based anonymous surveys, records collected from toxicology centers, and hospital emergency departments. The symptoms of acute SC intoxication (for comprehensive reviews, see Castaneto et al., 2014; Zawilska & Wojcieszak, 2014) can be divided into five categories:

- *Psychoactive*—hallucinations, psychoses with delusions, agitation, aggressive behavior, anxiety, panic attacks, short-term memory deficits, cognitive impairment, confusion, disorganized thoughts.
- *Neurological*—drowsiness, xerostomia, headache, motor incoordination, retarded sequence of movements, seizures, slurred speech.
- *Cardiovascular*—tachycardia, hypertension, chest pain, acute myocardial infarction, cerebral ischemia.
- *Ocular*—reddened conjunctivae, mydriasis, blurred vision.
- *Miscellaneous*—nausea, vomiting, diaphoresis, respiratory depression, acute kidney injury, muscle pains, dry mouth, hypokalemia, acidosis.

Given the ever evolving structure of available SCs, clinicians must be prepared for other unexpected adverse effects.

It should be emphasized that there are reports documenting cases of driving under influence of drugs with SCs (Musshoff et al., 2014; Tuv et al., 2014; Yeakel & Logan, 2013). The subjects displayed dizziness, appeared unstable and demonstrated a retarded sequence of movements, as well as somnolence; some of them were involved in traffic accidents. Hence, it is assumed that the consumptions of SCs, like the cannabis use (Hartman & Huestis, 2013), can lead to a potentially dangerous impairment of driving skills.

4. MANAGEMENT OF ACUTE INTOXICATION WITH NPS

There are no specific treatment guidelines for NPS intoxication. The management of patients consists of their stabilization combined with supportive and symptomatic care. Renal, muscular, cardiovascular, respiratory, and hepatic functions should be monitored. In patients with hyperthermia serial temperature checks should be done during hospitalization. Sympathomimetic complications, agitation, and seizures are treated with benzodiazepines (e.g., lorazepam, midazolam), while aggression and psychosis may require the use of antipsychotic drugs (e.g., haloperidol, fentanyl, risperidon) (Smith & Robert, 2014; Wood et al., 2012). However, as haloperidol may contribute to hyperthermia and cardiac arrhythmias, its use in cathinone-intoxicated patients should be restricted and carefully controlled (Musselman & Hampton, 2014). Management of hyperthermia and serotonin syndrome, in addition to cooling and benzodiazepines, includes cyproheptadine. When body temperature is higher than 41 °C, immediate paralysis with nondepolarizing agents (e.g., rocuronium, veronium), tracheal intubation, and ventilation are recommended. Antipyretics and dantrolene are ineffective (Dean et al., 2013; Musselman & Hampton, 2014; Smith & Robert, 2014). Treatment of hyponatremia in asymptomatic patients requires fluid restriction, while sodium correction with hypertonic saline is recommended in patients with neurological symptoms (Smith & Robert, 2014).

REFERENCES

Aarde, S. M., Angrish, D., Barlow, D. J., Wright, M. J., Jr., Vandewater, S. A., Creehan, K. M., et al. (2013). Mephedrone (4-methylmethcathinone) supports intravenous self-administration in Sprague-Dawley and Wistar rats. *Addiction Biology*, *18*, 786–799.

Aarde, S. M., Huang, P. K., Creehan, K. M., Dickerson, T. J., & Taffe, M. A. (2013). The novel recreational drug 3,4-methylenedioxypyrovalerone (MDPV) is a potent psychomotor stimulant: Self-administration and locomotor activity in rats. *Neuropharmacology*, *71*, 130–140.

Advisory Council on the Misuse of Drugs (ACMD). (2013). "NBOMe" compounds: a review of the evidence of use and harm. Available at https://www.gov.uk./goverment/uploads/system/uploads/attachment_data/file/204808/J_TCDP_report_on_5-6APB_and_NBOMe_compounds.pdf. Retrieved October 17th, 2014.

Antia, U., Lee, H. S., Kydd, R. R., Tingle, M. D., & Russell, B. R. (2009). Pharmacokinetics of 'party pill' N-benzylpiperazine (BZP) in healthy human participants. *Forensic Science International*, *186*, 63–67.

Antia, U., Tingle, M. D., & Russell, B. R. (2009). Metabolic interactions with piperazine-based 'party pills'. *Journal of Pharmacy and Pharmacology*, *61*, 877–882.

Araújo, A. M., Valente, M. J., Carvalho, M., Dias da Silva, D., Gaspar, H., Carvalho, F., et al. (2014). Raising awareness of new psychoactive substances: Chemical analysis and in vitro toxicity screening of 'legal high' packages containing synthetic cathinones. *Archives of Toxicology*. http://dx.doi.org/10.1007/s00204-014-1278-7.

Aung, M. M., Griffin, G., Huffman, J. W., Wu, M., Keel, C., Yang, B., et al. (2000). Influence of the N-1 alkyl chain length of cannabimimetic indoles upon CB_1 and CB_2 receptor binding. *Drug and Alcohol Dependence*, *60*, 133–140.

Auwärter, V., Dresen, S., Weinmann, W., Müller, M., Pütz, M., & Ferreirós, N. (2009). 'Spice' and other herbal blends: Harmless incense or cannabinoid designer drugs? *Journal of Mass Spectrometry*, *44*, 832–837.

Barratt, M. J., Cakic, V., & Lenton, S. (2013). Patterns of synthetic cannabinoid use in Australia. *Drug and Alcohol Review*, *32*, 141–146.

Baumann, M. H., Partilla, J. S., Lehner, K. R., Thorndike, E. B., Hoffman, A. F., Holy, M., et al. (2013). Powerful cocaine-like actions of 3,4-methylenedioxypyrovalerone (MDPV), a principal constituent of psychoactive 'bath salts' products. *Neuropsychopharmacology*, *38*, 552–562.

Bebarta, V. S., Ramirez, S., & Varney, S. M. (2012). Spice: A new "legal" herbal mixture abused by young active duty military personel. *Substance Abuse*, *33*, 191–194.

Bonar, E. E., Ashrafioun, L., & Illgen, M. A. (2014). Synthetic cannabinoid use among patients in residential substance use disorder treatment: Prevalence, motives, and correlates. *Drug and Alcohol Dependence*, *143*, 268–271.

Bosak, A., LoVecchio, F., & Levine, M. (2013). Recurrent seizures and serotonin syndrome following "2C-I" ingestion. *Journal of Medical Toxicology*, *9*, 196–199.

Brennan, K., Johnstone, A., Fitzmaurice, P., Lea, R., & Schenk, S. (2007). Chronic benzylpiperazine (BZP) exposure produces behavioral sensitization and cross-sensitization to methamphetamine (MA). *Drug and Alcohol Dependence*, *88*, 204–213.

Brents, L. K., Gallus-Zawada, A., Radominska-Pandya, A., Vasiljevik, T., Prisinzano, T. E., Fantegrossi, W. E., et al. (2012). Monohydroxylated metabolites of the K2 synthetic cannabinoid JWH-073 retain intermediate to high cannabinoid 1 receptor (CB1R) affinity and exhibit neutral antagonist to partial agonist activity. *Biochemical Pharmacology*, *83*, 952–961.

Brunt, T. M., Poortman, A., Niesink, R. J., & van den Brink, W. (2011). Instability of the ecstasy market and a new kid on the block: Mephedrone. *Journal of Psychopharmacology*, *25*, 1543–1547.

Buttler, R. A., & Sheridan, J. L. (2007). Highs and lows: Patterns of use, positive and negative effects of benzylpiperazine-containing party pills (BZP-party pills) amongst young people in New Zealand. *Harm Reduction Journal*, *4*, 18.

Carroll, F. I., Lewin, A. H., Mascarella, S. W., Seltzman, H. H., & Reddy, P. A. (2012). Designer drugs: A medicinal chemistry perspective. *Annals of the New York Academy of Sciences*, *1248*, 18–38.

Castaneto, M. S., Gorelick, D. A., Desrosiers, N. A., Hartman, R. L., Pirard, S., & Huestis, M. A. (2014). Synthetic cannabinoids: Epidemiology, pharmacodynamics, and clinical implications. *Drug and Alcohol Dependence*, *144*, 12–41.

Chen, C., Kostakis, C., Irvine, R. J., & White, J. M. (2013). Increases in use of novel synthetic stimulant are not directly linked to decreased use of 3,5-methylenedioxy-N-methylamphetamine (MDMA). *Forensic Science International*, *231*, 278–283.

Coppola, M., & Mondola, R. (2013). 5-Iodo-2-aminoindan (5-IAI): Chemistry, pharmacology, and toxicology of a research chemical producing MDMA-like effects. *Toxicology Letters*, *218*, 24–29.

Corazza, O., Demetrovics, Z., van den Brink, W., & Schifano, F. (2013). 'Legal highs' an inappropriate term for 'Novel Psychoactive Drugs' in drug prevention and scientific debate. *The International Journal on Drug Policy, 24*, 82–83.

Corazza, O., Valeriani, G., Bersani, F. S., Corkery, J., Martinotti, G., Bersani, G., et al. (2014). "Spice," "kryptonite," "black mamba": An overview of brand names and marketing strategies of novel psychoactive substances on the web. *Journal of Psychoactive Drugs, 46*, 287–294.

Corkery, J. M., Elliott, S., Schifano, F., Corazza, O., & Ghodse, A. H. (2012). 2-DPMP (desoxypipradrol, 2-benzhydrylpiperidine, 2-phenylmethylpiperidine) and D2PM (diphenyl-2-pyrrolidin-2-yl-methanol, diphenylprolinol): A preliminary review. *Progress in Neuropsychopharmacology and Biological Psychiatry, 39*, 253–258.

Corkery, J. M., Elliott, S., Schifano, F., Corazza, O., & Ghodse, A. H. (2013). MDAI (5,6-methylenedioxy-2-aminoindane; 6,7-dihydro-5H-cyclopenta[f][1,3]benzodioxol-6-amine; 'sparkle'; 'mindy') toxicity: A brief overview and update. *Human Psychopharmacology: Clinical and Experimental, 28*, 345–355.

Corkery, J. M., Schifano, F., & Ghodse, A. H. (2012). Mephedrone-related fatalities in the United Kingdom: Contextual, clinical and practical issues. *Pharmacology, 17*, 355–380. Available at: http://cdn.intechopen.com/pdfs/32134/InTech-Mephedrone_related_fatalities_in_the_united_kingdom_contextual_clinical_and_practical_issues.pdf, Retrieved December 9, 2012.

Cosbey, S. H., Peters, K. L., Quinn, A., & Bentley, A. (2013). Mephedrone (methylmethcathinone) in toxicology casework: A Northern Ireland perspective. *Journal of Analytical Toxicology, 37*, 74–82.

Dean, B. V., Stellpflug, S. J., Burnett, A. M., & Engebretsen, K. M. (2013). 2C or not 2C: Phenethylamine designer drug review. *Journal of Medical Toxicology, 9*, 172–178.

Deluca, P., Davey, Z., Corazza, O., Di Furia, L., Farre, M., Flesland, L. H., et al. (2012). Identifying emerging trends in recreational drug use; outcomes from the Psychonaut Web Mapping Project. *Progress in Neuropsychopharmacology and Biological Psychiatry, 39*, 221–226.

Dorairaj, J. J., Healy, C., McMenamin, M., & Eadie, P. A. (2012). The untold truth about "bath salt" highs: A case series demonstrating local tissue injury. *Journal of Plastic, Reconstructive & Aesthetic Surgery, 65*, e37–e41.

Drees, J. C., Stone, J. A., & Wu, A. H. (2009). Morbidity involving the hallucinogenic designer amines MDA and 2C I. *Journal of Forensic Sciences, 54*, 1485–1487.

Dresen, S., Ferreirós, N., Pütz, M., Westphal, F., Zimmermann, R., & Auwärter, V. (2010). Monitoring of herbal mixtures potentially containing synthetic cannabinoids as psychoactive compounds. *Journal of Mass Spectrometry, 45*, 1186–1194.

Elliott, S., & Evans, J. (2014). A 3-year review of new psychoactive substances in casework. *Forensic Science International, 243*, 55–60.

EMCDDA. (2011). *Report on the risk assessment of mephedrone in the framework of the Council Decision on new psychoactive substances*. Available at: http://www.emcdda.europa.eu/attachements.cfm/att_116646_EN_TDAK11001ENC_WEB-OPTIMISED%20FILE.pdf, Retrieved November 21, 2014.

EMCDDA. (2012). *Annual report 2012. The state of the drug problem in Europe*. Available at: http://www.emcdda.europa.eu/attachments.cfm./att_190854_EN_TDAC13001ENC_pdf, Retrieved June 9, 2014.

EMCDDA. (2013). *EU drug markets reports. A strategic analysis*. Available at: http://www.emcdda.europa.eu/publications/joint-publications/drug-markets, Retrieved June 9, 2014.

EMCDDA. (2014a). *European drug report 2014. Trends and developments*. Available at: http://www.emcdda.europa.eu/attachements.cfm/att_228272_EN_TDAT14001ENN.pdf, Retrieved October 22, 2014.

EMCDDA. (2014b). *EMCDDA—Europol joint report on a new psychoactive substance: MDPV (3,4-methylenedioxypyrovalerone)*. Available at: http://www.emcdda.europa.eu/attachements.cfm/att_222592_EN_TDAS14001ENN.%20pdf, Retrieved October 22, 2014.

EMCDDA. (2014c). *EMCDDA—Europol joint report on a new psychoactive substance: 5-(2-aminopropyl)indole*. Available at: http://www.emcdda.europa.eu/attachements.cfm/att_194430_EN_TDAS13001ENN.pdf, Retrieved October 16, 2014.

Fantegrossi, W. E., Moran, J. H., Radominska-Pandya, A., & Prather, P. L. (2014). Distinct pharmacology and metabolism of K2 synthetic cannabinoids compared to Δ^9-THC: Mechanism underlying greater toxicity? *Life Sciences*, *97*, 45–54.

Fantegrossi, W. E., Winger, G., Woods, J. H., Woolverton, W. L., & Coop, A. (2005). Reinforcing and discriminative stimulus effects of 1-benzylpiperazine and trifluoromethylphenylpiperazine in rhesus monkeys. *Drug and Alcohol Dependence*, 77, 161–168.

Fattore, L., & Fratta, W. (2011). Beyond THC: The new generation of cannabinoid designer drugs. *Frontiers in Behavioral Neuroscience*, *5*, 60.

Forrester, M. B., Kleinschmidt, K., Schwarz, E., & Young, A. (2012). Synthetic cannabinoid and marijuana exposures reported to poison centers. *Human & Experimental Toxicology*, *31*, 1006–1011.

Gallagher, C. T., Assi, S., Stair, J. L., Fergus, S., Corazza, O., Corkery, J. M., et al. (2012). 5,6-Methylenedioxy-2-aminoindane: From laboratory curiosity to 'legal high'. *Human Psychopharmacology: Clinical and Experimental*, 27, 106–112.

Gee, P., Richardson, S., Woltersdorf, W., & Moore, G. (2005). Toxic effects of BZP-based herbal party pills in humans: A prospective in Christchurch, New Zealand. *New Zealand Medical Journal*, *118*, U1784.

Gibbons, S. (2012). 'Legal highs'—Novel and emerging psychoactive drugs: A chemical overview for the toxicologist. *Clinical Toxicology (Philadelphia, Pa)*, *50*, 15–24.

Ginsburg, B. C., Schulze, D. R., Hruba, L., & McMahon, L. R. (2012). JWH-018 and JWH-073: Δ^9-Tetrahydrocannabinol-like discriminative stimulus effects in monkeys. *Journal of Pharmacology and Experimental Therapeutics*, *340*, 37–45.

Gregg, R. A., & Rawls, S. M. (2014). Behavioral pharmacology of designer cathinones: A review of the preclinical literature. *Life Sciences*, *97*, 27–30.

Gunderson, E. W., Haughey, H. M., Ait-Daoud, N., Joshi, A. S., & Hart, C. L. (2014). A survey of synthetic cannabinoid consumption by current cannabis users. *Substance Abuse*, *35*, 184–189.

Hartman, R. L., & Huestis, M. A. (2013). Cannabis effects on driving skills. *Clinical Chemistry*, *59*, 478–492.

Helander, A., Bäckberg, M., Hultén, P., Al-Saffar, Y., & Beck, O. (2014). Detection of new psychoactive substance use among emergency room patients: Results from the Swedish STRIDA project. *Forensic Science International*, *243*, 23–29.

Heltsley, R., Shelby, M. K., Crouch, D. J., Black, D. L., Robert, T. A., Marshall, L., et al. (2012). Prevalence of synthetic cannabinoids in US athletes: Initial findings. *Journal of Analytical Toxicology*, *36*, 588–593.

Hu, X., Primack, B. A., Barnett, T. E., & Cook, R. L. (2011). College students and use of K2: An emerging drug of abuse in young persons. *Substance Abuse Treatment, Prevention, and Policy*, *6*, 16.

Hudson, S., & Ramsey, J. (2011). The emergence and analysis of synthetic cannabinoids. *Drug Testing and Analysis*, *3*, 466–478.

Hunter, L. J., Dargan, P. I., Benzie, A., White, J. A., & Wood, D. M. (2014). Recreational drug use in men who have sex with men (MSM) attending UK sexual health services is significantly higher than in non-MSM. *Postgraduate Medical Journal*, *90*, 133–138.

Johnson, P. S., & Johnson, M. W. (2014). Investigation of "Bath Salts" use pattern within an online sample of users in the United States. *Journal of Psychoactive Drugs*, *46*, 369–378.

Johnson, L. A., Johnson, R. L., & Portier, R. B. (2013). Current "Legal highs" *Journal of Emergency Medicine, 44*, 1108–1115.

Katselou, M., Papoutsis, I., Nikolaou, P., Spiliopoulou, C., & Athanaselis, S. (2014). 5-(2-aminopropyl)indole: A new player in the drama of 'legal highs' alerts the community. *Drug and Alcohol Review, 34*, 51–57.

King, L. A. (2014). New phenethylamines in Europe. *Drug Testing and Analysis, 6*, 808–818.

Kronstrand, R., Roman, M., Dahlgren, M., Thelander, G., Wikström, M., & Druid, H. (2013). A cluster of deaths involving 5-(2-aminopropyl)indole (5-IT). *Journal of Analytical Toxicology, 37*, 542–546.

Loeffler, G., Hurst, D., Penn, A., & Yung, K. (2012). Spice, bath salts, and the U.S. military: The emergence of synthetic cannabinoid receptor agonists and cathinones in the U.S. Armed Forces. *Military Medicine, 177*, 1041–1048.

Maxwell, J. C. (2014). Psychoactive substances—Some new, some old: A scan of the situation in the U.S. *Drug and Alcohol Dependence, 134*, 71–77.

McElrath, K., & O'Neill, C. (2011). Experiences with mephedrone pre- and post-legislative control: Perceptions of safety and sources of supply. *International Journal on Drug Policy, 22*, 120–127.

McGraw, M., & McGraw, L. (2012). Bath salts: Not as harmless as they sound. *Journal of Emergency Nursing, 38*, 582–588.

Meyer, M. R., Du, P., Schuster, F., & Maurer, H. H. (2010). Studies on the metabolism of the α-pyrrolidinophenone designer drug methylenedioxypyrovalerone (MDPV) in rat and human urine and human liver microsomes using GC-MS and LC-high-resolution MS and its detectability in urine by GC-MS. *Journal of Mass Spectrometry, 45*, 1426–1442.

Meyer, M. R., & Maurer, H. H. (2010). Metabolism of designer drugs of abuse: An updated review. *Current Drug Metabolism, 11*, 461–482.

Meyer, M. R., Vollmar, C., Schwaninger, A. E., Wolf, E., & Maurer, H. H. (2012). New cathinone-derived designer drugs 3-bromomethcathinone and 3-fluoro-methcathinone: Studies on their metabolism in rat urine and human liver microsomes using GC-MS and LC- high-resolution MS and their detectability in urine. *Journal of Mass Spectrometry, 47*, 253–262.

Meyer, M. R., Wilhelm, J., Peters, F. T., & Maurer, H. H. (2010). Beta-keto amphetamines: Studies on the metabolism of the designer drug mephedrone and toxicological detection of mephedrone, butylone, and methylone in urine using gas chromatography-mass spectrometry. *Analytical and Bioanalytical Chemistry, 397*, 1225–1233.

Möller, I., Wintermeyer, A., Bender, K., Jübner, M., Thomas, A., Krug, O., et al. (2011). Screening for the synthetic cannabinoid JWH-018 and its major metabolites in human doping controls. *Drug Testing and Analysis, 3*, 609–620.

Monteiro, M. S., Bastos, Mde L., Guedes de Pinho, P., & Carvalho, M. (2013). Update on 1-benzylpiperazine (BZP) party pills. *Archives of Toxicology, 87*, 929–947.

Moore, K., Dargan, P. I., Wood, D. M., & Measham, F. (2013). Do novel psychoactive substances displace established club drugs, supplement them or act as drugs of initiation? The relationship between mephedrone, ecstasy and cocaine. *European Addiction Research, 19*, 276–283.

Motbey, C. P., Hunt, G. E., Bowen, M. T., Artissm, S., & McGregor, I. S. (2012). Mephedrone (4-methylmethcathinone, 'meow'): Acute behavioural effects and distribution of Fos expression in adolescent rats. *Addiction Biology, 17*, 409–422.

Musselman, M. E., & Hampton, J. P. (2014). "Not for human consumption": A review of emerging designer drugs. *Pharmacotherapy, 34*, 745–757.

Musshoff, F., Madea, B., Kernbach-Wighton, G., Bicker, W., Kneisel, S., Hutter, M., et al. (2014). Driving under the influence of synthetic cannabinoids ("Spice"): A case series. *International Journal of Legal Medicine, 128*, 59–64.

Paillet-Loilier, M., Cesbon, A., Le Boisselier, R., Jourgine, J., & Debruyene, D. (2014). Emerging drugs of abuse: Current perspectives on substituted cathinones. *Substance Abuse and Rehabilitation*, *5*, 37–52.

Papanti, D., Schifano, F., Botteon, G., Bertossi, F., Mannix, J., Vidoni, D., et al. (2013). "Spiceophrenia": A systematic overview of "spice"-related psychopathological issues and a case report. *Human Psychopharmacology: Clinical and Experimental*, *28*, 379–389.

Papaseit, E., Farré, M., Schifano, F., & Torrens, M. (2014). Emerging drugs in Europe. *Current Opinion in Psychiatry*, *27*, 243–250.

Pedersen, A. J., Petersen, T. H., & Linnet, K. (2013). In vitro metabolism and pharmacokinetic studies on methylone. *Drug Metabolism and Disposition*, *41*, 1247–1255.

Pedersen, A. J., Reitzel, L. A., Johansen, S. S., & Linnet, K. (2013). In vitro metabolism studies on mephedrone and analysis of forensic cases. *Drug Testing and Analysis*, *5*, 430–438.

Pertwee, R. G. (2005). Pharmacological action of cannabinoids. *Handbook of Experimental Pharmacology*, *168*, 1–51.

Presley, B. C., Jansen-Varnum, S. A., & Logan, B. K. (2013). Analysis of synthetic cannabinoids in botanical material: A review of analytical methods and findings. *Forensic Science Review*, *25*, 27–46.

Rojek, S., Kłys, M., Maciów-Głąb, M., Kula, K., & Strona, S. (2014). Cathinones derivatives-related deaths as exemplified by two fatal cases involving methcathinone with 4-methylmethcathinone and 4-methylethcathinone. *Drug Testing and Analysis*, *6*, 770–777.

Russo, R., Marks, N., Morris, K., King, H., Gelvin, A., & Rooney, R. (2012). Life-treating necrotizing fasciitis due to "bath salts" injection. *Orthopedics*, *25*, e124–e127.

Sacks, J., Ray, M. J., Williams, S., & Opatowsky, M. J. (2012). Fatal toxic leukoencephalopathy secondary to overdose of a new psychoactive designer drug 2C-E ("Europe"). *Proceedings (Baylor University. Medical Center)*, *25*, 374–376.

Schifano, F., Albanese, A., Fergus, S., Stair, J. L., Deluca, P., Corazza, O., et al. (2011). Mephedrone (4-methylmethcathinone; 'meow meow'): Chemical, pharmacological and clinical issues. *Psychopharmacology (Berlin)*, *214*, 593–602.

Seetohul, L. N., & Pounder, D. J. (2013). Four fatalities involving 5-IT. *Journal of Analytical Toxicology*, *37*, 447–451.

Shortall, S. E., Macerola, A. E., Swaby, R. T., Jayson, R., Korsah, C., Pillidge, K. E., et al. (2013). Behavioural and neurochemical comparison of chronic intermittent cathinone, mephedrone and MDMA administration to the rat. *European Neuropsychopharmacology*, *23*, 1085–1095.

Simmler, L. D., Buser, T. A., Donzelli, M., Schramm, Y., Dieu, L. H., Huwyler, J., et al. (2013). Pharmacological characterization of designer cathinones *in vitro*. *British Journal of Pharmacology*, *168*, 458–470.

Simmler, L. D., Rickli, A., Schramm, Y., Hoener, M. C., & Liechti, M. E. (2014). Pharmacological profiles of aminoindanes, piperazines, and pipradrol derivatives. *Biochemical Pharmacology*, *88*, 237–244.

Smith, C. D., & Robert, S. (2014). 'Designer drugs': Update on the management of novel psychoactive substance misuse in the acute care setting. *Clinical Medicine*, *14*, 409–415.

Spiller, H. A., Ryan, M. L., Weston, R. G., & Jansen, J. (2011). Clinical experience with analytic confirmation of "bath salts" and "legal highs" (synthetic cathinones) in the United States. *Clinical Toxicology (Philadelphia, Pa.)*, *49*, 499–505.

Strano-Rossi, S., Cadwallader, A. B., de la Torre, X., & Botrè, F. (2010). Toxicological determination and *in vitro* metabolism of the designer drug methylenedioxypyrovalerone (MDPV) by gas chromatography/mass spectrometry and liquid chromatography/quadrupole time-of-flight mass spectrometry. *Rapid Communications in Mass Spectrometry*, *24*, 2706–2714.

Stuart, D. (2013). Sexualised drug use by MSM: Background, current status and response. *HIV Nursing Journal, 13*, 6–10.

Tekulve, K., Alexander, A., & Tormoehlen, L. (2014). Seizures associated with synthetic cathinone exposures in the pediatric population. *Pediatric Neurology, 51*, 67–70.

Teske, J., Weller, J. P., Fieguth, A., Rothämel, T., Schulz, Y., & Tröger, H. D. (2010). Sensitive and rapid quantification of the cannabinoid receptor agonist naphthalen-1-yl-(1-pentylindol-3-yl)methanone (JWH-018) in human serum by liquid chromatography-tandem mass spectrometry. *Journal of Chromatography B, 878*, 2659–2663.

Tuv, S. S., Krabseth, H., Karinen, R., Olsen, K. M., Øiestad, E. L., & Vindenes, V. (2014). Prevalence of synthetic cannabinoids in blood samples from Norwegian drivers suspected of impaired driving during a seven weeks period. *Accident Analysis and Prevention, 62*, 26–31.

United Nations Office on Drugs and Crime (UNODC). (2013). Worlds drug report 2013. New psychoactive substances: Concepts and definitions, Vienna, pp. 60–115. Available at: http://www.unodc.org/unodc/secured/wdr/wdr2013/World_Drug_Report_2013.pdf. Accessed September 22, 2014.

Van Hout, M. C., & Bingham, T. (2012). "A costly turn on": Patterns of use and perceived consequences of mephedrone based head shop products amongst Irish injectors. *The International Journal on Drug Policy, 23*, 188–197.

Vandrey, R., Dunn, K. E., Fry, J. A., & Girling, E. R. (2012). A survey study to characterize use of Spice products (synthetic cannabinoids). *Drug and Alcohol Dependence, 120*, 238–241.

Vann, R. E., Warner, J. A., Bushell, K., Huffman, J. W., Martin, B. R., & Wiley, J. L. (2009). Discriminative stimulus properties of Δ^9-tetrahydrocannabinol (THC) in C57Bl/6J mice. *European Journal of Pharmacology, 615*, 102–107.

Vardakou, I., Pistos, C., & Spiliopoulou, C. (2010). Spice drugs as a new trend: Mode of action, identification and legislation. *Toxicology Letters, 197*, 157–162.

Watterson, L. R., Watterson, E., & Olive, M. F. (2013). Abuse liability of novel 'legal high' designer stimulants: Evidence from animal models. *Behavioral Pharmacology, 24*, 341–355.

Wiebelhaus, J. M., Poklis, J. L., Poklis, A., Vann, R. E., Lichtman, A. H., & Wise, L. E. (2012). Inhalation exposure to smoke from synthetic "marijuana" produces potent cannabimimetic effects in mice. *Drug and Alcohol Dependence, 126*, 316–323.

Wiley, J. L., Marusich, J. A., & Huffman, J. W. (2014). Moving around the molecule: Relationship between chemical structure and in vivo activity of synthetic cannabinoids. *Life Sciences, 97*, 55–63.

Winstock, A. R., & Barratt, M. J. (2013). Synthetic cannabis: A comparison of patterns of use and effect profile with natural cannabis in a large global sample. *Drug and Alcohol Dependence, 131*, 106–111.

Wood, D. M., Button, J., Lidder, S., Ramsey, J., Holt, D. W., & Dargan, P. I. (2008). Dissociative and sympathomimetic toxicity associated with recreational use of 1-(3-trifluoromethylphenyl)piperazine (TFMPP) and 1-benzylpiperazine (BZP). *Journal of Medical Toxicology, 4*, 254–257.

Wood, D. M., & Dargan, P. I. (2012). Use and acute toxicity associated with the novel psychoactive substances diphenylprolinol (D2PM) and desoxypipradrol (2-DPMP). *Clinical Toxicology (Philadelphia, Pa.), 50*, 727–732.

Wood, D. M., Puchnarewicz, M., Johnston, A., & Dargan, P. I. (2012). A case series of individuals with analytically confirmed acute diphenyl-2-pyrrolidinemethanol (D2PM) toxicity. *European Journal of Clinical Pharmacology, 68*, 349–353.

Yarosh, H. L., Katz, E. B., Coop, A., & Fantegrossi, W. E. (2007). MDMA-like behavioral effects of N-substituted piperazines in the mouse. *Pharmacology, Biochemistry, and Behavior, 88*, 18–27.

Yeakel, J. K., & Logan, B. K. (2013). Blood synthetic cannabinoid concentrations in cases of suspected impaired driving. *Journal of Analytical Toxicology*, *37*, 547–551.

Zawilska, J. B. (2011). "Legal highs"—New players in the old drama. *Current Drug Abuse Reviews*, *4*, 123–130.

Zawilska, J. B. (2014). Mephedrone and other cathinones. *Current Opinion in Psychiatry*, *27*, 256–262.

Zawilska, J. B., & Wojcieszak, J. (2013). Designer cathinones—An emerging class of novel recreational drugs. *Forensic Science International*, *231*, 42–53.

Zawilska, J. B., & Wojcieszak, J. (2014). Spice/K2 drugs: More than innocent substitutes for marijuana. *International Journal of Neuropsychopharmacology*, *17*, 509–525.

Zuba, D., & Byrska, B. (2013). Prevalence and co-existence of active components of 'legal highs'. *Drug Testing and Analysis*, *5*, 420–429.

Zuba, D., Byrska, B., & Maciow, M. (2011). Comparison of "herbal highs" composition. *Analytical and Bioanalytical Chemistry*, *400*, 119–126.

CHAPTER FOURTEEN

Psychostimulants and Artistic, Musical, and Literary Creativity

Iain Smith[1]
The Kershaw Unit, Gartnavel Royal Hospital, Glasgow, Scotland, United Kingdom
[1]Corresponding author: e-mail address: Iain.Smith@ggc.scot.nhs.uk

Contents

Abstract

This chapter explores links between psychostimulants and creativity in the arts. These links are set in the context of an overview of the association between mind-altering drugs in general and specific branches of the arts, particularly literature. The economic impact of the psychostimulants both historically and in today's world has been substantial and this is mirrored in the culture of the countries involved with the trade in these special commodities. As with other families of addictive drugs, the psychostimulants are sought out more frequently than is the norm by creative individuals who then may represent the drugs in their art or associate the drugs with their creativity. The creative process is outlined and it is noted that if a drug helps at all with creativity then the specific properties of the drug may link it to a particular stage of the creative process. Stimulants are particularly associated with the evaluation and elaboration stage of the creative process and in particular nicotine and caffeine have been used in this way by writers when putting words on paper. The ability of psychostimulants to boost

International Review of Neurobiology, Volume 120
ISSN 0074-7742
http://dx.doi.org/10.1016/bs.irn.2015.04.001

convergent thinking is the main mechanism at work but this is at a cost as divergent thinking is diminished. The other findings of note in this review are that particular venues based around the consumption of a psychostimulants can act as a creative hub-café culture in Paris and Vienna and early modern Europe—and that particular drugs can come to define an artistic grouping as with the Beats and the group around Warhol who had a preference for amphetamine.

1. INTRODUCTION

I'd hate to advocate drugs, alcohol or insanity to anyone, but they've always worked for me

Hunter S. Thompson

If we take as our starting point the broad classification of mind-acting drugs into sedatives, psychostimulants, opiates, hallucinogens, and drugs with mixed actions (Edwards, 2005), then the two main groups of drugs that one would logically turn to first to examine the claim that drugs enhance creativity are undoubtedly the psychostimulants and the hallucinogens. (There are, of course, some drugs such as MDMA—which we will consider here under psychostimulants—which blur the boundaries of these broad categories in our classification of mind-altering drugs e.g., drugs with mixed actions that combine psychostimulant and hallucinogenic properties.) Drugs with sedative properties, such as alcohol and benzodiazepines, and the opiates such as morphine which also sedate and slow cognition, are at first sight less likely candidates for enhancing creativity. Perhaps, an easier way to think of mind-altering drugs is as "Uppers, Downers and All Arounders" (Inaba & Cohen, 2011).

All mind-altering drugs have been examined to some degree in relation to creativity in controlled settings and all in addition have their links to artistic endeavor through visual, musical, and literary forms. In looking at psychostimulants in relation to creativity, we need to first consider some aspects of the psychology of creativity before looking at specific research on drugs in general in relation to creativity. We can then focus on the main psychostimulants in relation to cultural history and creativity. We will examine these in order of historical importance. This is, perhaps unsurprisingly, an order reflective of current levels of global usage. We will look, therefore, at caffeine, nicotine, cocaine, amphetamine, methamphetamine, MDMA/Ecstasy, and other psychostimulants including methylphenidate in turn.

It is worth noting here the general contribution of literary and historical studies to the field of addiction and to our understanding of mind-altering substances. Such studies can:

(a) Act as an adjunct to medical education.
(b) Foster an awareness of possible explanatory stories about drug use and drug effects.
(c) Produce lessons from history for policymakers. Addiction and drug taking are often portrayed as new phenomena and the past is suppressed.
(d) Show that the concerns of novels and biographies, including "biographies" of drugs themselves, can act as a mirror of the times. In this regard, there are many recent examples of this genre involving psychostimulants including recovery stories and "scare" stories. Books presenting "biographies," i.e., histories, of psychostimulants are also in vogue, as outlined below.

One interesting historical finding is that the use of the word "stimulant" was used more loosely in the past such that one can find literary and technical references to alcohol and opiates as "stimulants" (Historical Thesaurus: Home: Welcome, 2012). The initial disinhibition and mood enhancement produced by such drugs can produce the illusion of cognitive enhancement and stimulation while objectively the person is slowed and less reactive to stimuli. The review here confines itself to the drugs we would currently recognize under the rubric of stimulant/psychostimulant.

2. CREATIVITY RESEARCH

A simple definition of creativity is that it is the process of producing something new and worthwhile and that it involves an act of imagination.

Creativity is not confined to the Arts, but it is in the relationship with the Arts that the claimed association between creativity and drug use and the psychostimulants in particular comes to the fore.

There are many theories of creativity and it is an academic area that has brought together many disciplines from archeology through to zoology. The field is well reviewed in *The Encyclopedia of Creativity* (Runco & Pritzker, 2011). Modern neuroscience holds out the prospect of a neurobiological understanding of the creative process (Abraham et al., 2012) and this in turn opens up the prospect of a better understanding of how drugs might influence it (see various entries on cognitive enhancement in Nutt, Robbins, Stimson, Ince, and Jackson, (2007)).

As with most complex human psychological traits, there is an interplay between endogenous and exogenous factors in producing creativity in individuals. Of interest here are the propositions that:

(1) There is linkage between mental illness and creativity.

and

(2) There can be an influence of social groups on creativity with the group coalescing around a particular meeting place (e.g., a coffee house) or a particular drug (e.g., the Beats and the amphetamines).

The fact that individuals who are acknowledged to be particularly creative are more likely than controls to have other creative individuals in their family and also more likely to share particular forms of mental illness suggests a common genetic origin for creativity, psychosis, and affective disorder and possibly substance misuse. One hypothesis is that psychotic thinking, which is overinclusive and makes connections between ideas, which, to others, seem irrational, is an extreme example of creative thinking. Creativity is by definition the bringing together of elements that have not previously been connected in that particular way whether in a painting, song, or novel. (See Mednick, 1962, on the associative basis of creativity.)

The link between affective disorders and creativity is part of the explanation as to why alcohol and drug misuse and dependence are overrepresented in creative individuals and in their relatives, given the recognized comorbidity between the two types of disorder. The Bipolar II form of bipolar affective disorder, for example, has a particular association with substance use disorders.

As an illustration of this link, the American Psychiatrist Arnold Ludwig studied reviews of biographies in the New York Review of Books. Using reviews published between 1960 and 1990, he compared the lives of scientists with those of artists, writers, composers, and musicians. He found that the subjects who worked in the Arts were more likely than scientists to have suffered mental illness and to have used mind-altering substances (Ludwig, 1992).

Additionally, Ludwig showed differences within the creative arts. Unfortunately, he does not give us the fine detail of the drugs involved usually with alcohol misuse and mental illness clustering in the same individual, but given the European and American bias to the reviews undoubtedly amphetamines and cocaine will have featured alongside the opiates and to a lesser extent hallucinogens. Earlier the North American psychiatrist Andreasen (1987) had shown the link between creativity and mental illness. The British psychiatrist Felix Post in two widely cited papers further confirmed this association (Post, 1994, 1996).

3. STAGES OF THE CREATIVE PROCESS

Psychologists have identified that the creative process involves different stages and one common way to portray this is in a five-stage model as follows:

The Five Stages of Creativity

1. Preparation
2. Incubation
3. Insight
4. Evaluation
5. Elaboration

From Wallas, 1926 as cited in Runco and Pritzker (2011).

This idea of stages of creativity opens up the possibility that different types of drugs are more likely to be useful and, therefore, used at different stages of the creative process. This relates also to the concepts of Convergent Thinking and Divergent Thinking (Baird et al., 2012) and the differential effects of mind-acting drugs on these two forms of thought processes. Thus, hallucinogens, opiates, and sedatives are more likely to lead to divergent thinking and to be linked to the incubation and insight, and perhaps also the preparation stages of creativity.

This idea is well captured by this quote from Rimbaud:

> *The Poet makes himself a seer by a.... derangement of all the senses.*

The idea is often, also, illustrated in books linking drugs to creativity by quoting William Blake:

> *"If the doors of perception were cleansed, everything would appear to man as infinite*
> *For man has closed himself up, till he sees all things thro' narrow chinks of his cavern"*

And, also from Blake:

> *"The road of excess leads to the palace of wisdom"*

The titles of Aldous Huxley's "The Doors of Perception" (Huxley, Harper, & Brothers, 1954) describing his mescaline experiences and Marcus Boon's "The Road of Excess: A History of Writers on Drugs" (Boon, 2002) are both referencing Blake, the visionary poet and artist.

Psychostimulants are more likely to assist in the evaluation and elaboration stages of creativity and also with certain aspects of the preparation stage. They are recognized to bolster convergent and decrease divergent thinking.

Think of a writer who works in the morning fuelled by coffee and cigarettes and then socializes in the evening over copious amounts of alcohol. One can find many examples of famous authors who fit this pattern. Hemingway and Fitzgerald are good examples and the link between alcoholism and literary achievement among American writers has been discussed fully by Dardis (1989) in his book "The Thirsty Muse."

However, most laboratory-based studies suggest little or no benefit to creativity of using substances particularly those with depressant properties.

One study, for example, showed that when intoxicated individuals were asked to perform creative tasks they believed their work to be superior when in fact it showed a decrease in divergent thinking (Kowal et al., 2015).

There are many confounders in researching the effects of mind-altering drugs on creativity. One is that in a regular user of a drug, say caffeine or nicotine, an apparent improvement may be more down to a suppression of a withdrawal state rather than a direct effect of the drug. For some of the science behind this, see Iversen's Speed, Ecstasy, Ritalin (2006) and his chapter on the pharmacology of nicotine in Smoke (Gilman & Zhou, 2004). The evidence in relation to the ambiguous relation between caffeine and creativity is well reviewed also by Konnikova (2013). Another confounder is that all mind-altering drugs affect sleep and the stimulants in particular lessen sleep, which may be particularly bad for creativity, which has a link to REM/dream sleep (Killgore et al., 2008). Amphetamine research suggests a trade-off between cognitive enhancement and creativity in keeping with the convergent–divergent thinking model (Farah, Haimm, Sankoorikal, Smith, & Chatterjee, 2009).

4. DRUGS, CREATIVITY, AND CULTURAL HISTORY

The history of Western colonialism and Empire building is inextricably linked with the "discovery" and marketing of valued commodities. This trade produced great wealth and had major cultural and artistic resonance. Tea, coffee, cocoa, tobacco, sugar, opium, cannabis (Hemp), and Coca commerce, and the contemporaneous discovery of alcohol distillation were major forces in European and world history from the sixteenth through to the nineteenth century (see Devine (1975) for Tobacco; Mills (2003) for Cannabis; Porter and Teich (1995), Schivelbusch (1992), and Courtwright (2001) for all of the other addictive commodities).

Psychostimulants are well represented in this list of lucrative merchandise: caffeine (tea and coffee and cocoa/chocolate), nicotine (tobacco), and cocaine (coca) sit alongside theobromine (cocoa/chocolate). The wealth produced by this trade in mind-altering substances would support artistic endeavor through patronage and the creation of a culture with disposable income that valued art as commodity in all its forms. The merchants who with their families would be painted and represented by the artists they sponsored and commissioned would become the new aristocracy of the early modern world.

The first three drugs in our list of psychostimulants are all eventually extracted from plants: caffeine from tea and coffee, nicotine from tobacco, and cocaine from the coca plant. These plants were all nonnative to the Old World of European civilization. All continue to have major economic import today either legitimately (caffeine and nicotine) or illicitly in the case of cocaine.

Although no longer viewed in a technical sense as a "stimulant" any broad discussion on drugs and creativity needs to give a special place to alcohol. Alcohol is as old as human history and is well referenced in early Greco-Roman and Judeo-Christian written records.

The Bible famously treats wine with ambivalence. The prophet Isaiah warns, for example:

> *"Woe to those who rise early in the morning to run after their drinks, who stay up late at night till they are inflamed with wine. They have harps and lyres at their banquets, tambourines and flutes and wine, but they have no regard for the deeds of the Lord, no respect for the work of his hands."*
>
> ***Isaiah, Chapter 5, Verse 11.***

However, alcohol is also celebrated in other passages—e.g., the miracle at the wedding at Cana—and for Christians, it becomes part of the Eucharist. Overall though the scriptures warn against alcohol in excess and in Western culture beyond the Romans the pursuit of intoxication is condemned both socially and legally. This changes in the modern era where greater variation is seen in how alcohol is viewed by society. Consumption veers between extremes of prohibition and varying degrees of control within a liberal, free market.

It is with the Arts and modern bohemian writers that we get the idea of alcohol as an agent of mystical transport. Baudelaire instructs the writer to "Be drunk always." Absinthe drinking was particularly associated with a culture of creativity in Paris and Europe in the late nineteenth and early twentieth century, Celebrated imbibers included Emile Zola, Vincent van Gogh, Henri de Toulouse-Lautrec, James Joyce, and Ernest Hemingway. Hemingway is one of a group of American writers who combined alcoholism with high literary achievement. Dardis in The Thirsty Muse (1989) points to the fact that five of the eight Americans awarded the Nobel Prize for literature up to that date were alcoholics. He looks at three of the five in depth: Hemingway, Faulkner, O'Neill alongside F. Scott Fitzgerald who though not a Nobel prize winner is the paradigmatic writer of the Jazz age. (He leaves out John Steinbeck and Sinclair Lewis, the other two native born and alcoholic U.S. writers who were Nobel laureates.) For a short general review of alcohol and creativity, see Beveridge and Yorston (1999).

There is an even stronger association between opiates—again, today, no longer viewed as "stimulants"—and the creative arts through the association with the Romantics. The list includes the poets Coleridge, Keats, the composer Berlioz, and later the writers Marcel Proust and Edgar Allan Poe. Most notable and influential was the initially serialized then fully published account by Thomas De Quincey (De Quincey, 2013) of his addiction to opium. De Quincey declared boldly that:

> *"...upon all that has been hitherto written on the subject of opium...I have but one emphatic criticism to pronounce - Lies! Lies! Lies!"*
>
> ***Confessions of an English Opium-Eater (1822).***

Morrison (2009) in his biography emphasizes the extent of De Quincey's influence in both the British Isles and abroad. For example, a French translation ofDe Quincey influenced Berlioz in writing the *Symphonie Fantastique (1830)* and over a century later William Seward Burroughs, author of *Junky* (1977) and *The Naked Lunch* (1986), stated that "De Quincey wrote the first, and still the best, book about drug addiction."

For De Quincey, opium was a technique for parting the veils "between our present consciousness and the secret inscriptions on the mind." This statement is very similar to those made by the advocates of mescaline and LSD in the mid-twentieth century. (See Huxley (1954) on mescaline and Stevens (1988) and Lattin (2010) on LSD and American culture.)

De Quincey's account of the detail of his drug use—both good and bad—seems to have little resonance with the phenomenology of the experience of our current opiate-addicted patients. Few modern opiate addicts talk of wild dreams or visionary experience. Certainly, the emphasis by De Quincey as to the addictive nature of opium does accord with modern experience with heroin and the difficulties faced by addicts in giving up their habit.

This is, interestingly, challenged in "Romancing Opiates: Pharmacological Lies and the Addiction Bureaucracy" by Dalrymple (2006). Dalrymple asks if we have bought into a concept of heroin dependence that was produced by a literary tradition that has influenced public opinion and in turn the medical response to it. Undoubtedly, it can be hard to fully separate the effects of a drug from one's socially determined expectations of that drug's effect and experiments abound that use drug expectancy to show a response in particular contexts where no active drug is consumed (Dawkins, Shahzad, Ahmed, & Edmonds, 2011).

Despite attempts by some novelists and artists with alcohol or drug problems to mythologize and to claim that they created great works, while intoxicated most have been more honest in admitting, it was in the periods between intoxication that they were productive albeit drawing on their experiences around alcohol or drugs. There is good scholarship debunking some of the cases where authors or artists claimed to create under the influence of drugs—see John Sutherland—"Turns Unstoned," Times literary supplement, 30/10/98 (1998) and his "Last Drink to L.A."(2001).

There still exists an active prodrugs literature often reminding us of the long history of drug taking for creative and spiritual purposes—e.g., Pharmakon-Drugs and the Imagination by Vayne (2006)—with most of the drugs referenced having hallucinogenic properties. Arguably such drug use goes back into the depths of our evolutionary history (Hill & Newlin, 2002; Samorini, 2002) and our cultural history (Bancroft, 2009; Berridge, 2013; Davenport-Hines, 2002; Hillman, 2008; Jay & Wellcome, 2010; Walton, 2001b) and the persistence of such tribal traditions can be a challenge in our world of the global economy. The stimulant khat is one example of this (Anderson, 2007).

It is also important to realize that different types of narrative exist in memoirs and novels in terms of explanation of addiction and drug use and also of recovery from addiction (see "Narratives of Recovery from Addictive Behaviour," Hanninen & Koski-Jannes, 1999; Hurwitz, Tapping, & Vickers, 2007). The worldwide success of the AA and NA movement and other 12-Step programs has provided the predominant narrative for addiction and recovery. Thus, Cocaine Anonymous, for example, will portray cocaine addiction as a downward spiral to either death or an eventual realization from a personal "gutter" that total abstinence and spiritual renewal is the only answer in the knowledge that the next relapse might be the one that proves fatal.

5. DRUG DISCOVERY AND SYNTHESIS

Mike Jay who has written extensively on issues of drugs, culture, and creativity (Jay, 1999, 2011; Jay & Wellcome, 2010) makes an interesting observation in his Emperors of Dreams (2000). This is that the history of mind-altering drugs often follows the Frankenstein narrative:

Act one: the drug is discovered and its novelties and benefits celebrated.
Act two: the drug escapes from the laboratory and makes its journey in the world.
Act three: the powers that be unite in their attempt to extinguish it.

This narrative seems particularly pertinent to the psychostimulants and particularly those, which are more potent and have abuse potential and those, which have been rendered illegal. Cocaine, caffeine, and nicotine are all extracted from plant sources whereas the amphetamines and MDMA were synthesized in the laboratory. Cocaine, the amphetamines, and MDMA are the drugs, which most closely follow the narrative outlined by Jay. Also nicotine in the form of tobacco is belatedly subject to an Act three. It remains to be seen as to whether nicotine in its most recent incarnation of e-cigarettes, apparently untethered from the carcinogens in tobacco smoke, will suffer a similar fate or become as socially acceptable as caffeine.

Given that doctors—medical men, in particular, in the nineteenth century—were central to drug discovery and exploration they were also at greater risk of being seduced and subverted by drugs with addictive potential given their privileged access. Even the more recent history of medicine and in particular psychiatry has examples of this continuing dilemma particularly in relation to LSD (Dyck, 2008; Sandison, Spencer, & Whitelaw, 1954). The counter culture of the 1960s based around LSD again found voices from within the medical profession arguing against the prohibition of the drug and advocating its use (Lattin, 2010; Stevens, 1988). Doctors remain interested in the possibility that illicit mind-altering drugs may have therapeutic benefit, e.g., LSD, MDMA, and Ketamine, but remain constrained by restrictions on their use (Nutt et al., 2007; Sessa, 2012).

Literature on the sick doctor is also of interest in teaching and self-awareness for doctors. It reflects the predominance of alcohol and drug problems as the main cause of impairment in "impaired physicians" alongside mental illness. For a modern example of this read, "The Tennis Partner" (Verghese, 1998), a tragic account of a cocaine-addicted doctor written by an older mentor.

6. PSYCHOSTIMULANTS AND CREATIVITY

Two recent popular films—Limitless (2011) and Lucy (2014)—illustrate an interest in the possibility that drugs might be used for cognitive enhancement and to increase creativity and "brainpower." Both use fictional drugs but these appear to be stimulant as well as nootropic in nature

(Wijdicks, 2015, see pp. 246–247 for a discussion of Limitless). Generally psychostimulants increase convergent thinking and attention—at optimal doses—and decrease divergent thinking; however, in the worlds of these two science fiction films, the drugs seem to achieve the improbable feat of increasing divergent and convergent thinking simultaneously.

We will now look at the psychostimulants individually in relation to literature including drama and film followed by visual art and popular music. Inevitably, this is selective in nature given limitations of space.

7. PSYCHOSTIMULANTS, LITERATURE, AND LITERARY SCENES

There are now a large number of anthologies of drug "literature" with both historical and original, sometimes specially commissioned, pieces many of which are stimulant related. Worthwhile examples of the genre can be found with the following editors: Davidson (1998), Haining (1998), Jay (1999), Melechi (1997, 1998), Miller and Koral (1995), Rudgley (2001), Shannonhouse (2003), and Strausbaugh and Blaise (1991). The psychostimulants are referenced in around 20% of the stories and historical excerpts that are included in these selections albeit with some repetition of seminal sources such as Freud on cocaine. The broader field has been well analyzed in two books of literary criticism (Boon, 2002; Plant, 1999) and also more briefly in the review by Day and Smith in relation to medical education (2003).

7.1 Caffeine

Caffeine is the most ubiquitous of the psychostimulants. So much so that we tend to forget its status as a legal drug that is beyond regulation, other than those that pertain to food and nonalcoholic drinks. Caffeine is obtainable in many different formulations from coffee to tea to caffeinated soft drinks and over the counter tonics. The main formulation of interest in relation to culture and creativity is that of coffee. Historically coffee was viewed as a potentially dangerous substance in contrast to today's more benign viewpoint. This is illustrated here:

> *"[Coffee causes] an excessive state of brain-excitation which becomes manifest by a remarkable loquaciousness sometimes accompanied by accelerated association of ideas. It may also be observed in coffee house politicians who drink cup after cup ... and by this abuse are inspired to profound wisdom on all earthly events."*
>
> *Quoted in Lewin (1931): Phantastica: Narcotic and Stimulating Drugs*

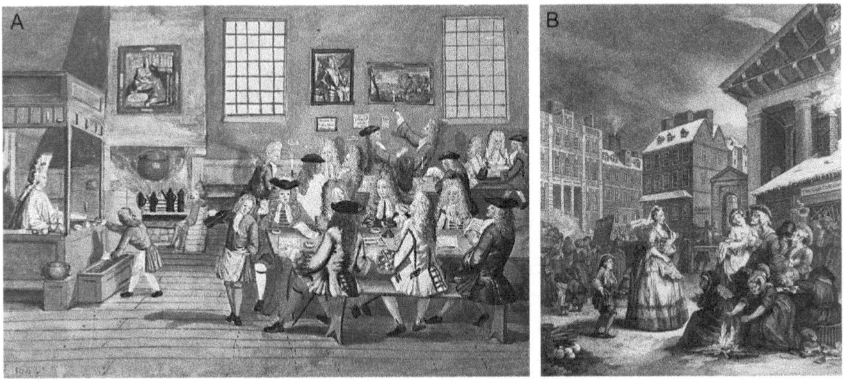

Figure 1 Coffeehouse Scenes. (A) Lordprice Collection/Alamy. (B) Public Domain-Tom King's Coffeehouse by William Hogarth, http://commons.wikimedia.org.

In early modern Europe, coffeehouses (Fig. 1) were viewed with some suspicion by the authorities of the day. They became important social hubs for commerce and creativity and a place to learn the latest news from home and abroad. In the great artistic and literary cities of Paris in the nineteenth and twentieth centuries and in fin-de-siècle Vienna, the café was of central importance for the creative individuals who gathered there.

An example is the French writer Balzac. He ingested what may have been 2–3 g of caffeine in a day in the form of ground coffee beans into an empty stomach. Balzac described this as "horrible, rather brutal," and only for men of "excessive vigor." He wrote of the consequences in relation to his writing in his 1839 essay "Traité des Excitants Modernes" ("Treatise on Modern Stimulants") thus:

> *"Sparks shoot all the way up to the brain" while "ideas quick-march into motion like battalions of a grand army to its legendary fighting ground, and the battle rages.*

Our modern expectation would be that such an overdose of caffeine would hinder rather than help writing. All hinges on the optimal dose of caffeine in keeping with the Yerkes–Dodson law. For more on how caffeine can "Cramp Creativity," see the article by Konnikova (2013) cited below.

The Jim Jarmusch film Coffee and Cigarettes (2003) gives us a series of fictional encounters between individuals, smoking and drinking coffee, in social and creative interaction. Thus, Iggy Pop meets Tom Waits and so on through a number of vignettes. The recent widespread banning of smoking in enclosed public places is breaking this connection with coffee to a degree, but it has been historically important in relation to literary and artistic communities and the social interchange that allowed such groups to come to prominence in particular locations at particular times.

There are two excellent "biographies" of coffee available (Pendergrast, 1999; Weinberg & Bealer, 2001). The coffeehouse remains widely visible in our modern society and most will still provide newspapers and on occasions promote works of fiction.

7.2 Nicotine

Nicotine was eventually purified and identified as the main psychoactive drug in tobacco in 1893. The name was given to the drug so identified in tobacco in honor of Jean Nicot de Villemain, who in 1560 introduced the plant (*Nicotiana tabacum*) to the court in Paris via Portugal where he was French ambassador. The seeds and tobacco had arrived from Brazil.

Nicotine like cocaine is viewed as one of the most potent and addictive of all drugs, and this potency has led to mass use of tobacco in all its forms with powerful cultural and creative associations being forged with smoking. This is well documented in The Faber Book of Smoking (Walton, 2001a), and the wonderfully illustrated Smoke (Gilman & Zhou, 2004).

The strength of the association for addicted writers is well illustrated in this Dennis Potter quote taken from The Faber Book of Smoking:

> *Nobody has yet been able to demonstrate to me how I can join words into whole sentences on a blank page without a cigarette burning away between my lips.*

This strong identification of creativity with smoking can be found with a number of famous writers. J.M. Barrie and his My Lady Nicotine is an example of a writer in love with tobacco and describe Barrie's difficulty in giving up pipe smoking at the behest of his wife-to-be. It is typical of a literature that was common between the 1880s and 1910s, which Umberger (Gilman & Zhou, 2004) describes as a "fumophile literature" (Fig. 2). These books were for pipe and cigar smoking men, usually bachelors, and associated pipe smoking in particular with hours of quiet contemplation, relaxation, and male bonding.

The playwright Simon Gray in his The Smoking Diaries confesses in his 66th year to a 65 cigarettes per day habit, but this use of cigarettes is a backdrop to a brutally honest literary diary which is both comedic and tragic in turn.

Richard Klein states in the Introduction to Cigarettes are Sublime, a more recent example of fumophile literature that "(his) aim in this book is to praise cigarettes, but certainly not to encourage smoking...." The book

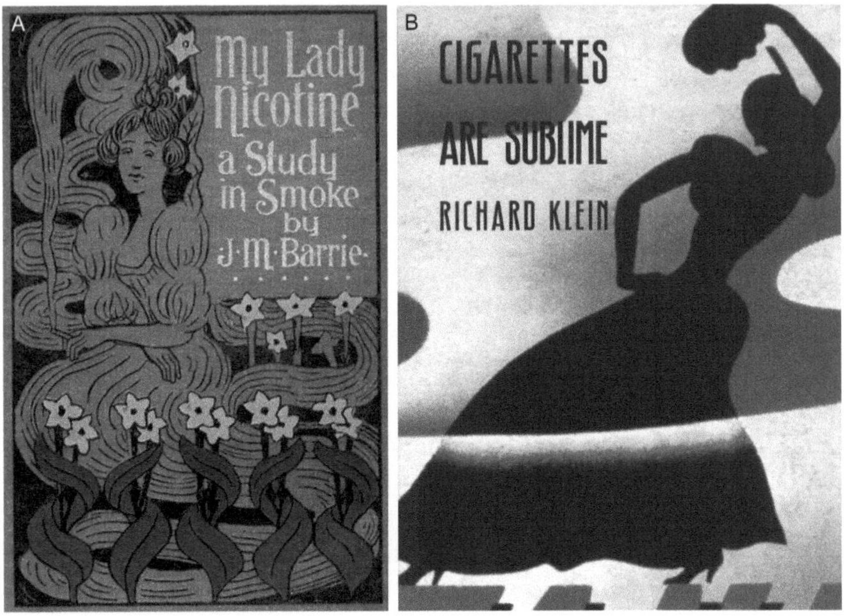

Figure 2 Examples of Fumophile Literature. (A) Public Domain, http://commons.wikimedia.org. (B) Republished by the permission of copyright holder www.dukeupress.edu.

then goes on to celebrate the use of the cigarette and the culture which "surrounds cigarettes and to which they gave rise" in what another author has branded "The Cigarette Century" (Brandt, 2007).

X20 (A Novel of Not Smoking) by Beard (1997) explores the difficulties of giving up cigarettes through the device of an author who has to write in a notebook every time he craves a cigarette in order to avoid succumbing to the urge to smoke. The novel is cleverly structured with a countdown over 20 days of the number of times the notebook is reached for, from 20 down to 1. It contains interesting subplots on the quest for a safe cigarette and the business of selling an addictive and lethal product. Each of the notebook entries is smoking related.

The novel Thank You For Smoking by Buckley (1994) is a black comedy centered on, Nick Naylor, a tobacco lobbyist in Washington. Along with lobbyists for alcohol and firearms he is part of the "M.O.D. Squad" with M.O.D. standing for the Merchants of Death. A moment of irony in the book is when Naylor is taken hostage and there is an attempt to kill him by covering him in nicotine patches, which he survives. However, he is rendered hypersensitive to nicotine and intolerant of smoking. The novel and the film based on it (2005) are superb at illustrating the doublethink of an industry trying to deny what had become obvious: the fact it is selling a poisonous and lethal product. The attempt of Naylor to deny that people continue to smoke because of choice rather than addiction has also fully unraveled over the last 20 years.

Based on an unpublished novel, another satirical film worth viewing in relation to Big Tobacco is Cold Turkey (1971). A small mid-American town attempts to win a huge financial prize offered by a tobacco company—in an ill thought out quest for publicity—for a town or city to become smoke free for 30 days. The mass nicotine withdrawal of the heavy smoking town and the prospect of excessive riches coming to the inhabitants have comedic expected and unexpected effects.

Tobacco also has its biographies. As well as Smoke and The Cigarette Century above there are works such as Gately's Tobacco (2001): A Cultural History of How an Exotic Plant Seduced Civilisation.

7.3 Cocaine

Boon (2002) comments, "the history of cocaine has been reviewed many times, a surprisingly large number of times in fact." Recent examples of such cocaine "biographies" include those by Constable (2002), Durlacher (2000), Karch (1998), Madge (2001), Naish and Scott (2013), Streatfield (2001), and Strongman (1997). If we add these to those that Boon is referring to from 1901 onward, the list is "surprisingly" large indeed. Perhaps, addictive drugs are surveyed more than other types of commodity in this way.

The most famous example of an eminent creative genius and medical man becoming enchanted with a psychostimulant drug and then later disillusioned with it is that of Sigmund Freud's dalliance with cocaine (Markel, 2011). Freud himself published a scientific monograph on the subject in Über Coca (On Cocaine) (Freud, 1884). He became personally enamored with the drug but eventually realized his daily use was a form of addiction that he had to break free from as he observed its destructive ability in others.

From fiction, the obvious example of a cocaine-using genius is Sherlock Holmes. Here, Conan Doyle's narrator Dr. Watson describes the great detective thus:

> *.... Holmes, who loathed every form of society with his whole Bohemian soul, remained in our lodgings in Baker Street, buried among his old books, and alternating from week to week between cocaine and ambition, the drowsiness of the drug, and the fierce energy of his own keen nature.*
>
> ***(Scandal 1.2).***

The attribution of drowsiness to cocaine seems to show a surprising confusion with opium, which Holmes used only occasionally. Holmes also introduces the modern innovation of injecting the cocaine (a 7% solution) using a needle and syringe that he keeps in a Morocco leather case.

The fact that Watson later helps Holmes overcome his addiction in the Conan Doyle stories is used as a starting point for the novel and film The Seven-Per-Cent Solution written by Meyer (1974). In this novel, the imaginary meets the real in that through an introduction by Dr. Watson Holmes meets Freud who uses hypnosis to cure the cocaine addiction and a delusional state induced by the cocaine.

Also in fiction while we are left guessing as to what type of substance will turn a Dr. Jekyll into a Mr. Hyde, it is well documented that Stevenson produced a first draft of the story (1886) under the influence of cocaine, which his wife tore up. In a less intoxicated state, he reproduced the story that has become emblematic of character change brought about by the ingestion of a drug.

The fictionalized autobiography Iced (Shell, 1993) is one of the most striking accounts of a descent into a personal hell due to crack cocaine addiction. Again, the stream of consciousness style is used in the narrative to reflect the mindset of the protagonist.

7.4 Amphetamine and Methamphetamine

Nicolas Rasmussen's "On Speed—The Many Lives of Amphetamine" (2008) is an excellent history of the drug first synthesized and discovered in California by Gordon Alles. If any drug was going to fit with the American psyche in relation to entrepreneurship and hard work then these new "pep pills" seemed an ideal candidate. Marketed originally in the 1930s as antidepressants here we have another drug, amphetamine, which with its many derivatives again gives us an example of Jay's Frankenstein narrative.

Amphetamines also became significant in World War Two with troops and airmen issued with the drugs to be used as a way to sustain attention during periods of prolonged combat or during a long-range bombing mission. Rasmussen shows us, however, that the evidence for the combat enhancing effects of amphetamine remained ambiguous despite trials on U.S. troops at the time. The Germans abandoned methamphetamine due to unpredictable effects including "friendly fire" incidents (Ulrich, 2005).

When Jack Kerouac sat down to write the first draft of On The Road (1957) in April, 1951 fuelled by caffeine, nicotine, and Benzedrine

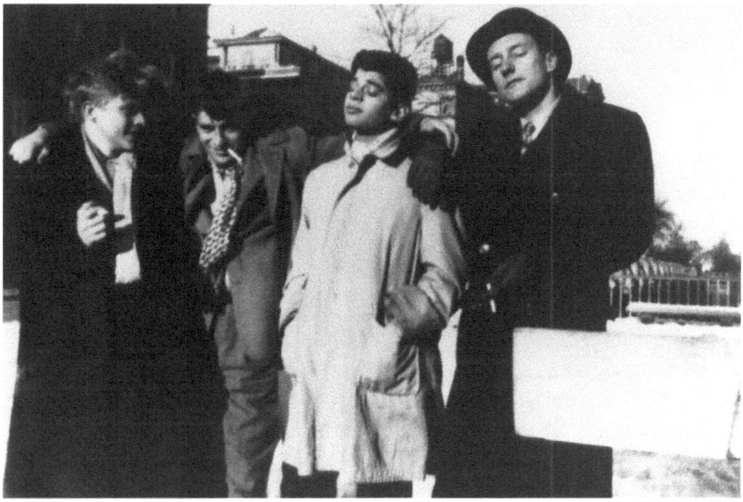

Figure 3 The key Beats as young men—Kerouac, Ginsberg, and Burroughs Sr. (L–R) with Hal Chase (far left). © *Allen Ginsberg/CORBIS.*

(dl-amphetamine) (and pea soup from his wife), it seems fitting that the first draft was produced in 3 weeks on a continuous 120 feet roll of paper called by Kerouac "The Scroll." This text produced without paragraphs or margins in a stream of consciousness fashion is typical of the genre of amphetamine-related literature that was to follow.

The literary and musical grouping that became known as the Beats (aka Beatniks) included William Burroughs and Allan Ginsberg (Fig. 3). Ginsberg's long poem Howl, written in a specific coffeehouse, refers to Benzedrine as a way to seek:

"the ancient heavenly connection to the starry dynamo in the machinery of night"

Amphetamine use also features in Junky by William Burroughs though heroin is the main drug being sought by William Lee, Burroughs' alter ego in the novel. The Beats experimented with many drugs but arguably the stimulants were the central drugs in this creative grouping.

William Burroughs Junior followed in his father's footsteps in producing drug-related autobiographical novels. Unlike his father, his life was cut short by his drug use at the tragically young age of 33 years. His two completed novels were Speed (1970) and Kentucky Ham (1973). The first recounts the progression of his methamphetamine addiction and the second starts with his admission to the Federal Narcotic Farm in Lexington, Kentucky.

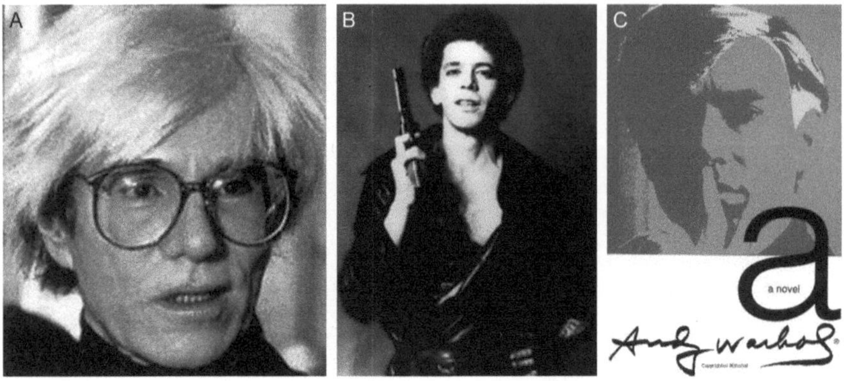

Figure 4 (A) Andy Warhol (Drella) and (B) Lou Reed (Lou) both feature in (C) a-A NOVEL. (A) wpclipart.com and (B) http://commons.wikimedia.org—both Public Domain; (C) © 2015 The Andy Warhol Foundation for the Visual Arts, Inc./Artists Rights Society (ARS), New York.

The association of the amphetamines with the arts in the United States was carried on into the 1960s with the various circles that formed around Andy Warhol in New York. The Factory was a center for the conjunction of popular music, visual, and cinematic art, and literature and amphetamine use. In Warhol's "a-A NOVEL," the "a" does indeed refer to amphetamine, and the book was initially conceived as a 24-h period in the life of Ondine, an actor, amphetamine addict and a Warhol Superstar captured on audiotape in a transcript also featuring Warhol, and 17 others including Lou Reed (Fig. 4). Four women including the drummer of the Velvet Underground later transcribed the tapes.

It is also speculated that Bob Dylan was referring to Edie Sedgwick, a Warhol associate, featured in the novel in these lines from "Just Like a Woman":

"Nobody has to guess
That Baby can't be blessed
Till she sees finally that she's like all the rest
With her fog, her amphetamine and her pearls"

Another novel based around the disaffected of New York is Hubert Selby Junior's Requiem for a Dream (1979), this novel, from the author of Last Exit to Brooklyn (1987), and also later a film, as well as showing the degradation brought about by heroin addiction shows us the danger of amphetamines as a legally prescribed diet aid when the mother of one of the protagonists becomes addicted and then suffers an amphetamine psychosis which leads to hospitalization.

Today, some of the best writing on drug-related topics is to be found in TV drama from the United States. The Wire, for example, showing the manifestations of the War on Drugs in Baltimore and, in particular, in Breaking Bad a series often approached through the medium of the "boxset." The main drug in Breaking Bad is methamphetamine in the form of crystal meth with the dying chemistry teacher anti-hero aiming to give his family financial security through his use of his synthetic skills to "cook" and sell the lucrative illicit product. The program is remarkably well informed on the chemistry of the amphetamines.

8. OTHER STIMULANT DRUGS

In our brave new world of "Legal Highs" or Novel Psychoactive Substances, it is very difficult to keep up with the proliferation of mind-altering drugs and many of the new drugs are stimulants or drugs of mixed action with some stimulant properties. The worlds of literature, music, and visual art has still to catch up with this exponential growth though the literature of the "Chemical Generation" or "Generation X" certainly took on board the earlier phases of this change with a particular interest in MDMA or Ecstasy. Generation X: Tales for an Accelerated Culture, a novel by Douglas Coupland (1991), and most of the work of Irvine Welsh, e.g., see "The Undefeated" in Ecstasy—Three Tales of Chemical Romance, in are reflective of the drug experimenting culture that has taken hold with a distrust of materialistic values and a scorn for authority. The Ecstasy Club (Rushkoff, 1997) is a novel that links the drug to other ways of questing for spiritual enlightenment.

MDMA has been most extensively studied given the prevalence of its recreational use (a minority seems to become dependent). Reference is made to some users experiencing enhanced creativity in the book, Pursuit of Ecstasy—The MDMA Experience (Beck & Rosenbaum, 1994, pp. 77–78) but again it is difficult to separate such subjective feelings from the objective reality of any drug effect on creativity. As always there is a price to pay and this is reviewed by Burgess, O'Donohoe, and Gill (2000) for MDMA.

Also in the 1990s, two books were published by Alexander and Ann Shulgin which along with the development of the Internet and social media became major catalysts to this change, PiHKAL—A Chemical Love Story (1991) and TIKHAL—The Continuation (1997). PIKHAL is short for

Phenethylamines I Have Known and Loved and TiKHAL for Tryptamines I Have Known and Loved. Again, we are in the territory of Breaking Bad in relation to the how to of drug synthesis, albeit with totally different motivation, and it is said that the police often finds the Shulgins' books in illegal drug laboratories. The Shulgins synthesized and tried most of the many compounds they list, "bioassaying," and in PiKHAL they list 10 "essential" amphetamines. The first section of PiKHAL is a fictionalized autobiography of the couple. Again, we are seeing here advocacy for stimulant and hallucinogenic drugs for mind expansion and life enhancement.

Methylphenidate in the form of Ritalin is the amphetamine that has expanded most in its usage in the past two decades with increased diagnosis and treatment of Attention Deficit (Hyperactivity) Disorder (ADHD). Again though the drug has escaped its intended usage with a thriving black market for the drug including a usage by students to sustain attention and prolong wakefulness in relation to course work and exam preparation. It is also being used recreationally for pleasure. This epidemic is starting to be mirrored in fiction: see for example, The Ritalin Orgy by Dexter (2013). The plot follows a male teacher in an American prep school in charge of the welfare of boys in a particular dorm. He comes to realize that the use of stimulant drugs is prevalent along with cannabis and alcohol and psychedelic mushrooms.

9. THE VISUAL ARTS

Less has been written about the relationship between the visual arts and artists and the use of drugs, and in particular the psychostimulants as compared to the relationship with writing and with popular music. Certainly, many depictions exist of smokers and coffee and tea drinkers over the centuries of modern Europe in paintings and drawings providing a social history of the progress of tobacco and coffee and tea and the café culture in Europe, the latter mirrors the concentration of artists in urban centers. Scholarship is beginning to look to these sources in more depth.

Take for example, the Ph.D. by Skelly (2010) later published in a shortened form as a monograph (2014). While mostly looking at alcohol and opiates it does have a chapter on cigarettes and cocaine and visual culture. The author presents the thesis that within visual culture artists seek to present outward signs of drug use as "legible on the body" but this can never be fully realized in such visual art as drug use is not always readable from a person's appearance. Sometimes, the art seems to get it wrong from our modern

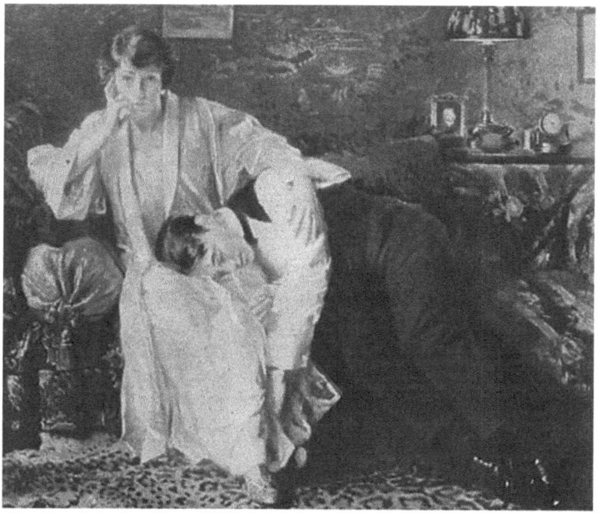

Figure 5 Cocaine by Alfred Priest, 1919 Alfred Priest, *Cocaine*, 1919, oil on canvas, location unknown. *Photo:* Graphic, *10 May 1919. © British Library Board. All rights reserved. LON MLD19 NPL.*

perspective. See for example Alfred Priest's Cocaine (1919) (Fig. 5) where again, as in Conan Doyle above, the effects of cocaine are presented as soporific rather than stimulant.

Another recent publication of interest is the book Addiction and Art (Santora, Dowell, & Henningfield, 2010), which picked the best of submissions of a U.S. wide competition to represent various forms of addiction visually in a way that accurately represented scientific knowledge of the specific drugs. There are striking images and explanations focused on tobacco and methamphetamine addiction among portraits touching on the whole gamut of addictive disorders and illustrating the fact that individuals are often multiply addicted.

10. PSYCHOSTIMULANTS AND POPULAR MUSIC

Harry Shapiro has provided two magisterial books on the links between drugs and the cinema (Shooting Stars, Shapiro, 2003a) and the links between drugs and the popular music industry (Waiting for the Man, Shapiro, 2003b). Drug history and popular music are inextricably linked and this goes back to Blues and Jazz music. Cocaine and cannabis are the main drugs associated. Many famous musicians were to spend time in the

Narcotic Farm in Lexington, Kentucky, with the concerts held there softening the time spent in this hospital penitentiary for drug rehabilitation.

Moving on to the last 60 years, we again find the association strengthening with the amphetamines, cocaine, and cigarettes featuring in the lyrics of many songs as well as in the habits of the musicians along with alcohol, cannabis, and opiates. The use of psychedelics also became a major influence in the 1960s on popular music and remains today albeit to a less obvious extent as at the peak of hippie culture. Also, the phenomenon of dance culture and "raves" in the 1980s and 1990s which linked the use of MDMA to rhythmic music and large gatherings for all night dancing has subsided but remains on a smaller scale as one of many subcultures in today's more varied and fragmented music scene (Collin, 2009).

The phrase "Sex, Drugs and Rock'n' Roll" has been used as a title for the recent publication (Cormier, 2014) that explores the scientifically researched connections and similarities between the effects music, drugs including stimulants and sexual activity have on the brains and biology of man and animals. It does seem that humans are "hardwired" to seek pleasure in the conjunction of the three activities.

11. CONCLUSION

Despite much research, the enhancement of creativity by stimulants remains to be established, but there is no doubt there is a strong association between their use and the creative arts. In exploring the links in the real world, we will have to look more carefully as to how different stages of the creative process are affected in different ways by particular families of drugs and specific drugs within a family such as the psychostimulants. The brief review above is by its nature impressionistic and reflective of my own reading and research in this area during a 25-year career working in an addiction clinic. Certainly, I would advocate that such supplementary reading away from the technical aspects of the field is a necessary corrective to a restrictive biomedical view of the addictive disorders.

The current explosion in new psychoactive substances through the Internet and clandestine laboratories, many with stimulant action, suggests a new chapter is opening in the story of the link among drugs, culture, and creativity. Undoubtedly, new literatures, new musical genres, and new visual cultures will result though given the numbers of drugs concerned these may be harder than in the past to discern.

REFERENCES

Abraham, A., Pieritz, K., Thybusch, K., Rutter, B., Kroger, S., Schweckendiek, J., et al. (2012). Creativity and the brain: Uncovering the neural signature of conceptual expansion. *Neuropsychologia, 50*(8), 1906–1917.

Anderson, D. (2007). *The khat controversy: stimulating the debate on drugs*. Oxford: Berg.

Andreasen, N. C. (1987). Creativity and mental illness: Prevalence rates in writers and their first-degree relatives. *The American Journal of Psychiatry, 144*(10), 1288–1292.

Baird, B., Smallwood, J., Mrazek, M. D., Kam, J. W., Franklin, M. S., & Schooler, J. W. (2012). Inspired by distraction: Mind wandering facilitates creative incubation. *Psychological Science, 23*(10), 1117–1122.

Bancroft, A. (2009). *Drugs, intoxication, and society*. Cambridge: Polity.

Beard, R. (1997). *X20*. New York: Arcade Pub, Distributed by Little, Brown & Co.

Beck, J., & Rosenbaum, M. (1994). *Pursuit of ecstasy: The MDMA experience*. Albany: State University of New York Press.

Berridge, V. (2013). *Demons: Our changing attitudes to alcohol, tobacco, & drugs*. Oxford, United Kingdom: Oxford University Press.

Beveridge, A., & Yorston, G. (1999). I drink, therefore I am: Alcohol and creativity. *Journal of the Royal Society of Medicine, 92*(12), 646–648.

Boon, M. (2002). *The road of excess: A history of writers on drugs*. Cambridge, Mass.: Harvard University Press.

Brandt, A. M. (2007). *The cigarette century: The rise, fall, and deadly persistence of the product that defined America*. New York: Basic Books.

Buckley, C. (1994). *Thank you for smoking*. New York: Random House.

Burgess, C., O'Donohoe, A., & Gill, M. (2000). Agony and ecstasy: A review of MDMA effects and toxicity. *European Psychiatry, 15*, 287–294.

Burroughs, W. S. (1970). *Speed*. London: Olympia Press Ltd.

Burroughs, W. S. (1973). *Kentucky ham*. New York: E.P. Dutton.

Burroughs, W. S. (1977). *Junky*. Harmondsworth, Middlesex, England: Penguin Books.

Burroughs, W. S. (1986). *The naked lunch*. London: Paladin Grafton books.

Collin, M. (2009). *Altered state*. London: Serpent's Tail.

Constable, N. (2002). *This is cocaine*. London: Sanctuary Pub.

Cormier, Z. (2014). *Sex, drugs and rock 'n' roll: The science of hedonism and the hedonism of science*. London: Profile Books.

Coupland, D. (1991). *Generation X: Tales for an accelerated culture*. New York: St. Martin's Press.

Courtwright, D. T. (2001). *Forces of habit: Drugs and the making of the modern world*. Cambridge, MA: Harvard University Press.

Dalrymple, T. (2006). *Romancing opiates: Pharmacological lies and the addiction bureaucracy*. New York: Encounter Books.

Dardis, T. (1989). *The thirsty muse: Alcohol and the American writer*. New York: Ticknor & Fields.

Davenport-Hines, R. P. T. (2002). *The pursuit of oblivion: A global history of narcotics*. New York: Norton.

Davidson, T. (1998). *Intoxication: An anthology of stimulant-based writing*. London: Serpent's Tail.

Dawkins, L., Shahzad, F.-Z., Ahmed, S. S., & Edmonds, C. J. (2011). Expectation of having consumed caffeine can improve performance and mood. *Appetite, 57*(3), 597–600.

Day, E., & Smith, I. (2003). Literary and biographical perspectives on substance use. *Advances in Psychiatric Treatment, 9*, 62–68.

De Quincey, T. (2013). *Confessions of an English opium eater*. Harmondsworth, England: OUP, Oxford.

Devine, T. M. (1975). *The tobacco lords: A study of the tobacco merchants of Glasgow and their trading activities, c. 1740–90.* Edinburgh: Donald.

Dexter, M. (2013). *The Ritalin orgy.* Cibolo, Texas: Perpetual Motion Machine Publishing.

Durlacher, J. (2000). *Heroin.* London: Carlton Books Ltd.

Dyck, E. (2008). *Psychedelic psychiatry: LSD from clinic to campus.* Baltimore, MD: Johns Hopkins University Press.

Edwards, G. (2005). *Matters of substance drugs—And why everyone's a user.* New York: Thomas Dunne Books/St. Martin's Press.

Farah, M. J., Haimm, C., Sankoorikal, G., Smith, M. E., & Chatterjee, A. (2009). When we enhance cognition with Adderall, do we sacrifice creativity? A preliminary study. *Psychopharmacology, 202*(1-3), 541–547.

Freud, S. (1884). *Über coca.* Wien: Verlag von Moritz Perles.

Gately, I. (2001). *Tobacco: A cultural history of how an exotic plant seduced a civilization.* New York, NY: Grove Press.

Gilman, S. L., & Zhou, X. (2004). *Smoke: A global history of smoking.* London: Reaktion Books.

Haining, P. (1998). *The walls of illusion: A psychedelic retro.* London: Souvenir Press.

Hanninen, V., & Koski-Jannes, A. (1999). Narratives of recovery from addictive behaviours. *Addiction, 94*(12), 1837–1848.

Hill, E. M., & Newlin, D. B. (2002). Evolutionary approaches to addiction: Introduction. *Addiction, 97*(4), 375–379.

Hillman, D. C. A. (2008). *The chemical muse: Drug use and the roots of Western civilization.* New York: Thomas Dunne Books/St. Martin's Press.

Historical Thesaurus: Home: Welcome (2012). From http://historicalthesaurus.arts.gla.ac.uk/.

Hurwitz, B., Tapping, C., & Vickers, N. (2007). Life histories and narratives of addiction Chapter 17. In D. J. Nutt, et al. (Ed.), *Drugs and the future: Brain science, addiction and society* (pp. 485–506). London: Academic Press.

Huxley, A. (1954). *The doors of perception.* New York: Harper & Brothers Publishers.

Inaba, D. S., & Cohen, W. E. (2011). *Uppers, downers, all arounders: Physical and mental effects of psychoactive drugs* (7th ed.). Ashland, OR: CNS Productions.

Iversen, L. L. (2006). *Speed, ecstasy, ritalin: The science of amphetamines.* Oxford: Oxford University Press.

Jay, M. (1999). *Artificial paradises: A drugs reader.* London: Penguin Books.

Jay, M. (2000). *Emperors of dreams: Drugs in the nineteenth century.* Gardena, CA: Dedalus Ltd.

Jay, M. (2011). *Emperors of dreams: Drugs in the nineteenth century.* Gardena, CA: Dedalus Ltd.

Jay, M., & Wellcome, C. (2010). *High society: Mind-altering drugs in history and culture.* London: Thames & Hudson.

Karch, S. B. (1998). *A brief history of cocaine.* Boca Raton, FL: CRC Press.

Kerouac, J. (1957). *On the road.* London: Penguin Books.

Killgore, W. D. S., Kahn-Greene, E. T., Lipizzi, E. L., Newman, R. A., Kamimori, G. H., & Balkin, T. J. (2008). Sleep deprivation reduces perceived emotional intelligence and constructive thinking skills. *Sleep Medicine, 9*(5), 517–526.

Konnikova, M. (2013). How caffeine can cramp creativity. *The New Yorker,* Retrieved 2013/06/17.

Kowal, M. A., Hazekamp, A., Colzato, L. S., van Steenbergen, H., van der Wee, N. J., Durieux, J., et al. (2015). Cannabis and creativity: Highly potent cannabis impairs divergent thinking in regular cannabis users. *Psychopharmacology, 232*(6), 1123–1134.

Lattin, D. (2010). *The Harvard psychedelic club: How four visionaries killed the fifties and ushered in a new age for America.* New York, NY: HarperCollins Publishers.

Lewin, L. (1931). *Phantastica: Narcotic and stimulating drugs [S.I.].* London: Kegan Paul, Trench and Trubner & Co. Ltd.

Ludwig, A. M. (1992). Creative achievement and psychopathology: Comparison among professions. *American Journal of Psychotherapy, 46*(3), 330–356.
Madge, T. (2001). *White mischief: A cultural history of cocaine*. New York: Thunder's Mouth Press, Distributed by Publishers Group West.
Markel, H. (2011). *An anatomy of addiction: Sigmund Freud, William Halsted and the miracle drug, cocaine*. New York: Pantheon Books.
Mednick, S. A. (1962). The associative basis of the creative process. *Psychological Review, 69*, 220–232.
Melechi, A. (1997). *Psychedelia Britannica: Hallucinogenic drugs in Britain*. London: Turnaround.
Melechi, A. (1998). *Mindscapes: An anthology of drug writings*. Baildon, West Yorkshire: Mono.
Meyer, N. (1974). *The seven-per-cent solution: Being a reprint from the reminiscences of John H. Watson, M.D.*. New York: Dutton.
Miller, J., & Koral, R. (1995). *White rabbit: A psychedelic reader*. San Francisco: Chronicle Books.
Mills, J. H. (2003). *Cannabis Britannica: Empire, trade, and prohibition, 1800–1928*. Oxford, New York: Oxford University Press.
Morrison, R. (2009). *The English opium-eater: A biography of Thomas De Quincey*. London: Weidenfeld & Nicolson.
Naish, N., & Scott, J. (2013). *Coke: The biography*. London: The Robson Press.
Nutt, D. J., Robbins, T., Stimson, G. V., Ince, M., & Jackson, A. R. W. (2007). *Drugs and the future: brain science, addiction and society*. Amsterdam, Boston: Elsevier/Academic Press.
Pendergrast, M. (1999). *Uncommon grounds: The history of coffee and how it transformed our world*. New York, NY: Basic Books.
Plant, S. (1999). *Writing on drugs*. London: Faber and Faber Ltd.
Porter, R., & Teich, M. (1995). *Drugs and narcotics in history*. Cambridge [England], New York: Cambridge University Press.
Post, F. (1994). Creativity and psychopathology. A study of 291 world-famous men. *The British Journal of Psychiatry, 165*(1), 22–34.
Post, F. (1996). Verbal creativity, depression and alcoholism. An investigation of one hundred American and British writers. *The British Journal of Psychiatry, 168*(5), 545–555.
Rasmussen, N. (2008). *On speed: The many lives of amphetamine*. New York: New York University Press.
Rudgley, R. (2001). *Wildest dreams: An anthology of drug-related literature*. London: Abacus.
Runco, M. A., & Pritzker, S. R. (2011). *Encyclopedia of creativity*. Boston, MA: Academic Press.
Rushkoff, D. (1997). *Ecstasy club: A novel*. San Francisco, CA: Harper Edge.
Samorini, G. (2002). *Animals and psychedelics: The natural world and the instinct to alter consciousness*. Rochester, VT: Park Street Press.
Sandison, R. A., Spencer, A. M., & Whitelaw, J. D. (1954). The therapeutic value of lysergic acid diethylamide in mental illness. *The Journal of Mental Science, 100*(419), 491–507.
Santora, P. B., Dowell, M. L., & Henningfield, J. E. (2010). *Addiction and art*. Baltimore: Johns Hopkins University Press.
Schivelbusch, W. (1992). *Tastes of paradise: A social history of spices, stimulants, and intoxicants*. New York: Pantheon Books.
Selby, H. (1979). *Requiem for a dream*. London: Boyars.
Selby, H. (1987). *Last exit to Brooklyn*. London: Bloomsbury.
Sessa, B. (2012). *The psychedelic renaissance: Reassessing the role of psychedelic drugs in 21st century psychiatry and society*. London: Muswell Hill Press.
Shannonhouse, R. (2003). *Under the influence: The literature of addiction*. New York: Modern Library.
Shapiro, H. (2003a). *Shooting stars: Drugs, Hollywood and the movies*. London: Serpent's Tail.

Shapiro, H. (2003b). *Waiting for the man: The story of drugs and popular music*. London: Helter Skelter.
Shell, R. (1993). *Iced*. New York: Random House.
Shulgin, A. T., & Shulgin, A. (1991). *Pihkal: A chemical love story*. Berkeley, CA: Transform Press.
Shulgin, A. T., & Shulgin, A. (1997). *Tihkal: The continuation*. Berkeley, CA: Transform Press.
Skelly, J. (2010). *The desire to fill: Addiction and British visual culture, 1751–1919*. Thesis (Ph.D., Art History), Belfast: Queen's University, 2010-07-21 13:31:48.788.
Skelly, J. (2014). *Addiction and British visual culture, 1751–1919: Wasted looks*. Farnham, Surrey: Ashgate.
Stevens, J. (1988). *Storming heaven: LSD and the American dream*. New York: Perennial Library.
Stevenson, R. L. (1886). *The strange case of Dr. Jekyll and Mr. Hyde and other tales of terror*. London: Penguin Classics.
Strausbaugh, J., & Blaise, D. (1991). *The drug user: Documents, 1840–1960*. New York, Baltimore: Blast Books, Dolphin-Moon Press.
Streatfield, D. (2001). *Cocaine: An unauthorised biography*. London: Virgin.
Strongman, P. (1997). *Cocaine: A novel*. London: Abacus.
Sutherland, J. (1998). Turns unstoned. *Times Literary Supplement, TLS, 4987*(October 30), 30.
Sutherland, J. (2001). *Last drink to LA*. London: Short Books.
Ulrich, A. (2005). *The Nazi death machine: Hitler's drugged soldiers*.
Vayne, J. (2006). *Pharmakon: Drugs and the imagination*. Oxford: Mandrake.
Verghese, A. (1998). *The tennis partner: A doctor's story of friendship and loss*. New York: HarperCollins.
Walton, J. (2001a). *The Faber book of smoking*. London: Faber.
Walton, S. (2001b). *Out of it: A cultural history of intoxication*. London: Hamish Hamilton.
Weinberg, B. A., & Bealer, B. K. (2001). *The world of caffeine: The science and culture of the world's most popular drug*. New York: Routledge.
Wijdicks, E. F. M. (2015). *Neurocinema: When film meets neurology*. Boca Raton: CRC Press.

CHAPTER FIFTEEN

Opium as a Literary Stimulant: The Case of Samuel Taylor Coleridge

Neil Vickers[1]
Department of English Literature, King's College London, London, United Kingdom
[1]Corresponding author: e-mail address: neil.vickers@kcl.ac.uk

Contents

Abstract

In our era, the idea of a stimulant is synonymous with its biochemical properties. A stimulant, we think, is a substance that enhances the activity of the central and peripheral nervous systems. But in the eighteenth century, a new family of theories about the workings of stimulants took shape, based on exciting but erroneous assumptions. Proponents of these theories thought that many more diseases were "nervous" in origin than had previously been supposed. They hoped that the workings of the "nervous power" could be aided by the judicious use of stimulants and narcotics. Practitioners working within this broad "neuropathological" paradigm equated the workings of stimulation with those of gravity. Stimulation, they believed, was a kind of master principle in nature. Some hoped it would help refound medicine on Newtonian, mathematical lines. For patients, the most visible legacy of the neuropathological revolution was the abandonment of bloodletting or "cupping" and the increasingly widespread use of opium and alcohol in medical treatments. In this chapter, I explore the career of one of the most famous writers of the Romantic era, Samuel Taylor Coleridge (1772–1834) who had the misfortune to live through this therapeutic revolution. I describe the circumstances under which he came to take opiates and the development of his opinions about their effect on him.

"Have you ever thought of trying large doses of opium in a hot climate, keeping your Body open by Grapes & the Fruits of the Climate?—Is it impossible, that by drinking freely you might at last produce the *Gout*, & that a violent Pain and Inflammation in the Extremities might produce new trains of motion & feeling in your Stomach and the Organs connected with it, the Stomach known and unknown?" (Griggs, ii, 1042). So begins a characteristically wheedling letter by the poet Samuel Taylor Coleridge to

International Review of Neurobiology, Volume 120
ISSN 0074-7742
http://dx.doi.org/10.1016/bs.irn.2015.02.007

his friend, benefactor, and fellow valetudinarian, Tom Wedgwood (1771–1805), dated 25 January 1804. Coleridge had resolved to try living in Madeira or Malta for a period and hoped Wedgwood would accompany him and perhaps meet the expenses associated with the trip. The two men had been very ill for years, plagued by mysterious stomach pains. As is well known, opiates inhibit the production of acetylcholine and gives rise to severe digestive difficulties. It is likely that opium was the cause of their pains—though we cannot say for certain. They lived in an era in which a medical concept of opium addiction did not exist (Sonnedecker, 1962–1963; Vickers, 2004). They were convinced that a penchant for metaphysics had made them peculiarly vulnerable to such infirmities. The Romantic period was perhaps the first in European history when a link was widely made between artistic and intellectual creativity of all kinds and the workings of psychostimulants. My aim in this chapter is to explain how men like Coleridge saw that connection. This is a subject that has been grievously misunderstood, at least by nonspecialists. In her beautifully written and widely read biography, *Samuel Taylor Coleridge: the Bondage of Opium* (1974) the late Molly Lefebure suggested that all of Coleridge's statements about opium could be dismissed as the lies of a "junkie" (pp. 13–14). The trouble with this view is that it credits him with knowledge he could not have possessed because no one in his lifetime possessed it. I want to redress the balance by focusing on what eighteenth-century medicine had to say about stimulation in general and opiates in particular before turning to Coleridge's case history.

One of the most significant turning points in medical history occurred during the 1660s when Dr. Thomas Willis (1621–1675), Sedleian Professor of Natural Philosophy at Oxford and at one time the tutor of the philosopher–physician John Locke, published two books containing the most comprehensive accounts of the brain and the nervous system in Europe to date (Willis, 1664, 1667). Willis discovered that the nerves of the animal body are lined with "conductors" which assist the movement of the humors in the veins and arteries. He came to the view that the brain and the nerves actually controlled all of the processes of health and disease. This led him to suspect that the brain and the nerves were the casing of the soul. Willis's hypothesis led to an explosion in the number of illnesses classified as nervous disorders at the end of the seventeenth century. As Robert Frank (1990) has observed, after Willis physicians "systematically attempted to convert diseases thought to be caused by the blood, viscera, or even supernatural agents, into diseases of the nervous system" (p. 141). Willis's ideas remained the preserve of an elite until they were given a popular inflexion by George Cheyne in *The English Malady* Cheyne (1733). *The English Malady* was nervous malady. Cheyne thought that up to a third of all diseases in England were nervous in origin and sought in his book to account for what he felt sure was an uncommonly high prevalence. According to Cheyne, when a person of unusually great virtue or ingenuity led a sedentary or luxurious life, his or her nerves would become exquisitely sensitive to stimuli. Virtue and ingenuity, on this view, bore witness to the soul's strength. Without the counterbalancing effects of exercise and spare diet, the soul's sensitivity—which he called "sensibility"—would become excessive, resulting in hypochondria, hysteria, and other nervous complaints. The English were exceptionally prone to these disorders because they were more virtuous and ingenious than other nations. "Nervous affliction," he assured his readers, "never happens, or can happen, to any but those of the liveliest and quickest natural Parts, whose Faculties are the brightest and most Spiritual, and whose Genius is most keen and penetrating, and primarily where there is the most delicate Sensation and Pain" (p. 54). Cheyne's book launched the cult of sensibility that fostered so much of the great literature of Europe. The novels of Richardson, Choderlos de Laclos, and even the young Goethe all drew upon it. Without Cheyne, there would have been no *Pamela* or *Clarissa*, no *Les Liaisons dangereuses*, and no *Sorrows of Young Werther*. It is even doubtful whether we would have had Austen's *Sense and Sensibility* which sends Cheyne's theory up. Moreover, in addition to Richardson, who was Cheyne's patient as well as a great exponent of his ideas in fiction, Cheyne's admirers included Hume, Boswell, and Dr. Johnson, all of whom sought to understand their own illnesses in the light of his theories (Rousseau, 2004).

There was of course nothing remarkable about animist medical theories in Enlightenment Europe. A more thorough-going animism, which held that the soul was diffused throughout the body, had been adopted by the great Swiss iatrochemist Georg Stahl (1659–1734) and his followers. What was new was Cheyne's claim—borrowed from Willis—that the soul resided in the brain and the nerves. This claim gave the nervous system a new salience and it explains the preoccupation of so many of the great medical innovators of the Enlightenment with what might be called "proto-neurology." Henceforth, the brain and the nervous system would be investigated on the assumption that they were the mediators of all the processes of health and disease. Therapeutically, the question was how to strengthen the soul. Cheyne's answer was to renounce luxury and to take regular exercise.

Alcohol too was to be avoided, along with any sedentary activity liable to excite the passions. "Assemblies, Musick Meetings, Plays, Cards and Dice" were especially perilous (p. 50).

If the Willis–Cheyne view presented the soul as engaging in an unequal contest with other parts of the body which predisposed it to illness, another hypothesis was put forward in Scotland by Robert Whytt (1714–1766), one of the most significant figures of the Edinburgh University Medical School. In a paper read before the Philosophical Society in Edinburgh in 1745 or 1746, Whytt postulated the existence of an immaterial "sentient principle" which he said could be treated synonymously with the soul, and which though present everywhere in the body operated most conspicuously through the nervous system. The sentient principle was not an autonomous force in the body in the manner of the soul in Georg Stahl's animist medical theory; but neither was it a weakly independent one in the manner conjectured by Willis and Cheyne; rather—and this is the most crucial point about it—it was *stimulated into activity* by external stimuli and stimuli arising within the body (French, 2004). It was this claim which made stimulation and stimulation such an important theme in eighteenth-century medicine.

Whytt's conception of the soul as a reactive organism was developed by the great Swiss physiologist Albrecht von Haller (1708–1777). Like Willis, Haller believed that the soul or "nervous power" was located exclusively in the brain and the nerves. He conjectured that the gluten in muscles adjacent to the nerves possessed a property to initiate changes in the nervous system which he termed irritability. Irritability was the capacity to respond to stimulation. Haller (1755) likened the workings of irritability in gluten to Newtonian laws over the material world. "What should hinder us," he wrote, "from granting irritability to be a property of the animal gluten, the same as we acknowledge gravity and attraction to be properties of matter in general?" (p. 60). Haller's compatriot, Samuel Tissot (1728–1797) made the Newtonian analogy even more forcefully in his Preface to the English translation of Haller's dissertation. "Attraction, the weight and elasticity of the air, shewed themselves to the senses every day; but it required a Toricelli or a Newton to illustrate them. Why may it not be the same with irritability?" Haller never tired of pointing out that his theories did not dispense with traditional Christian ideas about the soul; rather, they delineated the scope of the personal soul more precisely even as they threw into relief something akin to a world soul.

Most of the great medical systems dating from the second half of the eighteenth century are in fact footnotes to Haller. (Here I would include most of those included by Michel Foucault in *The Birth of the Clinic* (Foucault, 1973)). One of these deserves special mention: the so-called Brunonian system named after its originator, Dr. John Brown (1735–1788). Brown's admirers and followers included the two great radical physicians of the late eighteenth century, Thomas Beddoes (1760–1808) and Erasmus Darwin (1731–1802), and on the continent, Kant, Fichte, Schelling, and Novalis. According to Brown, all life was permeated by a life force which was given at birth as a "fixed share." This force Brown called "excitability." Excitability reacted with external stimuli to produce the phenomena of life. The fixed share was depleted by physical and mental exertion but we could draw on some of the excitability reserved for the future through the use of stimulants. Like Haller, Brown thought there were two classes of disease: those resulting from too little stimulation and those resulting from too much. Unlike Haller, Brown believed that most diseases fell into the first class. As Mike Jay (2009) has pointed out, Brown and his followers "offered patients the means to take over their own medical care without costly intermediaries. It treated the medical profession as an emperor with no clothes" (p. 33). It should be remembered that opiates at least had the merit of being effective analgesics. The therapy they replaced was that of bloodletting.

The tenet uniting all variants of irritability theory was that they reduced all illnesses into just a very small number. For Haller as for Brown, there were basically only two, diseases of irritability and diseases of sensibility. Diseases of irritability were caused by too little stimulation and diseases of sensibility by too much. Diseases of irritability could be treated with stimulants, those of sensibility with narcotics. However, here, great care is needed on the part of twenty-first-century readers. We think of stimulants in terms of their impacts on substances such as noradrenalin, dopamine, and serotonin, all of which were unknown in the eighteenth century. Eighteenth-century physicians and their patients understood it more simply as an affair of contractions in muscle tissue. It was because of irritability theory and its rivals that opium and alcohol began to be more widely used in medical treatments. But this was a consequence nobody foresaw. (Opium was a particularly vexed example because only Brunonians thought it was a stimulant. But non-Brunonian neuropathologists prescribed it readily as a sedative.) Extreme temperatures were commonly thought to constitute the most powerful stimulant (see e.g., Crumpe, 1793). A typical list of stimulants in a medical textbook would also have included meat, oxygen or "dephlogisticated air," exercise, and "the exciting passions of the mind."

Darwin and Beddoes were convinced that recent developments in chemistry had opened the way to a new form of therapy which they called pneumatic medicine. This took the form of getting patients to breathe in gases of various kinds. In 1800, a few months after his return from Göttingen, Coleridge went to Beddoes' Pneumatic Institution as a research subject in what is surely the most misrepresented scientific experiment of the Romantic period. The experiment into the effects of nitrous oxide which Humphry Davy oversaw (as Beddoes' "Chemical Superintendent") was an attempt to see whether that gas was the most powerful Brunonian "exciting power" that had yet come to light—in effect, whether it was the perfect stimulant. Biographer after biographer has represented this episode as if it were an investigation into the gas's psychotropic effects. The psychotropic effects of stimulants were always seen as a drawback in this period. What mattered was whether they restored a feeling of health. Beddoes and Davy abandoned pneumatic medicine in the early 1800s and for a time Beddoes experimented with Galvanism as an alternative stimulant force.

1. THE CASE OF COLERIDGE

In October 1800, at the age of 28, Coleridge lost his health for good (he lived for another 34 years). It all began with a bout of rheumatic fever, a condition he had contracted at the age of eight. The latest bout coincided with his arrival in Keswick in the Lake District where he had recently moved to be near his friend William Wordsworth. There is always a danger with accepting a diagnosis such as this one retrospectively. In this case, there is a great deal of circumstantial evidence to support Coleridge's view. Recurrences of rheumatic fever always follow a streptococcal infection. Shortly before coming down with the symptoms he recognized as rheumatic fever, Coleridge reported a severe infection of the eyes which prevented him from reading or writing alongside an attack of orchitis that caused his left testicle to swell to three times its natural size (Griggs, ii, 647; 667). Either of these could have been streptococcal. Soon afterward the symptoms of rheumatic fever appeared: "six large Boils in the back of the neck," pains in the back of the head, exhaustion, and of course the fever itself (Griggs, ii, 672). After several months, he decided he must have a different condition: "irregular gout."

We tend to think of gout as a disease of the joints so it seems odd that Coleridge should have diagnosed it in himself on the basis of stomach pains.

In doing so, he was in fact appealing to a new theory of gout first put forward by William Cullen (1778–1784). From ancient times, gout had been thought to arise when morbid humors "dropped" from the trunk of the body and collected in the joints giving rise to gout pains (the name gout, derived from *gutta*, the Latin for "drop," reflects this etiology). Cullen, arguing against this theory, suggested that gout occurs when pains originating in the stomach are conveyed to the extremities (especially the joints of the fingers, toes, and knees) through the medium of the nervous system by the sentient principle postulated by Whytt. In Cullen's view, "the gout is a disease of the whole system, or depends upon a certain general conformation and state of the body." It is "manifestly a disease of the nervous system." And "the stomach, which so universal an assent with the rest of the system, is the internal part that is most frequently and often very considerably affected by the gout" (pp. 380–382). Cullen was the first writer to distinguish regular from irregular gout. The basis of the distinction was that regular gout chiefly attacked the joints, whereas irregular gout assailed the stomach. Attacks of regular gout usually subsided after a few days, whereas the pains of irregular gout continued indefinitely. Cullen conjectured that the remissions characteristic of regular gout were due to the intervention of nervous "excitement" in the brain. The pains of irregular gout continued indefinitely because this mechanism of self-correction failed.

Although Coleridge had placed himself under the care of a surgeon apothecary, this diagnosis seems to have been his own. Near the end of March 1801, he announced he had "a sort of irregular gout" (Griggs, ii, 719). Within a month, his medical attendant was concurring (Griggs, ii, 726). In quick succession, he reported "three paroxysms of decided gout" (Griggs, ii, 739). His symptoms were "Swoln knees, a knotty fingers, a loathy Stomach, & a dizzy head" (Griggs, ii, 739). But the symptoms which caused him most suffering were stomach symptoms: as he told Sara Hutchinson in the summer, "for the first 10 days after my arrival at Stowey, I had every evening a Bowel attack—which layed my spirits prostrate—but by a severe adherence to a certain regular Diet & Regimen, I have, I hope, entirely got the better" (Griggs, ii, 780). To Southey, he complained that he was "often literally *sick* with pain" (Griggs, ii, 748).

In a rueful letter written some 13 years after these events, Coleridge described how he treated himself with opium:

> *I had been almost bed-ridden for many months with swellings in my knees—in a medical Journal I unhappily met with an account of a cure performed in a similar*

> *case ... by rubbing in of Laudanum, at the same time taking a given dose internally—It acted like a charm, like a Miracle! ... At length the unusual stimulus subsided—the complaint returned—the supposed remedy was recurred to—but I cannot get through the dreary history—suffice it to say, that effects were produced, which acted on me by Terror & Cowardice of PAIN & sudden death.*
>
> ***(Griggs, iii, 477)***

Wagner (1938) in an old but still valuable article conjectured that the "medical journal" from which Coleridge took this advice was none other than Brown's *Elements of Medicine* which Coleridge's friend Beddoes had edited in Beddoes (1795). Brown claimed to have formulated his discoveries while treating himself for this same condition:

> *The universal rule, suggested by the principles, and confirmed by the practice of this new doctrine, is to invigorate the whole system, and apply any diffusible stimulus, particularly laudanum, to the pained parts. By that practice I know not one cure, of some hundreds, that either I or my pupils have performed, that has failed. ... The effectual method of cure is to apply rags dipped in laudanum, volatile alkali, or ether, and renew them as often as they become dry, and to support [the patient] internally with durable and diffusible stimuli, proportioned in kind and quantity to the exigence of the case.*
>
> ***(Beddoes, i, pp. 191–192)***

Coleridge also made a number of statements about gout that have no warrant in Cullen's book, being based on Sydenham's view that gout was a "beneficial" disease whose symptoms were not the result of a pathological process but the expression of an attempt by the body to recover its natural powers. Thus, he talked of "ripening" his gout into a "fair Paroxysm" (Griggs, ii, 721) by undertaking a long walking tour, a cure endorsed by Sydenham in his famous essay on gout. (Sydenham believed that strenuous walking would drive the gouty matter to the extremities of his body where it would be shed via the skin of the fingers and toes.) In parallel, he paid close attention to his "nervous" symptoms: on April 18, he complained to Poole: "the Disease has seized the whole Region of my Back, so that I scream mechanically on the least motion" (Griggs, ii, 721).

And so we come full circle to the quotation at the beginning of this paper in which Coleridge urged Tom Wedgwood to try "large doses of opium in a hot climate," so as to "produce the *Gout*, & that a violent Pain and Inflammation in the Extremities might produce new trains of motion & feeling in your Stomach and the Organs connected with it, the Stomach known and unknown?" (Griggs, ii, 1042). All of this is consistent with what he knew of irritability treatments and with what he knew of stimulants.

In August of 1803, Coleridge went on a walking tour of Scotland with William and Dorothy Wordsworth during which he tried to use walking as a substitute for opium. He gave up opium because he thought it aggravated his psychological sufferings. The consequences were grievous. He reported prolonged shaking fits which he might equate with withdrawal. But that is not a word that Coleridge would have understood. I have argued elsewhere that he probably thought that his "gout" was taking on an epileptic dimension. He spoke, for instance, of "Epileptic winds and breezes, gusts from the bowels of the volcano upwards to the Crater of the Brain, rushings & brain horrors" (Coburn, i, 1822) and complained of "frequent paralytic feelings—sometimes approaches to Convulsion fit" (Griggs, ii, 975). Coleridge found that they stopped when he took opium again (though the nightmares and the hallucinations resumed).

Here, we come to one of the thorniest issues that beset historic analyses of addictions to psychostimulants. It is undeniable that some of the elements of what would subsequently become the theory of addiction had been discussed in detail by the close of the eighteenth century. Habituation was known about, as was tolerance and, in sketchier vein, some writers even ventured opinions about what we call "withdrawal." But these phenomena were not regarded as dangerous in themselves—indeed habituation was widely thought to make opium safer—and consequently did not warrant medical attention. Andreas-Holger Maehle, who has written the standard treatise on the history of opiates in the eighteenth century, has argued that habituation and the like were usually seen as "interesting pharmacological phenomena," rather than as fully fledged medical conditions (Maehle, 1999, 182). For someone in Coleridge's position, the challenge would have been to distinguish withdrawal phenomena from the symptoms from the condition for which he had begun taking the drug in the first place. If you think of diseases as protean entities, this was no small task.

Until he went to Malta, Coleridge believed that opiates were necessary because they enabled him to press his "inirritable" stomach muscles into action. After the Autumn of 1803, he was increasingly convinced that his stomach complaints were *psychically* caused. Opiates, he now began to think, were necessary in the first instance as a prophylactic against unendurably distressing nightmares and in the second, as a means of preventing his mind from thinking in ways that produced the gout-like, potentially fatal, stomach symptoms. He wanted to bring these "discoveries" to the attention of his loved ones but did not dare to. As he put it in a Notebook entry of 1807:

> *Meanwhile the habit of inward Brooding daily makes it harder to confess the Thing I am, to any one—least of all those, whom I most love & who most love me—and thereby introduces & fosters a habit of negative falsehood, & multiplies the temptations to positive, Insincerity. O God! let me bear my whole Heart to Dr B, or some other Medical Philosopher.*
>
> ***(Coburn, ii, 3079)***

"Dr B" was in all probability Thomas Beddoes whom Coleridge resolved to consult in January 1808 only to discover that he was dead. He then called for John Abernethy who was unable to see him. (Abernethy was a close friend of Beddoes' colleague and brother-in-law, John King.) Finally, he laid his case before a country practitioner near December. Coleridge struggled with opiates for the rest of his life and eventually died of a heart condition that was caused by the rheumatic fever that first afflicted him as a child.

Some readers will want to object that I have ignored the evidence of one of Coleridge's most celebrated poems, "Kubla Khan" which is prefaced by an explanation of how the poem came to be written which gives no small role to opiates.

> *In consequence of a slight indisposition, an anodyne which had been prescribed, from the effects of which he feel asleep in his chair at the moment that he was reading the following sentence, or words of the same substance, in "Purchas's Pilgrimage:" "Here the Kubla commanded a palace to be built and a stately garden thereunto. And thus ten miles of fertile ground were inclosed within a wall." The author continued for about three hours in a state of profound sleep, at least of the external senses, during which time he had the most vivid confidence, that he could not have composed less than two or three hundred lines; if that indeed can be called composition in which all the images rose up before him as things, with a parallel production of the correspondant impressions, without any sensation or consciousness of effort.*
>
> ***(Coleridge, p. 511)***

On the strength of this "Preface" Coleridge has sometimes been presented as someone who advocated the use of opium as a stimulant to literary creativity. And this "Preface" with its euphemistic reference to an "anodyne" appears to confirm that image. In fact in one of the manuscripts of the poem he says that the poem was written "in a sort of Reverie brought on by two grains of Opium taken to check a dysentery". And the poem should certainly be seen as a curiosity detailing the effects of opiates on the mind. But three further things should be borne in mind when considering "Kubla Khan." The first is that it seems to be the only instance in Coleridge's works in which opium is presented positively. If he really was committed to using opium to write experimental verse, we might expect to find more. In fact, there was a very good reason for not doing so. Precisely because there was no medical concept of addiction to opiates, a moral one prevailed: people who habitually took opium were thought to be "sensuous" and were compared with Orientals. The second is that at the time the poem was composed—1797 or 1798—Coleridge was not chronically ill and probably was not addicted to opiates. He himself dated his "enslavement" to the Spring of 1801. Third, Coleridge's *oeuvre* abounds in *negative* references to the impact of opiates on his creativity. These are less well known but no less fascinating. Some of the most powerful are to be found in his Notebooks. Coleridge's Notebooks rank alongside Virginia Woolf's Diaries as one of the richest accounts of the minutiae of a writer's subjectivity in English that we have. Here he is on the state of craving (opiates are very much on his mind in this connection):

> *When the spirit is forced back on itself to find another, as the exclusion and supersession of itself, and in the intensity of simple self-perception finds itself losing the actuality of Self, and sinks towards the aboriginal Craving . . . and Pain I believe to be in it's (sic) essence a dark Craving—a Desideratum sine formâ, sine Objecto ad extra [longing without form, without an external object]*
>
> ***(Coburn, v, 6559)***

Paragraphs like this one do not have the same hold on the public imagination because they stem from a much more complex set of preoccupations that seeks to place the phenomena of addiction in a spiritual and psychological context as well as a pharmacological one.

In conclusion, then, Coleridge, should not be remembered, let alone celebrated, as someone who used a literary stimulant. Rather, he should be seen as an unfortunate victim of the primitive state of research into opiates in his time. Coleridge's motive for taking the drug was shared by thousands if not tens of thousands of his contemporaries. Opium was a powerful analgesic and an alternative to bloodletting which often had no beneficial effect. Coleridge did not see his reliance on opiates in physiological terms alone. The "dark Craving" it initiated was connected with some of the obscurest and deepest mysteries of human nature. There lay its abiding interest. He saw too little to praise in it for its own sake.

REFERENCES

Beddoes, T. (Ed.). (1795). *The elements of medicine of John Brown M. D. 2 Vols.* London: J. Johnson.

Cheyne, G. (1733). *The English malady; or, a treatise of nervous disease of all kinds. With the author's own case, etc.* London: G. Strahan.

Coburn, K. (Ed.). (1957–2002). *The notebooks of Samuel Taylor Coleridge: 5 Vols*. London: Routledge.

Coleridge, S. T. (2001). Poetical works. In J. C. C. Mays (Ed.), London: Princeton University Press.

Crumpe, S. (1793). *An inquiry into the nature and properties of opium*. London: G. G. & J. Robinson.

Cullen, W. (1784). *First lines of the practice of physic: 4 Vols*. Edinburgh: C. Elliot & T. Cadell.

Foucault, M. (1973). *The birth of the clinic: An archaeology of medical perception*. (A. Sheridan-Smith Trans.). London: Tavistock Publications.

Frank, R. G. (1990). Thomas Willis and his circle: Brain and mind in seventeenth-century medicine. In G. S. Rousseau (Ed.), *The languages of psyche: Mind and body in enlightenment thought* (pp. 107–146). Berkeley: University of California Press.

French, R. (2004). Whytt, Robert (1714–1766), physician and natural philosopher. In H. C. G. Matthew & B. Harrison (Eds.), *Oxford dictionary of national biography*. Oxford: Oxford University Press. http://dx.doi.org/10.1093/ref:odnb/29345.

Griggs, E. L. (Ed.). (1956–1971). *The collected letters of Samuel Taylor Coleridge. 6 Vols*. Oxford: Oxford University Press.

Haller, A. (1755). *A dissertation on the sensible and irritable parts of animals*. London: J. Nourse.

Jay, M. (2009). *The atmosphere of heaven: The unnatural experiments of Dr Beddoes and his sons of genius*. London and New Haven: Yale University Press.

Lefebure, M. (1974). *Samuel Taylor Coleridge: A bondage of opium*. London: Gollancz.

Maehle, A.-H. (1999). *Drugs on trial: Experimental pharmacology and therapeutic innovation in the eighteenth century*. Amsterdam: Rodopi.

Rousseau, G. S. (2004). *Nervous acts: Essays on literature, culture and sensibility*. Houndmills: Palgrave.

Sonnedecker, G. (1962–1963). Emergence of the concept of opiate addiction. *Journal Mondial de Pharmacie*, *5*, 275–290 (continued 6 27–34).

Vickers, N. (2004). *Coleridge and the doctors*. Oxford: Oxford University Press.

Wagner, L. (1938). Coleridge's use of laudanum and opium as connected with his interest in contemporary investigations concerning stimulation and sensation. *Psychoanalytic Review*, *25*, 309–324.

Willis, T. (1681a). Of the anatomy of the brain. In *The remaining medical works of T. W. [Thomas Willis]: 3 Vols*. (pp. 52–136). London: T. Dring (Samuel Pordage Trans.) [1664].

Willis, T. (1681b). Of convulsive diseases. In *The remaining medical works of T. W. [Thomas Willis]: 3 Vols*. (pp. 137–192). London: T. Dring (Samuel Pordage Trans.) [1667].

INDEX

Note: Page numbers followed by "*f*" indicate figures and "*t*" indicate tables.

R

S

CONTENTS OF RECENT VOLUMES

Volume 39

Volume 40

Volume 41

Volume 42

Volume 43

Volume 44

Volume 45

Volume 46

Volume 47

Volume 48

Volume 49

Volume 50

Volume 51

Volume 52

Volume 53

Volume 54

Volume 55

Volume 56

Volume 57

Volume 58

Volume 59

Volume 60

Volume 61

Volume 62

Volume 63

Volume 64

Volume 65

Volume 66

Volume 70

Volume 71

Volume 72

Volume 73

Volume 74

Volume 75

Volume 76

Volume 77

Volume 78

Volume 79

Volume 80

Volume 81

Volume 82

Volume 83

Volume 84

Volume 85

Volume 86

Volume 87

Volume 88

Volume 89

Volume 90

Volume 91

Volume 92

Volume 93

Volume 94

Volume 95

Volume 96

Volume 97

Volume 98

Volume 99

Volume 100

Volume 101

Volume 102

Volume 103

Volume 104

Volume 105

Volume 106

Volume 107

Volume 108

Volume 109

Volume 110

Volume 111

Volume 112

Volume 113

Volume 114

Volume 115

Volume 116

Volume 117

Volume 118

Volume 119

FSC
www.fsc.org
MIX
Papier | Fördert gute Waldnutzung
FSC® C083411

Kolibri 360 GmbH
Ferdinand-Jühlke-Straße 7
99095 Erfurt, Deutschland
produktsicherheit@kolibri360.de